Public Health for the 21st Century

Public Health for the 21st Century

NEW PERSPECTIVES ON POLICY, PARTICIPATION AND PRACTICE

Editors: Judy Orme, Jane Powell, Pat Taylor, Tony Harrison and Melanie Grey

Open University Press

Open University Press
McGraw-Hill Education
McGraw-Hill House
Shoppenhangers Road
Maidenhead
Berkshire
England
SL6 2QL

email: enquiries@openup.co.uk
world wide web: www.openup.co.uk

and

Two Penn Plaza
New York, NY 10121-2289, USA

First Published 2003
Reprinted 2005
Copyright © Orme, Powell, Taylor, Harrison and Grey, 2003

A catalogue record of this book is available from the British Library

ISBN 0 335 21193 3 (pb) 0 335 21194 1 (hb)

Library of Congress Cataloging-in-Publication Data
CIP data has been applied for

Typeset by RefineCatch Limited, Bungay, Suffolk
Printed in the UK by Bell & Bain Ltd, Glasgow

Contents

Notes on contributors   x
Foreword   xiv
Acknowledgements   xvi
Introduction   1

PART 1
Policy for 21st century public health   13

Editors' overview   13

  1 **DAVID J. HUNTER**   15
     Public health policy

         Introduction   16
         The state of public health policy   16
         Public health: constraints on implementation   23
         The future of public health   26
         Conclusion   30

  2 **CHRIS MILLER**   31
     Public health meets modernization

         Public health meets Labour's modernization agenda   32
         The legacy of Thatcherism and the fear of 'old' Labour   34
         Modernization as a container   35
         Modernizing the democratic institutions   36
         The common threads of modernization   40
         The Modernization Agency   45
         Conclusion   46

  3 **GABRIEL SCALLY**   47
     Public health: a vision for the future

         Learning for the future from the past   48

A shared power world   49
Public health management and leadership   50
Public health services   51
Health protection   52
Regionalism and internationalism   54
Conclusion   56

PART 2
Participation and partnerships in 21st century public health   57
Editors' overview   57

4   STEPHEN PECKHAM   59
Who are the partners in public health?

Introduction   60
What are partnerships?   60
Why partnerships for public health?   65
Who are the partners in public health?   70
Conclusion   78

5   JENNIE NAIDOO, JUDY ORME AND GILL BARRETT   79
Capacity and capability in public health

Introduction   80
The public health workforce   80
Public health skills and competencies   81
The public health professional project   83
Conclusion   86
Case study: asylum seekers   87

6   STEPHEN PECKHAM AND PAT TAYLOR   93
Public health and primary care

Introduction   94
Re-evaluating primary care   94
Re-evaluating public health: developing a primary care perspective   96
Public health and primary care: making new connections   97
Current developments in primary care and public health   100
Current realities influencing the development of public health in
primary care   106

7   MELANIE GREY AND JOYSHRI SARANGI   107
Protecting the public's health

Health threats and emerging health protection policy   108
Organizations and structures for health protection   113
Health protection: principles and practice   119
Overview: the challenges   126

8 PAT TAYLOR   128
   The lay contribution to public health

   Introduction   129
   Why is lay involvement important to public health?   129
   The changing nature of public involvement in the NHS   130
   Lay perspectives in the history of public health   132
   Understanding lay perspectives   135
   Medical perspectives on lay involvement   137
   Promoting an effective lay contribution to public health   140
   Conclusion – challenges and opportunities   143

9 ALISON GILCHRIST   145
   Community development and networking for health

   Introduction   146
   Networks and community participation   147
   The 'community' dimension to health   148
   Networking and partnerships   152
   The community and voluntary sectors   154
   Community networks and health   155
   Networking in practice   156
   Conclusions   159

PART 3
Major contemporary themes in public health   161
Editors' overview   161

10 DAVID EVANS   163
   New directions in tackling inequalities in health

   Introduction   164
   The evidence for socio-economic inequalities in health   165
   The UK policy response   167
   UK policy effectiveness   169
   Potential policies for reducing inequalities in health   170
   Conclusion   175

11 MURRAY STEWART   177
   Neighbourhood renewal and regeneration

   Urban policy and neighbourhood renewal: historical context   178
   The development of the neighbourhood focus   180
   Neighbourhood policies and health inequalities   183
   Public health and the neighbourhood   187

12 COLIN FUDGE   192
   Implementing sustainable futures in cities
   Introduction   193

Urbanization, urban change, development and policy 193
Swedish cities case study 202
Strategic issues for the future of sustainability 205
Acknowledgements 208

13 **STUART McCLEAN** 210
Globalization and health

Introduction 211
The globalization debate 211
Key features of globalization in relation to public health 213
The promoters of economic globalization and other key players 214
Global trade policy and the UK health care context 217
Global inequalities in health: the local impact of global divisions 218
Globalization and emerging public health risks 220
Conclusion: the challenges for public health in a global era 223

PART 4
Evidence and evaluation in 21st century public health 225
Editors' overview 225

14 **TONY HARRISON** 227
Evidence-based multidisciplinary public health

Introduction 228
Defining evidence-based multidisciplinary public health 229
The development of evidence-based public policy and public health 231
Main problems of evidence-based systems for multidisciplinary
public health 237
The role of theory in evidence-based public health 243
Conclusion 245

15 **JON POLLOCK** 246
Epidemiology in 21st century public health

Defining the scope 247
Identifying appropriate epidemiological approaches for contemporary
public health 248
How has epidemiology changed to support contemporary public health? 251
Future developments in public health epidemiology: concepts and methods 255
Conclusion 261

16 **JANE POWELL** 263
Health economics and public health

The role of economics in 21st century public health 264
Key concepts, tools and techniques in health economics 264
Economic evaluation 268

New directions for health economics in public health action   274
Conclusion   276

17   STUART HASHAGEN   278
Frameworks for measuring community health and well being

    Introduction   279
    Community health and well being action   279
    Achieving Better Community Development (ABCD)   282
    Measurable outcomes from community health and well being action   283
    Public health programme evaluation   284
    Learning Evaluation and Planning model (LEAP)   289
    Conclusions   295

18   JACK DOWIE   296
Health impact: its estimation, assessment and analysis

    Introduction   297
    Health impact assessment   297
    Health impact estimation and health impact analysis   303
    Summary   308

Glossary   310
References   323
Index   356

Notes on contributors

The editors

The editors are all members of academic staff at the University of the West of England, Bristol. The idea for this book sprang from discussion and delivery of modules on our established postgraduate programme in public health (MSc in Public Health).

Judy Orme is Principal Lecturer in Public Health and Director of the Research Centre in Public Health and Primary Care Development in the Faculty of Health and Social Care at the University of the West of England, Bristol. Her research interests include young people and risk, particularly relating to drug prevention and alcohol use, the sociology of public health and primary care.

Jane Powell is Senior Lecturer in Health Economics in the Faculty of Health and Social Care at the University of the West of England, Bristol. Her research interests are the identification and quantification of alcohol misuse in adults and young people and its relationship with quality of life. Other strong interests include the application of economics and social science in public health programme evaluation, impact of priority setting in NHS organizations and reduction of health inequalities in public health practice.

Pat Taylor is Senior Lecturer in Community Care in the Faculty of Health and Social Care at the University of the West of England, Bristol. Her research interests include community development and public involvement in public health.

Tony Harrison was, until recently Principal Lecturer in Housing and Urban Studies in the Faculty of the Built Environment at the University of the West of England, Bristol. He is a social scientist whose main research interests include evidence-based policy and practice, planning and healthy cities. He now lectures part-time at the University of the West of England, Bristol, and combines this with consultancy work.

Melanie Grey is Head of the School of Environmental and Interdisciplinary Sciences in the Faculty of Applied Sciences at the University of the West of England, Bristol, and lectures in Environmental Health. Her research interests include assessment of environment and health risks, and evaluation of interventions. Other interests are the development and training for capability in the public health field for health protection.

Other contributors

Gill Barrett is Senior Lecturer in Health Promotion at the University of the West of England, Bristol. She has a background in nursing and health promotion. Gill's research interests include health promotion, interprofessional education and health communication.

Jack Dowie is Professor of Health Impact Analysis, London School of Hygiene and Tropical Medicine. Jack took up the newly created chair in Health Impact Analysis at the London School of Hygiene and Tropical Medicine on 1 October 2000, leaving the Open University where he had been a member of the Faculty of Social Sciences since 1977. While at the Open University he designed and ran the multimedia courses on risk (from the late 1970s) and professional judgement and decision making (from the late 1980s).

David Evans is Director of Community Development and Public Health for Bristol North Primary Care Trust. His primary care trust covers the inner city, north and east of the city of Bristol and includes communities with high levels of deprivation and relatively poor health as well as some of the most prosperous areas of the city. With a background in social science, health promotion and nursing, David is one of the first NHS directors of public health from a background other than medicine. His research interests include the evaluation of initiatives to tackle inequalities in health and the development of multidisciplinary public health.

Professor Colin Fudge is Dean of the Faculty of the Built Environment and Pro Vice Chancellor at the University of the West of England, Bristol. He fulfils a number of key roles in the field of urban design and sustainable development. Internationally these include the Royal Professor of Environmental Science appointed by the Swedish Academy of Sciences for 2002–03, the Chair of the EU Urban Environment Expert Group, the Chair of the European Sustainable Cities and Towns Campaign and Urban Environment Sustainable Development Adviser to the European Commission.

Nationally his roles include Member of the UK Department of the Environment, Transport and Regions Research Committee, Member of the UK Ministerial Working Group on Urban Design. Regionally, he is a member of a number of bodies in Bristol and the south-west of the UK including Sustainability South West, the South West Regional Development Agency working group on Europe and the South West Regional Development Agency Steering Group on the Regional Centre of Excellence.

He has extensive experience of working internationally including in Sweden, Finland, Australia, New Zealand, Zimbabwe and Japan, as well as for the EU, WHO, UNESCO, UN Development Programme, OECD and Swedish International

Development Agency. He has written several books on public policy, government and planning, and edits a book series, Public Policy and Politics, for Macmillans. His recent books include: *Implementing Sustainable Futures in Sweden* (2000) with Dr Janet Rowe; *City and Culture* (1999) with Dr Louise Nyström; and *European Sustainable Cities* (1996) with Dr Liz Mills, D. Ludlow and S. Pauli.

Alison Gilchrist worked for many years as a community development worker in inner-city neighbourhoods in Bristol and chaired the Executive Committee of the Standing Conference for Community Development between 1995 and 1998. For 11 years she taught community and youth work at the University of the West of England, Bristol, and during this period undertook research into the value of networking for community development. In 1999 she joined the Community Development Foundation as their Regional Links Manager, responsible for the Foundations work with regional levels of government. She has a particular interest in promoting genuine community involvement in cross-sectoral partnerships and equal opportunities strategies.

Stuart Hashagen is Scotland Manager with the Community Development Foundation and Co-director of the Scottish Community Development Centre. He works in most of the Scottish Community Development Centre programmes, working with a cross-section of community and public organizations to help develop good practice in community development. As well as working with community health projects and programmes, he is also involved in social inclusion, community planning and environmental issues. Scottish Community Development Centre programmes include training and support on skills in planning and evaluation, developing effective partnerships and promoting participation. He is a past convenor of the Poverty Alliance and currently a management committee member of a community-based housing association in Glasgow.

David Hunter is Professor of Health Policy and Management in the School for Health, University of Durham. His interests are in public health policy and practice, and health policy and management; he has published extensively in these areas. His latest book, *Public Health Policy*, is to be published in September 2003 by Polity Press. He is Honorary Member of the Faculty of Public Health Medicine and Fellow of the Royal Society of Physicians (Edinburgh).

Stuart McClean is Lecturer in Health Science (sociology and social anthropology) at the University of the West of England, Bristol. His research interests include the resurgence of alternative medicine in Western societies, and the global dimensions surrounding health. Stuart is currently completing his PhD, which is an ethnographic study of spiritual healing in the north of England.

Chris Miller is Principal Lecturer in Applied Social Studies and Director for the Research Centre for Local Democracy at the University of the West of England, Bristol. He is Editor of the international *Community Development Journal*. His research interests include participation and democratic theory, local governance, and public service organizational development.

Jennie Naidoo is Principal Lecturer in Public Health, in the Faculty of Health and Social Care at the University of the West of England, Bristol. She has a background in sociology, health promotion and education. Jennie worked in health promotion and research prior to taking up her post at the University of the West of England, Bristol. Her research interests include gender and health, and health promotion in primary care. She has written extensively on health promotion, theory and practice.

Stephen Peckham is Reader in Health Policy and Head of the Department of Sociology and Social Policy at Oxford Brookes University. He has been involved in health and social policy research and teaching for 12 years and previously worked in the voluntary and local government sectors. He has particular research interests in the areas of health policy analysis, interagency collaboration, public involvement, young people and sexual health, governance, primary care, and public health. He is currently leading a three year project for the UK Public Health Association examining the links between community organizations and primary care on public health issues. He is also working on the relationship between carers and primary care and an evaluation of the Oxfordshire Bodyzone school-based health clinics. He has published widely on primary care and health policy and his most recent book, *Primary Care in the UK: Policy, Organisation and Management* was co-written with Mark Exworthy.

Jon Pollock is Principal Lecturer in Epidemiology. His interests are in health services research and the contribution of epidemiology to studies of child health, care of the elderly, service provision and the evaluation of health and social care interventions.

Joyshri Sarangi is a consultant public health physician who works as Consultant in Communicable Disease Control and Regional Epidemiologist in the south-west region. She has extensive practical experience in the management of health protection incidents and in policy issues, and is a visiting lecturer at the University of the West of England, Bristol.

Gabriel Scally is Regional Director of Public Health for the south-west region of England. Gabriel has undertaken a number of assignments abroad for British and Irish governmental agencies including projects in Nigeria, Zambia, Zimbabwe and Seychelles. He was a member of the General Medical Council for the UK from 1989 to 1999 and has served on the Professional Conduct, Education, Health and Standards Committees. He is also a former member of the Northern Ireland Board for Nursing, Midwifery and Health Visiting. He has published papers on poorly performing doctors and most recently on clinical governance. He has edited a book on public health and is currently Joint Editor of *Clinical Governance Bulletin*, a journal published by The Royal Society of Medicine.

Murray Stewart is Visiting Professor of Urban and Regional Governance in the Cities Research Centre at the University of the West of England, Bristol. His interests are in urban policy, regeneration and renewal, and the evaluation of public policy.

Foreword

At the start of the twentieth century, public health as a discipline seemed to be emerging from a deeply and sharply political past, to establish itself as a mainstream medical specialty. It also seemed to be gaining ground with its techniques and methods. Health gains for the population were tangible and improving and as the new century dawned, not with standing existing public health problems, there was a genuine optimism about the possibilities of improvement and reform, an optimism shared across many spheres of life in Imperial Britain as the Edwardian era began. While the Edwardian dreams may have died for many on the battlefields of France during the First World War, the optimism for public health did not, and the twentieth century witnessed very important improvements in the health of the public. However, today that optimism has to be tempered. Health gain has continued. But at the heart of public health in Britain, lies a conundrum. The conundrum may be briefly stated. As a whole the health of the population is better than it was a hundred years ago, but the health of the most disadvantaged has not only not kept pace with the overall health gains of the population, but in some cases is actually static or getting worse. So while health improves, inequalities in health become greater.

This book provides important insights into the policies, practices and methods that are available to attack this problem. The structure of the book reflects the important linkages between the role of evidence, the role of interventions and their impact on inequalities These three things are in turn linked to broad policy and political processes and frameworks, the global and regional context and the importance of a multidisciplinary perspective with methods derived from the social as well as the biomedical and statistical sciences.

This book takes an historical perspective on the development of public health and the population approach to health improvement. It explores both the undoubted successes of the early public health movement, and the tensions arising from the approaches of the pioneers that were at times top down and authoritarian and became deeply enmeshed within a biomedical approach. Interestingly, these tensions remain at the heart of public health today. The book's explorations of contemporary public health and recent innovations and service developments demonstrate the ways in which such tensions permeate contemporary practice.

It is sometimes said that while public health is extremely sophisticated in its description of the problem of inequalities and it has been much more muted in its ability to define with precision what can be done to reduce them. This book looks at the some of the recent initiatives that have been put in place to address the question of inequalities in health. In so doing the book considers some of the tools that may assist the practitioner including data, evidence, health economics, measurement and health impact.

Public health has always been political and has always been multi disciplinary. This book demonstrates the depth of the political history and current political context of public health as well as the breadth of its disciplinary coverage. As we begin the next hundred years' journey in public health, this book is a timely reminder of both the ever presence of the political and the importance of interdisciplinary working.

Professor Mike Kelly
Director of Research and Information
Health Development Agency

Acknowledgements

Our thanks go to Linda Ewles from Headspring Consulting for joining us at a late stage and at a crucial point – when the size of the project and our available time seemed to be far apart. She brought superb editing skills together with a knowledge of the subject area which has been invaluable. Also thanks to Lynne Lilburn for flexible and efficient administrative support, to Jane Wathen for her technical support and to Selena Gray for her contribution to our work.

Thanks go to all the contributors for their cooperation, support and enthusiasm for this project.

Our thanks also go to our colleagues at the University of the West of England, Bristol, who have given encouragement and practical support at key times in the development of this book.

Finally, thanks go to our families for putting up with our absences, both mental and physical.

INTRODUCTION

Twenty-first century public health

The start of the 21st century is an exciting era for public health theory and practice.

Improving the public's health and well being is now a high profile feature of government policy. Public health action has expanded into a far wider arena as it recognizes that factors in people's social, economic and physical environment have a profound impact on their health. It involves a wider range of people than ever before from many different disciplines and professions working in partnership with the lay public and across agency and organizational boundaries. There is a growing need for a diverse public health workforce with an expanded range of expertise and skills.

Public health action now embraces work on major areas such as addressing inequalities in health, tackling challenges of urban renewal and sustainability, and taking on board the impact of globalization on health. It seeks to find better ways of finding out what works in public health and why it works, evaluating effectiveness and measuring outcomes.

About this book

Public health can be conceptualized in two ways: public health as *action* and public health as *resource*. Public health action refers to activities to improve health by professionals and lay people, and by individuals, groups and communities. It is within this idea of public health action that the rationale for partnership and multidisciplinary practice is established. Public health resources refer to the sources of information and expertise that contribute to public health action. There is clearly a strong interdependent relationship between public health activity and public health resources; in this book we deal with both aspects.

The task of this book is to raise and develop the debate about different contributions from the various partners in multidisciplinary public health practice. Public health action is, and should continue to be, approached in a different way from the traditional practice of expert domination, and local political and economic tensions highlighted in Ibsen's play, *An Enemy of the People* (see Box I.1). Although the

---

Box I.1   Setting the scene – Ibsen's *An Enemy of the People*

In Heinrich Ibsen's play *An Enemy of the People*, written in 1882, a doctor discovers that bacterial contamination of a small town's bathing complex poses a serious risk to the health of the public. The doctor tries to get support to close the facilities in order to sort out the problem of infection, but as the only meeting place for the local population the complex is seen as fundamental to the town's well being and economy.

Powerful local interests (including his brother, the mayor) resist closure on the grounds of cost and inconvenience. A full blown conflict of local and personal politics ensues with the former characterized by suspicion because of their closed nature. Accusations that the moral stand of the doctor is a front for personal gain are made by a number of individuals including his brother. A local newspaper becomes involved, the doctor's home is vandalized and both he and his sister lose their posts in the town.

This story can be seen to represent, in dramatized form, many of the components of a traditional public health problem that requires public health action. Without closure of the baths, the bacteria will impact on the health of an 'at risk' aggregate, the local population; but if the doctor takes public health action to close the baths, the population will be disadvantaged socially and economically.

An Enemy of the People reminds us that action in public health can lead to fundamental discord between different interest groups within a local community, and in this case in the same family. The knowledge and authority of the expert (the medical doctor) is set against a more general understanding of what is best for the town that comes from the mayor and others, who in turn either do not understand or distrust 'expert' knowledge.

The play illustrates the relative power, influence and perspectives of different groups in society which influence health outcomes. At another level, *An Enemy of the People* reveals a tension between economic activity and environmental and public health concerns that present trade-offs for society. Pragmatic economic interests are set against the absolute moral stand of the doctor. At the end of the play he defies authority and remains in the town.

---

problems of local politics, conflict and economic activity remain, contemporary public health acknowledges a multiplicity of interests and experts all of whom have a legitimate place in improving the health and well being of the public.

In this book, we analyse and reflect upon public health history, theories, research and practice. We explore the meaning of public health for the 21st century within the current debates and policy changes that are reshaping its context. We examine the vital connections between the public health body of knowledge and other professional discourses, and the rationale for the current commitment to the multidisciplinary nature of public health. We demonstrate how different disciplines (such as epidemiology and health economics) make important contributions to public health.

Our book also offers insight into current controversies and contradictions that will influence the way forward for public health. For example, not everyone agrees on the best way to assess the effectiveness of public health programmes, with different disciplines bringing a rich range of perspectives to bear on the issue.

Scope

In this book, we seek to define multidisciplinary public health in terms of its professional scope and discipline basis. Our core aims are to analyse the who, why, what and how of multidisciplinary public health for the 21st century.

The book's content is intended to be a scoping exercise for partnerships of agencies and organizations, professionals, managers, practitioners, students, policy-makers and service users, all engaged in the task of improving and studying the health of the public. It explores a range of perspectives from the many different disciplines that contribute to public health theory and practice.

An important development in scoping public health practice is the recently published *National Standards for Specialist Public Health* (Skills for Health 2002a). The key areas of work which need to be undertaken to achieve these objectives are set out in Table I.1. Scrutiny of these ten key areas of competence and their sub-areas provides a guide to the range of skills needed to work in contemporary specialist public health. A similar mapping has also been developed for scoping skills for public health practitioners. These national standards for specialist public health and public health practice and the breadth of activity that is encompassed within these provide a framework for this book. We have referred to this breadth of activity in order to scope and define our view of public health in the 21st century. Skills for Health (2002b) assert that public health action aims to:

- improve health and well being in the population;
- prevent disease and minimize its consequences;
- prolong valued life; and
- reduce inequalities in health.

Structure

This book has been developed and edited as a resource for the development of future public health with contributory chapters by authors in public health academia and practice.

Table I.1 National standards for specialist public health

A	Surveillance and assessment of the population's health and well being
B	Promoting and protecting the population's health and well being
C	Developing quality and risk management within an evaluative culture
D	Collaborative working for health and well being
E	Developing health programmes and services and reducing inequalities
F	Policy, strategy development, implementation to improve health and well being
G	Working with and for communities to improve health and well being
H	Strategic leadership for health and well being
I	Research and development to improve health and well being
J	Ethically managing self, people and resources to improve health and well being

Source: Skills for Health (2002a)

It is structured into four parts. In order to give overall coherence to this wide ranging book, each of the four parts has its own Editors' overview. We hope that readers will find that reading this Introduction to the whole book, and the overview of each part is, in itself, a useful exercise for getting to grips with the scope of 21st century public health. Each chapter also has an Editors' introduction, intended to enable readers to see the relevance of the chapter to their own situation, and to be introduced to the chapter's subject matter.

There is likely to be an audience for the book as a whole, but there will also be readers who are interested in particular parts and chapters. Each chapter can stand alone for those wishing to dip into a specific issue, for example, to find guidance in how to complete and interpret an economic evaluation study or to learn more about the field of regeneration and health.

Contents

In Part 1 the authors consider three aspects of the public health policy context that are a precursor to effective multidisciplinary action. Public health policy including modernization and its implementation is evaluated critically and the future of public health is mapped out using a historical perspective for reference.

In Part 2 the authors identify the partners in public health and assess the capacity and capability of the public health workforce, including lay people and communities, to meet new objectives of building social capital and community networks. The new roles for primary care trusts and health protection professionals are evaluated and assessed.

Public health resources and action have to address some all pervasive public health problems. For example, socio-economic inequalities in health, improving health and health inequality at a neighbourhood level, improving health in the cities of the world, and looking at the wider picture of global influences on health and health inequalities, all underpin recent change in public health policy, participation and practice. Each of these themes is considered in Part 3.

In Part 4 the authors suggest ways in which professions and disciplines can work together and move forward in the difficult challenge of providing evidence for the impact and effectiveness of public health action. The authors outline four separate disciplinary approaches to evaluation from epidemiology; economics; community health and well being; and health impact assessment, estimation and analysis. They highlight the growing requirement for robust, theory-based evaluation frameworks appropriate for complex, context specific public health programmes. They discuss the move from the traditional, medically dominated 'hierarchy of evidence' towards 'evidence informed public health'.

Figure I.1 provides an overview of the book's structure and the major themes of the chapters.

Who this book is for?

This book is intended for all those people for whom developing and implementing policies for health improvement and the reduction of inequalities in

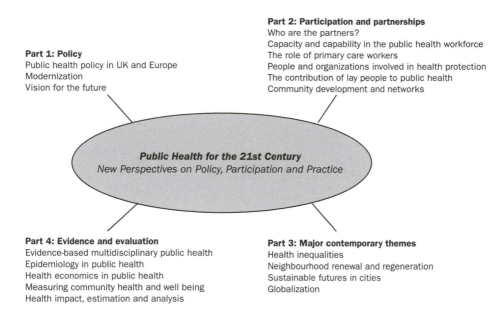

Part 1: Policy
Public health policy in UK and Europe
Modernization
Vision for the future

Part 2: Participation and partnerships
Who are the partners?
Capacity and capability in the public health workforce
The role of primary care workers
People and organizations involved in health protection
The contribution of lay people to public health
Community development and networks

Public Health for the 21st Century
New Perspectives on Policy, Participation and Practice

Part 4: Evidence and evaluation
Evidence-based multidisciplinary public health
Epidemiology in public health
Health economics in public health
Measuring community health and well being
Health impact, estimation and analysis

Part 3: Major contemporary themes
Health inequalities
Neighbourhood renewal and regeneration
Sustainable futures in cities
Globalization

Figure I.1 Structure and major themes of this book

health is the central focus of their practice. This would include people working in the fields of health and social care, environmental health and in community regeneration.

Our intended readership also includes a wider audience of professionals and lay people who would not immediately label their work as 'public health', but who would see that they contribute to the wider health and well being of their communities (see Figure I.2). This wider audience includes people involved in leisure, education, employment, housing, transport and community safety. One of the aims of this text is to explore the similarities and overlap in the core public health agenda and the wider agenda of contributing to well being, as well as to identify barriers to working together.

The main audience for this book is likely to be UK-based, as discussion on policy making and administrative arrangements is largely drawn from UK practice. But this book will also be of interest to an international audience in so far as it deals with global public health concerns, for example, health inequalities, sustainability, evidence-based public health, regeneration and renewal, partnership working and the impact of the forces of globalization on public health.

Historical perspectives on public health

Contemporary public health has not been written on a blank slate, but has evolved and developed through centuries. History informs practice, so it is useful to consider briefly the roots and development of today's public health theory and practice.

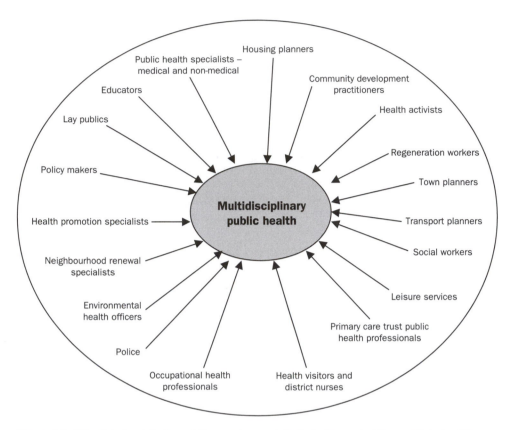

Figure I.2 Who this book is for: all those who contribute to improving the public's health

The 19th century origins of public health practice

The history of public health illustrates the interrelationship between public health information and public health action. In the mid-1800s, outbreaks of disease were thought to be spread through odours in the air (the miasma theory) until one physician, John Snow, treating an outbreak of cholera in Broadgate, a poor area of London, observed that the disease also affected a single patient in a more affluent area some distance away. Snow discovered from the patient's maid that the patient did not visit the Broadgate area but preferred to drink the water from the Broadgate pump. Snow hypothesized that cholera was transmitted through water rather than by 'bad smells'.

So began the basis of evidence-based public health, with a physician observing events and taking time to engage with ordinary people to find out about their habits and practices. Snow linked the data on sources of disease with mortality data in London, established an association and then a causal link between the events, taking action to close the water pump which was 6 feet from a cesspit contaminated with cholera.

Public health practice began with recognition by some Victorians of the importance of clean water and sanitation to health. Chadwick and other medical colleagues and social campaigners were engaged in campaigns to achieve environmental improvements in, for example, sewers and clean drinking water. Contemporary observers have argued that these reforms led to greater improvements in population health than anything subsequently achieved by the NHS (Baggott 2000). These early public health campaigners, who included the trade union movement, worked to persuade politicians and municipal authorities to make environmental improvements; such action required political motivation and public support.

The realization that disease was no respecter of social class or wealth, and that the health of the most deprived members of society had to be of concern to the population as a whole, was a strong factor in the growing momentum of public health action. These 19th century reforms created the basis for the system of public health located at the level of municipal or local authorities; inevitably they were influenced by the local politics of the time, as illustrated in Ibsen's play (Box I.1).

Early 20th century public health

Concerns about the state of the population's health appeared throughout the early 20th century, significantly at times of war when the poor state of army recruits revived concerns about the conditions influencing the health of the working classes. The approach to population health at this time was essentially paternalistic. Communities were expected to receive public health expertise and intervention gratefully in the form of immunization, screening or hygiene advice. The rationale for public health action was a societal 'common good' and those who did not comply were seen as feckless or undeserving.

By the mid-20th century, due to improvements in sanitary conditions and specific preventative and curative measures, the impact of infectious diseases had reduced markedly, and was superseded by 'preventable' medical and psychiatric disorders, such as diseases of the circulatory system, cancers and depression.

1948 and 1974: significant milestones

The creation of the National Health Service (NHS) in 1948 was a response to the concerns of war and was a direct result of pressure from trade unions to provide better conditions for workers who had contributed to the war effort as soldiers and civilians. Debates at that time showed a clear expectation that providing a free and accessible illness service for the whole population would result in a reduction of the need for such services in the long term. The NHS appeared to be based on a clear distinction between services for ill health and the preventative health activities.

Until 1974 the public health structure was left untouched within the local authority. A medical officer of health headed up a team of public health workers including environmental health officers, health visitors and welfare officers dealing with population health issues. But in 1974, the medical officer of health was moved into the NHS thereby severing the link from locally based public health action. This also meant that public health was viewed within a medically dominated health service model.

20th century perspectives on 'health'

The World Health Organisation (WHO) has been influential in broadening out the concept of health and establishing appreciation of the range of determinants of health and disease. The original and classic definition of health as 'a state of complete physical, mental and social well being, not merely the absence of disease and infirmity' (WHO 1946) with its holistic emphasis on health and well being, underpinned the later Health for All movement and the declaration of Alma Ata (WHO 1978). This clearly acknowledged the gross inequalities between advantaged and disadvantaged peoples as politically, socially and economically unacceptable (Tones 2001).

'New' public health in the 1980s

A significant shift in public health thinking occurred during the 1980s, with acknowledgement of a broader ecological perspective on health, and the emergence of the 'new public health' (Ashton and Seymour 1988). Significant developments in this period included the Healthy Cities movement (Ashton 1992; Davies and Kelly 1992) and the 1985 Targets for Health for Europe (WHO 1985). This was followed by the Ottawa Charter in 1986 (WHO 1986) with its five main strategies for health improvement. The developing environmental movement at this time resulted in the agreement of Agenda 21 which sets out how developed and developing countries could work towards sustainable development (United Nations 1992; Allen 2001).

Another significant event in the 1980s was the publication of a report on public health in England (Acheson 1988). In his report Acheson, the Chief Medical Officer for England, defined public health in a much wider context than before as:

> the science and art of preventing disease, prolonging life and promoting health through the organised efforts of society. These efforts will address policy issues at the level of the population's health and will tackle the role of health and disease, as well as considering the provision of effective health care services. Public health works through partnerships that cut across disciplinary, professional and organisational boundaries, and exploits this diversity in collaboration, to bring evidence and research based policies to all areas which impact on the health and well being of populations.
>
> (Acheson 1988)

Acheson's definition reveals key ideas embedded in much contemporary public health, identifying partnership and multidisciplinary working, collaboration, an evidence-based approach and the width of action from population health gain through to the provision of health care services. It also illustrates the complex and contested nature of public health. The term public health is generally understood as a nebulous concept; attempts have been made at a more precision result in a continuum of definitions between science and art which are far from compatible. But one generally agreed characteristic is that the basis of public health information is *population* focused and in contrast to the *individual* patient focus of most health professionals.

The Acheson Report recommended that a director of public health should be appointed in each health authority. The director would act as a chief medical advisor and 'would advise on priorities, planning and evaluation, co-ordinate the control of communicable disease and develop policy on prevention and health promotion' (Baggott 2000: 47).

'New Labour' in 1997 and a new focus on health inequalties and public health

Following the change of government in 1997, the late 1990s witnessed growing governmental concern with health inequalities and the first minister for public health was appointed. (The history of public health since 1997 is discussed in detail in Chapters 1 and 2.) The 'new Labour' government commissioned Sir Donald Acheson to report on inequalities in health and this marked a significant resurgence of interest in addressing the 'health gap' between richer and poorer people and tackling the root causes of poor health and health inequality such as poverty, homelessness, lack of life chances and unemployment (Acheson 1998). (Tackling health inequalities is discussed in Chapter 10.)

Into the 21st century: public health in primary care

The publication of *Shifting the Balance of Power: Next Steps* (Department of Health 2002b) sets out clearly the government's intention to make primary care trusts (PCTs) the local focus for health development within the NHS including public health. (We examine the role of PCTs in depth in Chapter 6.)

PCTs carry the main responsibility for leading the development of health improvement and modernization plans. They are expected to achieve specific targets for health gain and partnership, and are required to work with a range of initiatives, including New Deal, Sure Start, Neighbourhood Renewal, health action zones and healthy living centres, all introduced by the government in their commitment to tackling inequalities in health. (These initiatives are discussed more fully in Chapter 11.)

This move to put primary care at the centre of public health development has the potential to maximize public health activity at a local and community level. This will be an important starting point for other local statutory, voluntary and community agencies and local publics to develop their understanding of health issues, and to make connections between local concerns and public health issues. It also has the potential for local communities to influence the nature and content of the public health agenda, including research and priorities, giving a wider meaning to the term public health action.

Multidisciplinary public health

Fundamental to this book is the notion of *multidisciplinary* public health. So finally, as part of the Introduction, it is helpful to consider it briefly.

A diversity of disciplines

It is easy to label 21st century public health blithely as 'multidisciplinary', but much less easy to explain what this means. What is more certain is that the multiple disciplines that underpin contemporary public health have different traditions in terms of philosophy, approaches and methods ranging from 'positivist/quantitative' to 'interpretivist/qualitative'. A 'discipline' can be defined as a way of thinking and a set of tools and techniques that complement that thinking. Given this definition, the disciplines of contemporary public health are not easily listed as they include many levels of contribution from a wide range. One of the related challenges is the use of different languages by different disciplines.

A multidisciplinary evidence base

Discussions about the constitution of a multidisciplinary public health are linked strongly with contentious issues about the evidence base for public health. Public health action should be predicated upon evidence and a number of disciplines, such as epidemiology, health impact assessment, health impact analysis, health impact estimation and economics come into play here through the 'hierarchy of evidence'. But there is much contention regarding the 'hierarchy of evidence' that informs public health debate and how this is disseminated and applied in current practice.

The challenge of developing an evidence-based multidisciplinary public health is considerable. It involves, among other things, complex theoretical and methodological debates across disciplines, realignments of power and influence within the public health profession and community, an open mindedness combined with rigour about evidence among those training for public health practice and the development of accessible mechanisms for the dissemination of evidence. (Part 4 of this book addresses these issues in depth.)

One of the challenges of this book could be to explain how the separate disciplines of multidisciplinary public health are to be brought together 'as disciplines and not just people' (Dowie 1996), in order to move the public health movement forward. We argue that the complexity of this task is so great, particularly for creation of a multidisciplinary public health evidence base, and that it is not really necessary. Given that all the disciplines that contribute in some way to the health of the public are, in themselves, being influenced by the evidence-based movement in its broadest sense, there may be an argument for leaving specialists in different fields to 'do their own thing'. The argument for evidence-based multidisciplinary public health is not an argument against specialisms and the benefits these bring. It is an argument for recognizing the contributions of different disciplines to public health and for incorporating these into a framework that does not exclude potential contributors. This approach would allow partnerships and other multidisciplinary teams in public health to appraise and use evidence on the basis of its fitness for purpose rather than its adherence to specific methodological traditions.

This is not to say that an evidence-based approach should dominate all aspects of public health. Public health is a complex activity, involving long-term goals and fundamental shifts in both policy and practice. This means that it is 'both an art and a science, but it should not be an act of faith' (Gowman and Coote 2000). It should make risks of failure clearer, encourage monitoring of outcomes and add to the constant improvement of the evidence base which will inform future decisions.

A multidisciplinary model of health

A biomedical, economic, psychosocial model of health, rather than a medical model, forms the basis of our 21st century view of public health. This creates a new public health practice, characterized by 'open politics' in which different interests are transparent and governance allows for open negotiation to resolve conflict. It replaces the idea of irreconcilable conflict (between, for example, environmental health and economy) with the possibility of resolving differences through openness and understanding. Improvements in the health of the public will occur through 'open' partnership, with government policy and public health action working in tandem. Across professional boundaries of health, social care, crime, regeneration and renewal, partnerships acting upon 'appropriate' and independent evidence will help to resolve the deep seated health-related problems of society: health inequalities, poverty, low quality of life and social exclusion. This is the vision for 21st century public health, with all its constraints and opportunities, discussed by the contributors to this book.

Conclusion

This Introduction has set out our vision of 21st century public health. We have outlined this book's content, scope and purpose, and who it is for. We have summarized the history of public health in the past 200 years, so that readers can understand how current practice has developed from the pioneering work of public health thinkers and practitioners in the past. Finally, we have explored the fundamental concept of the multidisciplinary nature of public health.

We hope that readers will find this book thought provoking, informative and above all helpful in taking public health forward to meet the challenges of the 21st century.

PART 1

Policy for 21st century public health

Editors' overview

What is the broad policy framework for public health at the start of the 21st century? How has it evolved, and what may happen in the future?

These are the fundamental question addressed in Part 1. It provides readers with an overview of the development and context of public health policy and its potential scope in contemporary society. It explores current debates in relation to the influences of social, political and cultural factors. It takes a critical look at how public health fits into current government policy and uses a historical perspective to help inform a vision for the future of public health.

Understanding the context of policy development in public health is an essential precursor to effective multidisciplinary public health activity. Overall this part of the book engages readers in an interdisciplinary context through the analysis of, and reflection upon, public health theories, research and practice. It includes reference to wider international developments in public health.

The chapters focus on three aspects of the public health policy context: current public health policy and its implementation; public health and the government's modernization agenda; and a vision for the future of public health.

In Chapter 1 David Hunter takes a critical look at current public health policy and its implementation. Hunter questions whether the current and developing administrative and policy framework is appropriate for the problems which need to be tackled in the development of multidisciplinary public health. His chapter briefly considers the policy context in Wales, Scotland and Northern Ireland. First, he reviews the present state of public health policy and its recent history since 1997, then he examines the constraints on implementing public health policies, before considering the future of public health policy. He provides public health professionals with suggestions about what needs to happen if there is to be a sustained shift in policy towards health as distinct from health care.

In Chapter 2 Chris Miller reflects on the government's modernization agenda and its importance in the development of public health in the 21st century. He examines the precursors to modernization, how it has happened, why it has happened and the dilemmas it has created for public health. The implications of the modernization agenda are then examined focusing on generic threads that affect public health work. These include partnership working, user involvement, community focus, leadership and quality of service provision. Miller provides unique insight into political processes and their impact on the health of the public.

In Chapter 3 Gabriel Scally presents a vision for the future of public health in the 21st century. He focuses on several core themes which include learning from historical public health, the need to function in a shared power world, the importance of public health management and leadership, the prospect of dedicated public health services, the importance of health protection and the impact of regionalism and internationalism. This discussion provides public health professionals with important issues to consider which are likely to be of central importance for public health development.

1

DAVID J. HUNTER
Public health policy

Editors' introduction

Government policy on public health, along with related policy on issues which affect health such as education, employment, food and transport, provide the broad framework for action to improve the health of the population; policies can facilitate new opportunities for health improvement but they may also hinder progress.

It is therefore crucial that public health workers develop a critical understanding of current public health policy and programmes at both national and local level. In this chapter, the author provides a refreshing insight and critique into the important area of public health policy development and implementation, which should prove useful for everyone working in the field of public health, in whatever capacity.

The government's commitment to public health is evidenced by a range of policy initiatives since 1997. The author takes a critical look at current policy developments and examines how they have been put into action. He questions whether the current and developing policy and administrative framework are 'fit for purpose' and appropriate for the problems and challenges posed by the development of multidisciplinary public health in the 21st century. He identifies and discusses barriers and difficulties posed by the breadth of policy development.

The chapter is in three sections. The first section reviews the present state of public health policy and its recent history since 1997. In particular, it assesses the tension in health policy between a 'downstream' agenda fixated on acute health care and an 'upstream' agenda centred on public health interventions designed to maintain and improve health, and avoid or delay contact with the NHS.

The second section examines the constraints on implementing public health policies and the bias in public health towards the NHS and health care. It questions how far this can be influenced and changed.

The final section and conclusion consider the future of public health policy and make suggestions for what needs to happen if there is to be a sustained shift in policy towards health as distinct from health care.

Introduction

This chapter takes a critical look at current public health policy and its implementation. It questions whether the current and developing policy and administrative framework are 'fit for purpose' and appropriate for the problems and challenges posed by the development of multidisciplinary public health and concludes that they pose major barriers and other difficulties which, if not addressed, will seriously impede implementation. Though centred on the position in England, the chapter briefly considers the differing policy contexts elsewhere in the UK post-devolution. The impact of devolution affords opportunities for policy learning.

The chapter is in three sections. The first section reviews the present state of public health policy and its recent history since 1997. In particular, it assesses the deep rooted tension in health policy between an 'upstream' agenda centred on public health interventions, and a 'downstream' agenda fixated on acute health care. The second section examines the constraints on implementing public health policies and the bias in public health towards the NHS and health care; it questions whether this is inevitable. The third section considers the future of public health policy and makes suggestions for what needs to happen if there is to be a sustained shift in policy towards health as distinct from health care.

The state of public health policy

The new Labour government May 1997: public health renaissance

Public health underwent something of a renaissance following the election of the Labour government in May 1997. The new government acted quickly to appoint the first ever minister for public health as a member of the ministerial team in the Department of Health. Her remit only extended to England as plans for devolution to Scotland, Wales and Northern Ireland were already well advanced. The new minister was anxious to map out a new approach to health policy to demonstrate the government's commitment to a more socially equitable and cohesive society.

There was a recognition that improving health and narrowing the widening 'health gap' between social groups were policy challenges that transcended any single department's responsibilities. They were cross-cutting issues and therefore key features of the government's concern that there should be 'joined up' solutions to 'joined up' social problems. The minister for public health immediately set in progress three initiatives:

- the development of a new health strategy to replace *The Health of the Nation*, the first ever health strategy for England which existed from 1992 to 1997 (Secretary of State for Health 1992);
- an evaluation of the impact of *The Health of the Nation* at local level, the findings from which would inform the new strategy (Department of Health 1998b); and
- an inquiry into inequalities chaired by a former chief medical officer, Sir Donald Acheson, to demonstrate where the scientific evidence showed interventions to be effective in tackling inequalities (Acheson 1998).

The Acheson inquiry made 39 recommendations only three of which directly concerned the NHS. This only confirmed the government in its view that improving the public's health and tackling inequalities had to be part of concerted action across government. (See Chapter 10 for a detailed discussion of tackling inequalities in health.)

Table 1.1 lists key policies, reports and initiatives in public health since the Labour government came to power in 1997.

Table 1.1 Key policies, reports and initiatives in public health 1997–2002

1997	Election of new Labour government; commitment to public health action to reduce health inequalities.
1998	Acheson *Independent Inquiry into Inequalities in Health* published.
1999	New national strategy for health in England published: *Saving Lives: Our Healthier Nation*. Initiatives such as health action zones, healthy living centres and Sure Start started to be launched to improve health and reduce inequalities in health.
2000	Health Development Agency set up; remit included strengthening the evidence base of public health. *The NHS Plan* published; signalled organizational change and attracted criticism about the lack of emphasis on public health.
2001	National targets on health inequalities published. *Shifting the Balance of Power* published – devolving NHS responsibility to the 'front line'. House of Commons Select Committee reports on public health published, which criticized the lack of government emphasis on public health. *The Report of the Chief Medical Officer's Project to Strengthen the Public Health Function* also published. Two reports: *Tackling Health Inequalities* (consultation document) and *Vision to Reality* (progress report on tackling health inequalities) published.
2002	Wanless Report published on future health trends and resources required; it supported public health action to bring health and economic benefits. *Tackling Health Inequalities* report published on action needed. HM Treasury and Department of Health *Tackling Health Inequalities: Summary of the 2002 Cross-Cutting Review* published, which committed the government to placing tackling health inequalities at the heart of public service delivery.

New health strategy and other initiatives

A new health strategy finally appeared in 1999 after some delay (Secretary of State for Health 1999). Entitled *Saving Lives: Our Healthier Nation*, it attempted to take on board at least some of the lessons from the evaluation of its predecessor, *The Health of the Nation*. The strategy was widely welcomed although some commentators felt it remained rather too firmly wedded to a health care model which was less about supporting communities to remain healthy than about keeping individuals alive (Fulop and Hunter 1999). The strategy focused mainly on disease-based areas. To this extent, therefore, there were limits on how far it represented a move 'upstream'. A key finding from *The Health of the Nation* evaluation was that the dominance of the medical model underlying the strategy 'was a major barrier to its ownership by agencies outside the health sector, notably local government and voluntary agencies' (Department of Health 1998c). Commenting on the new health strategy, the Local Government Association and the UK Public Health Association in a joint report concluded that 'the traditional concerns of public health medicine focused primarily on alleviating sickness and preventing premature death' remained a 'dominant and overly narrow perspective' (Local Government Association and UK Public Health Association 2000: 2).

Almost simultaneously with these policy developments, the government launched a bewildering array of other new programmes and initiatives. These included health action zones (HAZs), healthy living centres (HLCs), Sure Start (with its pledge to end child poverty within a generation), New Deal for Communities and health improvement programmes. Judging by the sheer number of announcements and their scope and range there could be no doubting the government's resolve and drive in respect of raising the priority attached to improving the public's health and narrowing the gap between rich and poor.

At the same time, the Health Education Authority was replaced by a virtually new body, the Health Development Agency, charged with strengthening the evidence base for public health in line with similar developments that were already underway in respect of evidence-based medicine. The new Agency's remit included a commitment to disseminate the evidence about what interventions worked and those that did not work, as well as to provide developmental support to those organizations struggling to apply the evidence in practice.

The government's commitment to evidence-based public health reflected the 'new scientism' that had invaded government during the late 1980s and early 1990s (Klein 1996). There was a view that if only the evidence were available to point policy makers in the right direction then it would be possible to answer those critics who believed public health interventions were ineffective and based on rhetoric rather than solid evidence. Indeed, this is the opinion of the Minister for Public Health, Hazel Blears. In one of her first major speeches following her appointment, she stressed her enthusiasm for the evidence of what works. 'Evidence is vital, not least because I am well aware that there are sceptics who suggest that none of this effort makes any difference to the health of the public' (Blears 2002). But perhaps the sceptics simply choose to ignore the evidence that already exists. In any event, the evidence will always be imperfect and incomplete. In this respect the position is no different for public health than for any other area of policy.

While welcoming the government's commitment to public health evident in the outpouring of policy statements, ministerial speeches and so on, critics accuse the government of suffering from 'initiativitis'. This actually makes the job of 'joining up' policy and management more difficult because each initiative tends to operate in isolation and receives its own dedicated funding and its success is judged according to criteria specific to that particular initiative (Hunter 2003). Rather than simplifying partnership working, which the government claims it wants to do by, for instance, abolishing the NHS internal market, the plethora of initiatives only increases fragmentation. It has introduced a new kind of market as agencies compete against each other in bidding for funds to become a HAZ, HLC and so on.

The NHS plan

It was the appearance of *The NHS Plan* in July 2000 that gave an indication that the government's attention and energy were being progressively directed towards the NHS and its problems, the extent of which the government had underestimated during its initial years in office (Secretary of State for Health 2000). Aware that the NHS was a key electoral issue and that it must remain an asset for Labour rather than becoming a liability, ministers prepared for major changes in the system of delivering health care. Initially opposed to 'big bang' structural reform the type of which the NHS had become weary over decades of successive structural changes, the government embarked on the most comprehensive and complex organizational changes the NHS had witnessed (Department of Health 2001a). The NHS is still coming to terms with these changes but one of their effects has been to put at risk the government's early focus on public health.

A slim chapter buried deep in *The NHS Plan* was devoted to improving health and reducing health inequalities. Rightly or wrongly, this signalled to those outside the Department of Health that the main business of health policy was sorting out the NHS, since success on this front would determine the government's future at the next general election. Indeed, in an unprecedented move, the government and the prime minister personally, have staked their survival on the NHS being 'modernized'. (See Chapter 2 for a comprehensive discussion of Labour's 'modernization' agenda and what it means for public health.)

A debate on the merits of national health inequalities targets that was never resolved in *Saving Lives: Our Healthier Nation* was brought to an end with a promise in *The NHS Plan* to produce national targets. These duly appeared in March 2001. They are intended to complement the local targets called for in the health strategy and are to be delivered by a combination of specific health service policies, broader government policies, including abolishing child poverty through Sure Start, and action on cancer and coronary heart disease, to be taken through the appropriate national service frameworks. A problem with the targets was that while they were produced by the Department of Health and directed at the NHS for implementation, their realization actually depended on the activities of other bodies, especially local authorities. But these bodies were not engaged in the production of the targets and saw them as directed at the NHS rather than at them.

Public health – 'off the boil'?

As the government became more embroiled in sorting out the NHS through its *Shifting the Balance of Power* initiative aimed at devolving responsibility to the front line and intervening less from the centre, there was a growing sense of despondency in the public health community that the government had reverted to form in being preoccupied with urgent 'downstream' issues affecting the NHS. It merely indulged in a lot of symbolic posturing around the important 'upstream' determinants of health but was seemingly less committed to putting its own policies into action. Policy resembled what Bachrach and Baratz (1970) termed 'decisionless decisions'.

Many of these sentiments around public health having gone 'off the boil' were given added impetus when expressed by the House of Commons Health Committee in a critical report on public health in March 2001 (House of Commons 2001a, b). The Committee was critical of the imbalance in government policy in favour of health care as distinct from health. Even in respect of those initiatives, like HAZs and health improvement plans, intended to promote health the Committee was critical of the way in which they had been implemented. The difficulties arose principally from the sheer number of initiatives and their lack of integration. Although welcoming the Plan's commitment to health inequality targets, the Committee felt that 'a great opportunity to give public health a real impetus has been lost by the lack of emphasis on this area in the Plan' (House of Commons 2001a). The Committee noted the contrast with the equivalent plans in Wales and Scotland which both led with a strong commitment to the public's health (see below).

Reviews and reports strengthening public health

As if sensing the change of mood about its commitment to public health, the government, in addition to producing the national targets, published a number of other policy documents and reports testifying to its determination to fulfil its public health objectives and possibly seeking to reassure its critics that its eye had not been taken off the health ball altogether. The much delayed final report of the chief medical officer's review of the public health function appeared simultaneously with the Health Committee's report in March 2001 (Department of Health 2001b). It restated the government's wish to strengthen the public health workforce, although the report was light on the cost of such an exercise or where the resources would come from; consequently, action following the report has been limited.

Later the same year two further reports appeared from the centre. The first, *Tackling Health Inequalities*, was produced to consult on the action needed to achieve the two national health inequalities targets (Department of Health 2001c). To deliver the targets, six priority themes were proposed:

- providing a sure foundation through a healthy pregnancy and early childhood;
- improving opportunity for children and young people;
- improving NHS primary care services;
- tackling the major killer diseases: coronary heart disease and cancer;
- strengthening disadvantaged communities; and
- tackling the wider determinants of health inequalities.

The report made the point, yet again, that effective action required joined up working across government and across sectors at national, regional and local levels. A follow up report was published in June 2002 (Department of Health 2002a). It provided feedback on the consultation exercise on the government's six priority themes. They were generally supported, but those consulted were critical of the document's largely NHS and medical focus. In particular, there was concern that the contribution to be made by local government had been given insufficient attention and weight and needed to be made more explicit. This should include its duty to develop strategies and its health scrutiny role. Local strategic partnerships (LSPs) were seen as key vehicles for involving both the NHS and local government. Again, in delivering the agenda the feedback was generally critical of the prominence given to the NHS to the virtual exclusion of other agencies. Finally, there was criticism of the heavy reliance on short-term projects and initiatives. They distracted staff and too often mainstream activities and services remained unaffected or unchallenged by any lessons the projects had to offer.

The second report to appear in 2001 (mentioned above), *Vision to Reality*, took the form of a progress report from the minister for public health and chief medical officer on developments since the Acheson inquiry on health inequalities, the *Saving Lives: Our Healthier Nation* strategy, *The NHS Plan* and the chief medical officer's public health function review (Department of Health 2001d). As such, it did not contain any new policy thinking but served as a reaffirmation of the government's commitment to a modernized health service and public health service that 'will lay even greater emphasis on the protection and improvement of the population's health, and which will at last start to reduce the gap between the best and worst off in society'. There was an acknowledgement that 'for too long the NHS has been seen as a sickness service not a health service'. The intention was to see the NHS acting in partnership with others 'to prevent sickness and ill health, as well as treating problems once they arise' (Department of Health 2001d).

While health policy was traditionally the preserve of the Department of Health, the Chancellor of the Exchequer, Gordon Brown, announced a long-term review of the challenges facing the NHS over the next 20 years. He appointed the former chairman of the National Westminster Bank, Derek Wanless, to lead a review to examine future health trends and the resources required over the next 20 years to close gaps in performance and to deliver *The NHS Plan*. The review team published an interim report in late 2001 and a final report in April 2002 (Wanless 2001, 2002). Rather unexpectedly, it gave an important boost to public health and certainly acknowledged its importance.

The review team argued that 'better public health measures could significantly affect the demand for health care' (Wanless 2002: paragraph 1.27). On top of any health benefits, a focus on public health was also seen to bring wider benefits by increasing productivity and reducing inactivity in the working age population. The review team expressed concern that the poor evidence base in public health demonstrating the effectiveness of interventions made it difficult to conclude that investment in public health should be significantly increased. In its final report, it revised this conclusion and was more optimistic in its assessment of the potential for public health interventions. 'Despite methodological difficulties and the length of time needed for research, there is evidence suggesting that some health promotion interventions are not only effective, but also cost-effective over both short and longer time periods' (Wanless 2002). It quoted research findings showing that 25 percent of all cancers and 30 percent of coronary heart disease are preventable through public health measures (McPherson 2001).

Most important, especially coming from a hard nosed banker, was a conviction that good health is good economics and that far from being a cost, investment in health is a benefit to individuals, employers and the government. Healthy communities attract investment, while unhealthy ones do not (Hunter 2002). What was required, according to Wanless, was a better balance between curing sickness on the one hand and preventing disease on the other. The review team expressed concern that perhaps too much effort and emphasis was being placed on 'downstream' acute care services in preference to 'upstream' interventions designed to maintain and improve health, and avoid or delay contact with the NHS. The Wanless review therefore gave an important and timely boost to those advocating a more assertive approach to public health interventions both inside and outside government.

The Treasury's commitment to tackling health inequalities was reflected in the 2002 cross-cutting review published jointly by it and the Department of Health in November 2002 (HM Treasury and Department of Health 2002). Launching it in a speech to the Faculty of Public Health Medicine, the Secretary of State for Health, Alan Milburn, stated that the review committed the whole of government 'to place tackling health inequalities at the very heart of public service delivery' (Milburn 2002). Perhaps of greater significance given the health secretary's preoccupation with the NHS and delivery of health care, he astonished his audience by conceding that 'the health debate in our country has for too long been focused on the state of the nation's health service and not enough on the state of the nation's health'. It was time for 'a sea change in attitudes' and 'to secure a better balance between prevention and treatment'.

This section has briefly reviewed the impressive volume of documentation establishing the case for rebalancing policy so that it gives proper attention and weight to health as distinct from health care. But, if there has been a common complaint running through the various policy pronouncements that have appeared since 1997 it has been that there remains an unhelpful bias in favour of the NHS and of avoiding ill health and disease rather than maintaining good health. The contribution other sectors and agencies can clearly make to the public health effort is too often overlooked or treated as an add on. It has been a recurring theme over many years and one that has been repeated ad nauseam in countless reports from numerous quarters. Hardly surprising, therefore, to find that other key stakeholders have not been engaged in ways that are essential if the wider public health agenda is to be addressed. The section below – Public health: constraints on implementation – probes a little further the implementation gap in respect of public health.

Devolution and public health policy

None of the policy documents reported above apply to Wales, Scotland and Northern Ireland. Nor is there a separate public health minister in these countries. Some documents, notably the health strategy, *Saving Lives: Our Healthier Nation*, and *The NHS Plan* have their equivalents in the other three countries. But it is still early days as far as devolution and its impact are concerned. Policy divergence is a slow process and although some evidence for it can be seen in respect of the various policy statements produced, how far any differences will get translated into practice remains to be seen.

In contrast to England, the Welsh and Scottish Plans both open with a strong commitment to putting health first (Northern Ireland has been omitted from this discussion because its circumstances are rather different from elsewhere in the UK). But there is scepticism in some quarters over whether this really signals a break with the past. Greer, for instance, who has studied the progress of public health across the UK asserts that the English Plan is 'primarily focused on health care services organisations'; Scotland is 'speaking of public health but still focusing on health care services'; and Wales is 'focusing on integrated public health activities and promotion' (Greer 2001: 21). Both Wales and Scotland appear to be addressing the public health infrastructure deficit more directly having established new bodies dedicated to the strengthening of the public health function. Nothing comparable has emerged in England. However, as Greer also points out, it makes little sense to take England as a baseline for intra-UK comparative purposes, tempting though this may be. Including Northern Ireland, there are now four policy arenas with four health policies. Each of these arenas is likely to display a mix of convergence and divergence. Perhaps one of the more interesting developments will be the impact of devolution on English regionalism. The final section below – The future of public health – returns to this issue.

Public health: constraints on implementation

Reasons advanced for the lack of effective implementation of policies favouring public health are many and include:

- lack of clarity of the public health function especially as performed by public health medicine specialists;
- a policy stance that seems to be more symbolic and concerned with gesture politics rather than with real change;
- the absence of clear boundaries – improving health is everybody's business (the risk being that it becomes nobody's responsibility);
- the results of interventions to improve health take many years to take effect and it becomes difficult to establish cause and effect;
- giving the lead role for public health to the NHS which, many would claim, is preoccupied with ill health rather than health; health care services have an insatiable appetite for growth and expansion and they are where the powerful vested interests in health policy are located; and
- poor evidence about the effectiveness of public health interventions in contrast to the alleged acceptance of evidence-based medicine.

Public health: core purpose?

It is possible to contest some of these explanations, like the issue of the evidence base where comparisons with evidence-based medicine are not sensible or valid. But a key factor in public health's failure to deliver, it is suggested, has its roots in confusion about its core purpose and the multiple roles it is expected to perform. These are:

- health promotion, including the wider public health;
- improving the quality of clinical standards; and
- protection of public health and management of risk: communicable disease control and so on. (See Chapter 7 for more about health protection.)

The weakening of public health's leading role in health improvement is not confined to the UK. Julio Frenk, Mexico's Minister for Health and until recently a senior official in WHO, claims that 'public health is experiencing a severe identity crisis, *as well as a crisis of organisation and accomplishment*' (Frenk 1992: 68, my italics). The US Institute of Medicine in 1988 claimed that 'public health, as a profession, as a governmental activity, and as a commitment of society is neither clearly defined, adequately supported nor fully understood' (Institute of Medicine 1988). The situation is little different throughout most of Europe.

Periodically, public health medicine has found itself at a crossroads in terms of the opportunities and challenges facing it. Yet, on each occasion, despite repeated attempts to refocus public health on its core business, the specialty has continued since the early 1970s to be buffeted by successive NHS reorganizations and has found itself more and more at the mercy of general managers who have strengthened their grip on the NHS and on its priorities. Few managers have been advocates for public health and have sought instead to use expensive clinically trained public health professionals to pursue their own agendas around evidence-based medicine, contracting, commissioning and clinical governance. For the most part, public health specialists appear to have been willing accomplices. Or, for whatever reason, they have felt unable to speak out.

Of course, all these essentially health care tasks are included in the mix of roles listed above and ascribed to public health practitioners but it is arguable whether such a complex and varied set of tasks can easily be vested in a single specialty or individual. Little wonder, then, that the practice of public health has 'shifted uneasily between the analysis of health problems and the administration of health services' (Berridge 1999: 45). While the commitment to tackling poor health and health inequalities may be genuine, the energy and resources appear to be directed to other more immediate and pressing concerns thereby dashing hopes of implementing national policy locally (Exworthy *et al.* 2002).

Too little emphasis on practice?

But there are other aspects of the public health function which have hampered implementation. There has always been a tension between public health *science* and public health *practice*. Both are essential to improving health but public health practice remains a much neglected area of the public health function. A similar conclusion is reached by Nutbeam and Wise (2002) when they assert that public health medicine has been more concerned with knowledge acquisition than with its application to change practice. At issue here is the training available to public health trainees and the balance between competencies and skills designed to equip them with an ability to acquire and handle evidence on the one hand and manage change on the other. Too little emphasis is placed on change management skills. The final section of this chapter, on the future of public health, returns to this theme.

Insufficient joining up

Another impediment to implementation is the compartmentalization of policies and structures mentioned earlier. The government has rightly argued that complex problems demand complex solutions and that there is a premium on ensuring that policy and management is joined up both horizontally across departments and agencies, and vertically between levels of government.

The rhetoric has been impeccable, while the reality has been disappointing. In practice, the government has approached policy and its implementation from exactly the opposite, 'reductionist', point of view – breaking a problem down into its component parts and then attempting to solve them in a linear fashion. The accompanying preoccupation with endless targets, performance management systems and all the other paraphernalia of modern managerialism has prevented the very 'joined upness' that the government says it seeks. There is a curious mismatch between ends and means with the chosen means almost certainly making the desired ends less, rather than more, likely to be achieved.

Moreover, despite the mantra of 'joined up' policy emanating from the prime minister's office, the persistence of departmentalism is evident all around. Nor is it denied within the Cabinet Office where reports from the Performance and Innovation Unit pull few punches in their critique of the government's approach to implementation (Cabinet Office 2001a, b).

In particular, the Performance and Innovation Unit is critical of the linear model of policy delivery which dominates thinking in central government (Cabinet Office 2001a). In important respects it does not describe the real world that governments inhabit, and its application often leads to failure and frustration. The Performance and Innovation Unit also notes that 'too many new policies and initiatives can wreck delivery by diverting management time – carrying out instructions gets in the way of better outcomes' (Cabinet Office 2001a: 6). In another report on leadership the Performance and Innovation Unit commented on the need for 'horizontal' leadership within and across sectors. There was a need for leaders 'who are able to see the whole picture, and create a common vision with other agencies' (Cabinet Office 2001b). The emphasis on targets was criticized too, since it could 'stifle innovation and initiative with leaders concentrating on centrally-set targets' to the exclusion of more important issues affecting their organizations.

Politics and power

Finally, if there is genuine concern about implementation failure and its causes then attention has to be given to the politics of change and the power plays that exist. It is incorrect to allege that if only the evidence existed in regard to which interventions worked then implementation would follow. Impediments to change often owe more to political than technical factors. 'Unless and until we are willing to come to terms with organisational power and influence, and *admit that the skills of getting things done are as important as the skills of figuring out what to do*, our organisations will fall further and further behind' (Pfeffer 1992: 12, my italics).

The future of public health

Given the present state of public health policy and the problems affecting its implementation, many of them, it has to be said, being far from new or of recent origin, this final section looks to the future and considers likely developments which will help guide and shape public health policy. Because the problems over lack of 'joined up' policy and organization, and the difficulties of establishing effective partnerships, are both long standing and deep seated, it is easy to be pessimistic about the future and to conclude that the government is practising a form of 'decisionless decision making' whereby the policy may be sound enough but fails to lead to real sustainable change. A continuation of such a style of policy making is indeed conceivable but would constitute a worst case scenario. There are many high risk elements evident in current health policy, notably the key role accorded primary care trusts (PCTs) to improve the health of their local populations. It is proving difficult for PCTs to take population health seriously when the pressures on them to deliver on the NHS acute health care agenda are so great and expectations of improved performance so high.

However, a more optimistic scenario may be envisaged, too. The Wanless Report, described earlier, may have an important bearing on future policy as it affects public health. The review developed three scenarios in order to identify the cost drivers and to help estimate the resources required to deliver a high quality health service. Of the three scenarios, the Treasury has accepted the 'fully engaged scenario'. It contains the most significant implications for public health since it assumes it will improve dramatically with a sharp decline in key risk factors such as smoking and obesity, as people actively take ownership of their own health. 'People have better diets and exercise much more . . . These reductions in risk factors are assumed to be largest where they are currently highest, among people in the most deprived areas. This contributes to further reductions in socio-economic inequalities in health' (Wanless 2002: 39).

The scenario is the most optimistic of the three and therefore the most challenging. If all goes according to the model and effective public health measures are applied, then NHS spending in 2022–23 will be £154 billion. Under the least optimistic 'slow progress' scenario, spending will be £184 billion – a gap of £30 billion. In respect of the gain to be achieved in reduced spending on the NHS there is clearly an incentive to ensure the 'fully engaged' scenario becomes a reality.

Other developments might contribute to such an outcome and some of the key ones are considered briefly below.

Regionalism

The impact of regionalism in England, especially the creation of elected assemblies, could give a new focus to public health. The link between regionalism and public health is widely supported by those working in public health but has not hitherto developed particularly vigorously. There is limited evidence to suggest that regional bodies have finally discovered public health and its importance to economic regeneration. *The NHS Plan* began the process of strengthening the wider regional role. It stated

> by 2002 there will be single, integrated public health groups across NHS regional offices and government offices of the regions. Accountable through the regional director of public health jointly to the director of the government office for the region and the NHS regional director, they will enable regeneration of regions to embrace health as well as environment, transport and inward investment.
>
> (Secretary of State for Health 2000: paragraph 13.25)

The move was widely welcomed, especially by those concerned with the wider public health and keen to remove its sole locus from within the NHS. However, as was reported earlier, *The NHS Plan* unexpectedly got overtaken by *Shifting the Balance of Power* and the major restructuring of the NHS it heralded. Part of the move towards devolution was the demise of the eight NHS regions to be replaced by four directorates of health and social care that were arms of the centre, which is the Department of Health.

The regional public health function as articulated in *The NHS Plan* has survived the *Shifting the Balance of Power* changes. Regional directors of public health, relocated to each of the nine regional offices of government, are to provide the public health function. Their role is wide ranging. Among their tasks, they are to tackle the root causes of ill health and inequalities through the health component of cross-government policies in the regions (for example, transport, environment and urban regeneration). For the first time, regional directors of public health will be able to work with other government departments in the regions to build a strong health component into regional programmes.

The Minister for Public Health, Hazel Blears, told the Faculty of Public Health Medicine's annual scientific meeting in June 2002 that the new regional arrangements 'will help spread the influence of public health across the business of the regions . . . The co-location between public health and the other regional functions is a very exciting prospect' (Blears 2002). Part of the appeal of the regional dimension is that it provides an opportunity to remove public health from the constant pressure on waiting lists that damages NHS public health.

A note of caution must be sounded. The remit of the regional directors of public health is very broad and, as was argued earlier, it may be asking too much of one person to perform such a range of tasks effectively. At least one senior public health practitioner now working in a regional government office has suggested that it might have been better to break down the regional role into its component parts, retaining the more medical health service elements within the NHS while confining the new regional public health function, involving the work of the regional offices of government, to a dedicated senior post.

Finally, the future of regional government remains uncertain although the government has at last published proposals to introduce elected assemblies where there is public support for them (Department of Transport, Local Government and the Regions/Cabinet Office 2002). As in the case of the Greater London Authority, public health is not to be an executive function but an influencing one. Nevertheless, the White Paper, *Your Region, Your Choice*, notes that regional assembly responsibilities in the fields of housing, transport and economic development have important links with public health. It also emphasizes the need for a joined up approach to drive improvements in public health outcomes.

(See Chapters 2 and 3 for further discussion on regionalism.)

Local government

It has been a long standing complaint that local government's significant contribution to public health – certainly greater overall than the NHS's – has been ignored or marginalized. Despite all the talk of 'joined up' government local government has always played second fiddle to the NHS, which has retained its lead role on public health matters. Part of the blame lies with local government itself. The President of the Society of Local Authority Chief Executives admits that 'local government is not very good at talking about health and the role it plays in achieving good health for its citizens' (Duggan 2001: 4). The new policy context, especially the development of local strategic partnerships, provides 'opportunities for local authorities to reclaim their original role as champions of the health of local communities' (Duggan 2001). In a significant, but little reported, development the cross-cutting spending review on health inequalities led by the Treasury and completed in July 2002 has given local authorities a lead role in achieving new targets designed to improve health and tackle inequalities (HM Treasury and Department of Health 2002).

There are also numerous examples of new joint arrangements in place where local authorities have taken the lead in exercising greater influence over public health. There are many joint directors of public health in post between the NHS and local government. In Manchester, a joint health unit has been established within the City Council by the Council and Greater Manchester Health Authority in a move to pass the lead role for public health to the local authority. These may be isolated examples but if they succeed they will point the way for others to follow.

Finally, the new local authority overview and scrutiny committees offer an opportunity for local government to assess the extent to which the NHS is concerned with improving the health of local populations rather than with treating ill health.

Europe

The concern in this chapter has principally been with developments in England although these are largely mirrored elsewhere in the UK. However, there is a European dimension which ought not to be overlooked. It is likely to become more significant in the years to come. The European Union was principally conceived to develop a single economic market. Social policy, including health, issues have tended to receive little attention and have remained the strict preserve of member states. But recent public concern over food safety and other issues like the environment has raised the importance of public health on the EU agenda. For many years, the UK has been 'in a state of active denial about the influence of Europe' (Mossialos and McKee 2002: 991). This is no longer a tenable position to adopt.

Public health issues have never been accorded much prominence in the EU but the situation has begun to change for the reasons noted above and a new public health programme is close to being adopted. The proposed programme 'takes a horizontal and policy-driven approach on the basis of a broad view of public health' (Commission of the European Communities 2001: 2). It focuses on three strands of action:

- improving information and knowledge for the development of public health;
- responding rapidly to health threats such as those arising from communicable diseases; and
- addressing health determinants and tackling the underlying causes of ill health.

The new public health policy represents a significant departure from the EU's approach to public health hitherto. No longer will public health be seen as a series of separate action programmes, largely disease orientated. In its place, a more structured approach linked to clearer policy objectives will be introduced (Merkel and Hubel 1999). The focus will be on health determinants, health status and health systems rather than specific diseases or conditions.

It remains to be seen how far the EU is really prepared to pursue a vigorous public health policy since to do so may conflict with the overriding aim of the EU which is the creation of a single market. Anything which could interfere with its smooth running has not been accorded priority. Yet, a change of climate about the importance of health in a well run economy does appear to have occurred. Only time will tell whether this is more than a rhetorical flourish.

(See also Chapter 3 for discussion about Europe in the future of public health.)

The management of change

Before concluding this section, there is a more general issue in regard to the success of public health which concerns the change management model the government has adopted. Its essentially mechanistic, reductionist nature is proving dysfunctional. As was suggested earlier, the transmission of policy into practice is more complex than perhaps the government appreciates or is even prepared to acknowledge. This is despite criticisms of its approach from no less an authority than the Cabinet Office, located at the heart of government. There are serious, and often neglected, issues about whether, and how, national policy can be effectively implemented locally and what needs to be in place for this to occur.

In a recent booklet from DEMOS (an independent think tank) on system failure, Chapman (2002) argues that a major impediment to 'joined up' management and organization (in other words, implementation of 'whole systems' policy making) is the adherence to a linear rational model of policy making that is no longer a guide to the policy maker. He asserts that 'a new intellectual underpinning for policy is required' (Chapman 2002: 23). The complexity and breadth of the public health agenda is not in any doubt. It may therefore be more fruitful to start from this point and to view the various moves to tackle health, as distinct from ill health, as resembling a complex adaptive system (Plsek and Greenhalgh 2001). Such a system has been described as 'a collection of individual agents with freedom to act in ways that are not always totally predictable, and whose actions are interconnected so that one agent's actions changes the context for other agents' (Plsek and Greenhalgh 2001: 625). Complexity based organizational thinking is concerned with the whole system rather than with artificially viewing the system as comprising discrete parts or sectors. There is growing awareness that if sustainable progress is to be made in securing an 'upstream' change agenda, then moving away from current models of implementation is an essential prerequisite. However, the precise nature and shape of whatever might replace these models remains unclear.

(See also Chapter 3 on public health management and leadership.)

Conclusion

The problem in public health does not lie in the lack of sound policy but in its follow through and implementation, where progress has been less impressive. Contributing to the problem is a tendency in all health care systems for resources and effort to be concentrated on health care services. However, there is also a need for government to adopt a new model of policy and implementation if progress is to be made. Treating public health as a complex adaptive system would herald such a new approach and it would then be possible to devise new management systems and skills with which the public health workforce could then be equipped. But it is not simply a case of advocating a set of skills devoid of context. Context is all important, especially in a field like public health which transcends so many organizations and professional groups.

Unfortunately, we are some way from achieving such an outcome. But unless the capacity for public health practice is strengthened, policy in this area will for ever remain symbolic.

2

CHRIS MILLER
Public health meets modernization

Editors' introduction

People working in all parts of the public sector, including public health workers, have felt for many years that change and reorganization are permanent features of their working lives. New government policies and directives, and new plans and programmes, are introduced frequently and rapidly as part of the government's agenda of 'modernization'. What does it mean? And more specifically, what does it mean for people who work in the field of public health?

In this chapter, the author takes a critical look at the government's modernization agenda and explains why public health is part of this. He argues that the government's commitment to reform and to the modernization of health and social care services provides a real opportunity to give visibility to the breadth of public health. He provides a concise history of the roles that different political parties have played in the modernization of health and social welfare, examining the complex relationship between public health and politics.

The author discusses new Labour's journey through its commitment to reform of public institutions, relationships between citizens, the promotion of community relations and the reform of social policy. He examines the precursors to modernization, how it has happened, why it has happened and the dilemmas it has created for public health. The discussion helps readers to understand what is expected of modernized services and how modernization affects professions and agencies upon whom the success of public strategies depend.

The author moves on to consider the impact on public health of three new arenas outside of the health sector: regional government offices, elected regional assemblies and local strategic partnerships, arguing that these developments provide new opportunities for public health.

The author then examines the implications of the government's modernization agenda for public health, focusing on the common threads of partnership working, user involvement, community focus, leadership and quality of service provision. He concludes by considering the very practical implications of current modernization activity for front line public health professionals. He recognizes the potential for public health to emerge as a powerful lever for change within the modernization agenda.

Public health meets Labour's modernization agenda

The 1997 general election brought a 'new' Labour government to power and with it a higher profile for public health. This followed 18 years of neoliberal Conservative rule, during which the value of 'the public' was diminished. 'Modernization' was central to Labour's electoral platform, a large part of which focused on public services. Labour restated its traditional commitment to public services but not to 'old' ways of providing such services. Labour's commitment to fostering the 'active citizen', preventative services, opportunity rather than dependence – or 'positive welfare' (Giddens 1994) – gave some services, including public health, a higher profile than previously. However, all services would be modernized. Some features of modernization are common to all services while others are service specific. Public health is both a creator of a modern health service and the object of modernization. Alan Milburn, when he was Health Minister, articulated the former view 'the time has now come to put renewed emphasis on prevention as well as treatment so that we develop in our country health services and not just sickness services' (Milburn 2002:1).

Milburn presents three reasons why it is appropriate to 'up our nation's game on public health':

1   the government's commitment to invest extra resources within a ten year reform plan;

2   the emergence of new health problems that make health improvement more challenging, but also more important; and

3   the need to address the widening health gap between the better off and the worst off which denies basic life opportunities and economic prosperity to too many people.

This is good news for professionals long committed to demonstrating the potential of public health in the fight against ill health and for a healthier society. However, public health professionals will themselves be subjected to a process of modernization, some aspects of which will be more challenging. Just as it is important to understand what is expected of the service it is also important to know how modernization impacts upon those other professionals and agencies upon whom the success of public health strategies depends. As Milburn states 'The job of improving health then, is not just for one department of government but for the whole government – and not just between government departments but between government, business, local communities and individuals to provide real and lasting opportunities for better health' (Milburn 2002: 6).

It is important, too, to understand what lies behind an otherwise sensible desire to provide a 'modern' service.

Labour and modernization

Labour offers a pragmatic 'modern' welfare package – a 'new deal' (Powell 2000; Lister 2001). This 'third way', distinctive from both 'old Labour' and the 'new right', as unfolded during the first four years of office, defines a welfare system based upon:

- increased coordination, through 'joined up' policy, strategic thinking and professional practice;
- a plurality of service providers working in partnership to address complex problems;
- service user and public involvement in the planning, delivery and monitoring of policy;
- greater efficiency and accountability through national service standards and targeting of provision on identifiable vulnerable or challenging groups;
- increased service quality, continuous improvement, performance management and the identification and dissemination of good practice;
- an emphasis on evidence-based practice combined with the adoption of 'common sense' pragmatism;
- strong leadership and good public sector management; and
- a revised sense of public sector professionalism and a public sector ethos.

Early in his second term Tony Blair (2002) summarized four key principles of reform, namely:

- a national framework of standards with minimum floor targets;
- an increase in devolved power or 'earned autonomy' to providers who demonstrate a capacity to meet national targets, allowing for greater local diversity and more effective consumer pressure at the front line of service delivery;
- a reform of public service professionals; and
- greater choice between service providers and within each service.

The juxtaposition of 'new' Labour and 'modernization' is not coincidental but signals the party's attempt to redefine itself from previous incarnations (Levitas 1998) and as the political party of our time prepared to face the challenges that this brings (Driver and Martell 1998). In a pre-election paper Tony Blair argued for a programme of national renewal (Blair 1996). In it he referred to 'a new language of social justice' (Blair 1996: 22), arguing that 'the force of change outside the country is driving the need for change within it' (Blair 1996: 23). The way ahead lay in building a cohesive stakeholder society built on opportunity, responsibility, fairness and trust (Deacon 2000).

Modernization has meanings beyond those related to specific policy measures. The desire to create and maintain a new party image, in the belief that this is essential to its electoral success, has intruded into the policy discourse. It rules out the use of any language associated with 'old' premodern practices. Modernization is concerned with the reform of public institutions, the relationship between them and the citizen, the promotion of particular instruments and social relationships in the delivery of social welfare, and the reform of specific policy areas. Public services needed modernizing 'to create better government to make life better for people . . . brings services to the people, is more accountable and brings more power to local communities' (Cabinet Office 1999).

The legacy of Thatcherism and the fear of 'old' Labour

To understand Labour, the damage inflicted by successive defeats by a neo-right Conservative party cannot be underestimated. During its opposition 'wilderness' years, 1979–97, Labour suffered four general election defeats and witnessed the decline of its traditional electoral base. Labour's journey of modernization began in earnest with Neil Kinnock's resignation, following the 1992 election defeat, and John Smith's election as party leader. His premature death and Tony Blair's subsequent election in 1994 accelerated the process.

Labour had grown anxious that it was 'unelectable', despite the popularity during the 1980s of many Labour held local authorities. Highly publicized support for minority groups and single issue causes suggested to some that Labour with its 'looney left' had lost direction. Internal divisions, culminating in the 1987 contest for the deputy leadership, were fuelled by the left's belief that the weakness of the Callaghan government under pressure from the International Monetary Fund, and its confrontation with public sector unions, led to Thatcher's election. Labour's relationship with the trade union movement, especially the use of the union bloc vote and its financial support, suggested that it was a party disproportionately influenced by a sectional interest. Resistance to the practice of 'one member, one vote' reinforced the impression that Labour was itself undemocratic.

Thus the first target of modernization was the party itself, and in particular the voices and faces projecting the party's image and message. Those associated with 'old' ways or who were hostile to the new project were sidelined and resources concentrated in the packaging of the message. This risk management strategy produced a culture of control centred around a handful of individuals (Rawnsley 2001).

For 18 years Thatcherite free market economic policies and morally Conservative social strategies dominated Britain. The value of state organized provision was undermined and any collective interdependence or mutual needs denied. Need, or rather wants, could only be truly satisfied by the market and the successful would be those committed to its competitive ethos. Individuals were responsible for the well being of themselves and their families while voluntarily contributing to that of neighbours and communities. When all else failed, the state would provide minimal and controlled support, set within a punitive framework, although charitable assistance was preferable.

Thatcherism asserted that an overreliance or dependency on the state coupled with the expectation that it could and should meet an ever expanding list of needs and desires had progressively undermined the UK's economic efficiency, sapped its morale and weakened its international position. Responsibility for this belief in the omnipotence of the welfare state was laid at the door of both politicians and health and welfare professionals. The latter were accused of pursuing their material interests from a monopoly position, extending their welfare empires by defining circumstances that, by dint of professional training, only they could resolve. The rhetoric of 'rolling back the state' was harder to implement in practice, but it was successful in restructuring, or 'marketizing', the management, organization and delivery of health and social welfare (Clarke and Newman 1997).

Whenever possible public provision was privatized and local authorities were required to place a growing list of services out for competitive tendering. The old state monopolies in which departments were responsible for the identification of need, the determination of how they were to be met and the actual provision and evaluation of such services were broken up. Functions were split within a quasi-market between 'purchasing' and competing 'provider' agencies. Private agencies, whether for-profit, not-for-profit or non-profit, were actively encouraged to compete, while in some policy areas, such as community care, local authorities were required to allocate a significant proportion of available funds to non-state agencies.

Services were subjected to a system of regulation, administered by external auditors, built around the three 'e's' of economy, efficiency and effectiveness. Alongside such competitive relations between agencies, they were each subjected to a process of managerialization. This marked a shift away from a bureau–professional culture, in which administrators coordinated the work undertaken by professionally qualified specialists. Generic managers were introduced, often recruited from the private sector, or senior practitioners were converted into managers, to challenge professional power and to undermine the public service ethos. However, the 'right to manage' could neither be assumed nor guaranteed. A variety of private sector practices, such as appraisal, performance management, target setting, incentives and performance related pay were introduced, alongside reducing budgets and the removal of job security, as a way of breaking the influence of trade unions and pressuring staff to be more compliant. While Labour has played down the centrality of the market and reduced the internal competitive relationships, replacing the latter with a collaborative framework, it has retained and even extended many of the features of Conservative strategy.

Modernization as a container

Government initiatives can never be entirely separated from a desire for electoral success in which appearance is often a substitute for substance. Labour's determination to secure a second term of office was extraordinarily influential in shaping its politics. The drive to retain power began on the day of the 1997 election victory with the promise that the government would adhere to previous Conservative spending plans during the first two years in office. Such a hunger for office can afford only a loose attachment to values and consistency. As a sign of just how modern it has become, Labour is increasingly proud of its pragmatism, encapsulated in the phrase, 'what works is what counts' (Powell 2000; Lister 2001). As a political strategy, being suitably vague but upbeat about the vision and cautious in relation to specific changes it has proved to be very successful.

Modernization does not reflect a grand strategy hammered out in caucus meetings but is a loose container in which to hold still embryonic policy ideas and a variety of meanings. To be identified as the modernizing party challenges the opposition to identify an equally compelling image. Modernization is emblematic of a thrusting, dynamic force that is at the forefront of everything, never complacent or left behind, but associated with all contemporary icons be they in sport, culture, technology, business, international relations or political change. Conversely, as such a force, everyone wants to be associated with it. However, it is one thing to claim to be 'modern' in everything, and another, more challenging thing to deliver it. It might also be unnecessary.

Labour's continuing anxiety with media management, in which feedback from focus groups has appeared disproportionately significant in political decision making, has exposed it to the charge of being strong on policy rhetoric and weak on substance. Modernization requires ambitious policy claims that can reveal large gaps between what is espoused and the resources offered to deliver the policy. The desire to be the embodiment of modernization risks neglecting previous achievements. There is a cynicism among front line professionals who see that there is something familiar with much of what is now projected as new. To distinguish the present from the past in too dramatic a fashion suggests that what was done had no value or that what is now required is so profoundly different that the transition is too onerous. Modernization implies a lack of trust in those responsible for policy implementation, a perception strengthened by a culture of detailed regulation focused on performance.

The rush to modernize has, despite a commitment to 'joined up' policy, produced both 'initiative fatigue' and a lack of coherence that is exhausting, frustrating and confusing to service providers, users and the public – including those active citizens Labour wishes to encourage (Ahmad and Broussine 2003 forthcoming).

Modernizing the democratic institutions

Labour has been concerned with the 'democratic deficit' as characterized by falling membership levels in political parties, low turn outs in local elections, the poor credibility of politicians, the perceived distance between those responsible for decision making and those affected by the decisions taken, and broad disenchantment with the political process.

Labour's response has been threefold. First, it has introduced specific reforms to particular institutions.

Second, it has attempted to recast the focus of attention at a local level towards issues of governance. This has included, for example, the creation of new overarching local stakeholder bodies, such as local strategic partnerships, concerned with strategic issues in relation to the area's well being and development. The NHS is described as part of a network of public bodies concerned with enhancing individual and collective well being (Secretary of State for Health 1999). New duties have been imposed upon local authorities that go beyond their traditional concerns for the delivery of specific services, to develop strategies to further the area's economic, social and environmental well being.

Third, it has emphasized the need to create a socially inclusive society by investing in the processes of engaging service users and citizens. Labour has given considerable weight to the concept of the active citizen who is fully engaged in the Labour market, in their communities and in democratic processes.

These three issues are explored below.

Reforming political institutions

The reform of political institutions has included, with various degrees of success:

- reforming the House of Lords;
- devolution in Scotland, Wales and Northern Ireland;
- the creation of a Greater London Authority; and
- regional devolution within England.

To date English regional devolution has largely been associated with strengthening the role of the regional government offices. These are responsible for the sponsorship and monitoring of regional development agencies, 'the economic powerhouse for the region', acting as champion for the Department of Trade and Industry's strategy on innovation and small businesses, and significantly for regional governance. The latter has involved a more proactive approach by the government offices to encourage the creation of regional representative assemblies as a forum for regional debate and identity.

The recent White Paper (Department of Transport, Local Government and the Regions 2002) brings together under the government offices all existing government regional offices, including the Department of Health's regional public health team, and provides it with an enhanced role in such areas as crime reduction and the community cohesion agenda. The White Paper provides for the possibility of an elected regional assembly, to be preceded by a referendum to establish local support for one. Elected regional assemblies will not be imposed, creating the likelihood of uneven development with some but not all regions opting for an elected regional assembly. There is a commitment that those regions that choose not to proceed should not suffer any detriment. Yet this could have an impact in the area of public health, one of the functions for which elected regional assemblies will have some responsibility.

Elected regional assemblies will be expected, as they take up responsibilities devolved from both central government and quangos, to work to an overall vision for the region, setting priorities for and delivering regional strategies. They have the potential to become key bodies in relation to government offices and both will be influential in relation to public spending reviews. The White Paper proposes that one-third of the seats within an elected regional assembly should be allocated as 'top up' seats to non-governmental organizations and the business community. Again there are opportunities here for regionally-based public health bodies. Elected regional assemblies will both receive a direct single government grant and have the power to spend and raise independent funds, either through imposing a regional tax or by borrowing. The process to be followed before an elected regional assembly can be constituted is lengthy. It is unlikely that much progress could be made before the end of 2006, but the government is committed to establishing at least one elected regional assembly within the life of this current parliament.

Local government reforms

The attempt to subject the health sector to greater direct democratic accountability, as evidenced in a limited way by the inclusion of public health within the regional structures, is expanded considerably within Labour's local government reforms. Again a number of measures have been introduced including locally elected mayors, a new internal system of cabinet and scrutiny committees designed to give back bench elected councillors greater authority and an enhanced role while making for a more effective and accountable decision-making process. As part of their remit in health improvement and reducing health inequalities, the new overview and scrutiny committees have been given powers to examine local NHS provision, including public health. Of greater significance for public health is the new duty imposed on local authorities, under the Local Government Act (2000), to take a lead role in the drawing up of a 'community strategy'. This is to be devised in relation to social, economic and environmental well being and thus closely linked to an inclusive public health agenda.

The Act also provides a power to local authorities, and is therefore permissive, 'to do anything which they consider is likely to achieve' the objective of local well being. Although local authorities are expected to take the lead, the strategy should be generated within the framework of a broad 'community partnership' providing an overarching framework within which other local initiatives can operate (Department of the Environment, Transport and the Regions 2000a). This is to be linked to both the sustainable development strategy, based on work undertaken through Agenda 21, and the local authority's 'duty of best value'. Local neighbourhood strategies are also expected to form part of the broader community strategy. The whole process is to be overseen by the local strategic partnership (see below). The Act states clearly that central to its purpose is that local communities can 'articulate their needs and priorities' (Department of the Environment, Transport and the Regions 2000a: 38). Further, 'community strategies must give local people a powerful voice in planning local approaches to economic, social and environmental well-being and in holding core public services and politicians to account' (Department of the Environment, Transport and the Regions 2000a: 16).

Local strategic partnerships

The Act outlined proposals for the creation of a new non-statutory and non-executive body, local strategic partnerships. Eventually, these are to be established in all local authorities and accredited by regional government offices, but initially they have been a requirement only in the 88 priority areas eligible for support under the Neighbourhood Renewal Fund. Authorities outside the designated priority areas are likely to create a local strategic partnership since there is little difference in the expectations as laid down for partnership development between the designated priority areas and the rest.

Local strategic partnerships are identified as the key mechanism to bring together under one umbrella local authorities, residents and private, voluntary and community sector organizations. They will be expected to act as the partnership overseeing all other partnerships, exercising a powerful influence over their constituent elements and beyond. Partnership strategies focused on specific policy areas, such as public health or children's services, will thus be subjected to scrutiny by the local strategic partnership. The extent to which a local strategic partnership will be able to require detailed changes to service specific strategies, however, is unclear, as the expertise will ultimately lie within the more specialized partnerships. It is more likely that service specific strategies will increasingly be constructed with reference to the broader strategy devised by the local strategic partnership. As local strategic partnerships grow in confidence and build up a knowledge base they will also be able to identify potential connections and gaps between the more service specific strategies.

The primary task of the local strategic partnership is to produce a community strategy for the area along with local neighbourhood renewal strategies that aim to bring improvements to health as well as securing greater employment, reducing crime, improving housing, providing better education and reducing the gap between disadvantaged neighbourhoods and the better off. Local strategic partnerships are expected to contain all other local partnerships and initiatives so as to facilitate greater effectiveness among service providers. Milburn's speech, *Tackling Health Inequalities, Improving Public Health* (Milburn 2002), in identifying this as the first priority for public health, announced the introduction of a new funding formula to direct greater resources to high need areas and it is likely to create greater incentives to work more closely with the local strategic partnership framework. The emphasis is on being strategic, inclusive, action focused, efficient, establishing clear links between the aims and objectives of the local strategic partnership with performance management systems of its individual organizational members, and building on best practice (Department of the Environment, Transport and the Regions 2001b).

Local strategic partnerships are seen as essential 'for developing new ways of involving local people in how public services work' (Neighbourhood Renewal Unit 2001: 5). Two funding mechanisms, the Community Empowerment Fund and Community Chests, accessible only to the designated areas, have been established to support community involvement. The link between the local strategic partnerships and the government offices is potentially important as the latter feeds directly into central government. *Shifting the Balance of Power* (Department of Health 2001a) makes much of the importance of regional accountability for public health to the Department of Health. A regional director of public health is to be appointed in each region and, working with a small team, will be co-located within the government offices. The importance of an integrated multisectoral approach in addressing the 'wider determinants of health' at this level is emphasized as is the role of the regional director in bringing a health perspective to other policy areas and raising the public health profile within local strategic partnerships.

New arenas for public health

Taken together, the regional government offices, the proposed elected regional assemblies and the local strategic partnerships present three new arenas outside of the health sector in which a broad strategic overview is identified as a core responsibility and in which public health is given specific mention. Local strategic partnerships will also have representation on the new local bodies created by and accountable to the Commission for Patient and Public Involvement in Health (see below). Such links widen the scope and range of those with a responsibility for or interest in public health. They provide new opportunities for those organizations with a public health remit, to raise the public health profile, direct attention to the public health implications of the work of other organizations, and ensure that public health secures a higher level of priority in neighbourhood, community and regional strategies.

At the very local level public health professionals should not encounter much resistance, as health matters have long been a concern to community and voluntary organizations, and especially within women's organizations (Health Education Unit and Open University 1991). The emphasis given to joined up policies and seamless services can also work in favour of those with a public health interest now that it has been specifically identified as a critical aspect of social, economic and environmental development.

However, the extent to which health sector professionals or organizations will be represented within local strategic partnerships is not clear. In such fluid circumstances it is important that professionals and civic organizations act both assertively and in collaboration to ensure a strong presence. Another concern is likely to be whether the learning that takes place within such deliberative bodies and the strategic priorities that emerge penetrates those agencies concerned with health provision so as to impact upon front line provision. There will, no doubt, be some resistance from within the medical profession to what might be seen as inappropriate 'interference' in health issues by external bodies lacking in expertise.

The common threads of modernization

Labour's modernization agenda contains a number of common threads in relation to the organization and delivery of public services. For those with a history of working within community-based public health there is much here that will be familiar. However, for those who now find themselves with an extended role that includes some responsibility for an element of public health these features will present some new challenges. While some aspects are reviewed in more detail in other chapters the purpose here is to highlight the key generic elements.

Mixed economy of welfare

Labour has continued with the mixed economy of welfare advanced by the Conservatives (Blair 1998b). The state is no longer to be the primary body responsible for both the identification of need and the delivery of services to meet them. The plurality of public service providers that had begun to emerge, operating across all sectors of social life, would remain and indeed flourish.

To facilitate this, Labour has sought to enter into a set of formal relationships with both representatives from the voluntary sector and the private corporate sector. The former have produced a 'compact' agreement (Home Office 1998) while the latter have seen 'concordats' and more controversially, the Public Private Partnership policy first introduced by the Conservatives in 1992 but embraced by Labour (HM Treasury 2000b; Ball *et al.* 2001; Pollock *et al.* 2001). The role of the local authority – historically the core provider – would now be that of enabling and leadership with a specific responsibility 'to weave and knit together the contribution of the various stakeholders' (Blair 1998a). The state acts as funder, regulator, facilitator and coordinator, concerned with governance, democracy, enabling others and providing the framework within which these multiple providers must operate.

In encouraging a further expansion in the number and diversity of providers Labour had to confront issues of fragmentation, poor communication and coordination, reinforced by the previously dominant competitive relationships between the players that characterized their drive to secure service contracts. Under the Conservatives the 'competitive contract' became the primary basis of the relationship between independent provider agencies and the state. Labour set about replacing what it saw as a destructive competitiveness with collaborative relationships based on partnerships.

Partnership and collaboration

The need for collaboration was reinforced by the acknowledgement that despite previous efforts the state was faced with the continuing and often growing presence of complex and seemingly insuperable social concerns. Single-handedly no agency or profession could be expected to address these. The desire to protect and extend organizational territory alongside the partiality of professional groupings had long been a problem to the detriment of the service user and the creation of a 'seamless service'. The envy, rivalry and sense of superiority that can be a feature within the pecking order of professionalism not only created unjustifiable divisions of Labour, especially from the user's perspective, but also fractured cross-boundary communications again to the detriment of the service user. *Shifting the Balance of Power* (Department of Health 2001a) stresses this point in relation to public health, stating: 'A modern public health function can only be delivered successfully by a workforce which is interdisciplinary in its orientation, training, remit and composition' (Department of Health 2001a: Annex B paragraph 3).

Partnership working sits at the heart of Labour's restructuring processes and is either required or assumed to be good practice (Department of the Environment, Transport and the Regions 2001b). The Health and Social Care Act (2001) placed a duty of partnership on both the NHS and local authorities. The 26 health action zones are expected to develop a variety of partnership models to tackle health inequalities and bring about improvements. Partnerships should involve all stakeholders, including service users (McArthur 1996) and expectations are high about what they might achieve (Maddock and Morgan 1997; Pugh 1997) although the requirements for success have often been neglected (Mayo 1997; Atkinson 1999). For example, political pressure for early success has militated against the long-term requirements of building trust and developing relationships that enable collaboration within complex and uncertain environments. For those within public health, and especially community health, collaboration has long been critical to success and is further reinforced in *Shifting the Balance of Power* (Department of Health 2001a). While modernization adds strength to this, the formalization of partnership working and the emergence of partnership structures could, ironically, undermine genuine collaborative work, especially between front line professionals. Partnership structures can be mistaken for partnership working. (Chapters 4 and 9 explore issues about partnerships and partnership working.)

Engaging service users and carers

Alongside the emphasis on collaboration, priority has been given to the engagement of service users and carers (Department of Health 2001e). The belief that service users and carers have a legitimate and distinct contribution to make to the policy process and should be involved in service planning and evaluation has never been stronger (Wilson 1998). The Commission for Health Improvement's paper *Nothing About Us Without Us* (Commission for Health Improvement 2002) identifies its espoused core principles and working practices to make it more effective in engaging with patients and the public to improve the quality of care.

Although there is a fear that this might lead to the incorporation of user voices (Forbes and Sashidharan 1997; Gilliatt *et al.* 2000) the overwhelming perception is that user involvement is the only secure basis for service improvement (Corrigan and Joyce 1997; Beresford 2001). The category of service user, however, is a complex one as is the basis of their involvement whether as consumer or citizen. Beyond the rhetoric, little effort has yet been made in defining who might be the user in any particular situation, how best to access them and how to ensure some notion of representation and accountability (Taylor 1995). To date there are few, if any, areas of public provision where the user voice is particularly robust or where user organizations feel satisfied with either the process or outcomes of involvement (Barnes 1999). (See Chapter 8 for more about the lay contribution to public health.)

This presents particular challenges for public health professionals with the broadest of user base. The health service has a poor track record in this respect, acknowledged in the White Paper, *Involving Patients and the Public in Healthcare* (Department of Health 2001e). New bodies have been created with the aim of ensuring that, 'the voices of patients, their carers and the public generally are heard and listened to through every level of the service, acting as a lever for change and improvement' (Department of Health 2001e: paragraph 2.1).

A patient advice and liaison service, offering a one stop advisory service, is to be established within each hospital and primary care trust. This will operate alongside an independent complaints advocacy service linked to the new Commission for Patient and Public Involvement in Health. Part of the Commission's remit will be to create local network bodies with outreach teams employed by and accountable to it and responsible for supporting community groups and promoting public involvement. Both the Commission and the local network bodies will have lay reference panels to 'drive' them forward. Membership will be drawn from the new patient forums, the local strategic partnerships, the voluntary sector and locally elected representatives.

The patient forums, again located within every NHS trust and PCT, with a place on the new strategic health authority boards, are expected to represent local community views on the quality and configuration of local health services. Strategic health authorities are to have a director of public health, working with a small team and responsible for performance management of local public health work. They are also charged with the creation of a public health network, designed to be 'flexible and responsive and . . . change and evolve over time', to include non-government agencies, and provide specialist support for local PCTs. Each PCT will have a director of public health and a public health team, expected to take the lead on improving health and reducing inequalities in local neighbourhoods, 'the engines of public health delivery up and down the country' (Department of Health 2001b: Appendix C, paragraph 3). Alan Milburn (2002: 8) described this as: 'a huge opportunity . . . to take a hands-on community-oriented role . . . to forge local alliances . . . necessary to tackle specific local health problems'.

Essential to this will be their capacity to work in partnership with local authorities, in relation to community and local neighbourhood strategies, and with local strategic partnerships. Appointments to the post of director can, for the first time, be made from non-medical as well as medical public health professionals. Moreover, they are expected to 'be well known, respected and credible with local people – particularly those in the most deprived communities, local authorities, general practitioners and other clinicians' (Department of Health 2001b: paragraph 5).

Community focus

Closely associated with service user involvement is the need to be community focused (Social Exclusion Unit 2001a), continuing the revival of interest in a concept previously written off as a worthwhile area of study (Stacey 1969). Writers such as Beck (1999) view citizen involvement in their communities as a benchmark of a healthy democracy and the basis of social inclusion and solidarity. Community is currently viewed as the site of service provision and a key place where needs are defined and met. It is both the recipient and provider of services, the context in which collaboration takes place, and the basis on which policy is constructed (Policy Action Team 17 2000).

Communities are expected to play a significant role in relation to the new community strategy. Yet in order to do so, communities must have the internal capacity to respond and must be experienced by their members as positive life affirming places. The need to invest in such capacity building is now acknowledged, although the time taken and skills required is sometimes neglected (Active Community Unit 2001; Social Exclusion Unit 2001a). There is still insufficient knowledge of the complexities and conflicts that lie within communities, how these can be negotiated or the skills and qualities required.

Public health professionals are expected to contribute to this process, as specified in *Shifting the Balance of Power* (Department of Health 2001a), although they might find they are insufficiently prepared to do so effectively. Recognition that, once created, local community-based organizations have a tendency to develop their own priorities will be critical. It is one thing to promote strategies to encourage powerful community voices to emerge and quite another to be able to respond to such voices, especially when they all do not express the same viewpoint. Well organized, assertive and independent local bodies do not sit comfortably with the centralizing and controlling aspects of Labour's modernization.

Two other common elements in the modernization agenda are worth highlighting in the context of public health: leadership and quality of services.

Leadership

The current emphasis on leadership suggests a gradual movement away from the managerial strategies that dominated the 1980s and early 1990s (Cabinet Office 2001b; Organisation for Economic Cooperation and Development 2001). The importance of being output driven, focused on demonstrable and measurable improvements, with the associated target setting and performance management has not disappeared. Performance targets continue to proliferate and many still deny the complexities of social interventions. An emphasis on the need for 'strong' almost heroic leadership especially at the top of the organizational hierarchy also continues. Conflicts still occur over a manager's attempts to secure 'the right to manage' (Pollitt 1993), and front line staff continue to resist managerial attempts to impose top-down solutions or coerce them into compliance (Horton and Farnham 2000). However, the attempt to introduce private sector values and practice through the crude and bludgeoning process of marketization and managerialization is being replaced by a more sophisticated process (NHS Executive 1999; Cabinet Office 2001a).

The combined effects of an extended mixed economy, the provider–purchaser separation, competitive funding regimes operating on an annual cycle, and internal decentralization, is now seen as inefficient and ineffective, creating an overly fragmented service (Cutler and Waine 2000). The imposition of private sector approaches ignores crucial differences arising from the political decision making and accountability frameworks within the public sector (Dixon *et al.* 1998). There is some evidence that in its second term Labour has recognized the need to develop a broader culture of organizational learning (Social Exclusion Unit 2001a) leaning towards the view that 'leading is learning' (Vaill 1999).

Within a learning organization leaders are expected to model the processes of learning and thereby expose their own lack of knowing. While Labour remains deeply pragmatic, there is some acknowledgement that learning is iterative and hence the potential for innovation and diversity. There are also signs of an acceptance of a more dispersed form of leadership, rather than one that equates it with hierarchical position (Senge 1999). Although lacking a commonly accepted meaning (Easterby-Smith 1997), concepts such as 'dialogue' (Isaacs 1993; Schein 1993) and 'communities-in-practice' (Cooke and Yarrow 1993) generated from within organizational learning, speak to Labour's emphasis on collaborative working. Public health professionals will need to take advantage of any such opportunities for leadership in shaping the broader health agenda and will need to allow leadership to be exercised by other constituencies beyond the health sector.

Quality of services

Central to Labour's modernization agenda is the emphasis given to the quality of service provided (Department of Health 1997a; Department of the Environment, Transport and the Regions 1998; Bovaird and Halachmi 2001). The judgement of quality, however, is a negotiated process between service providers and users (Gaster and Deakin 1998) and made difficult by the intangible, heterogeneous and inseparable nature of public provision (Lewis and Hartley 2001). *The New NHS White Paper* (Department of Health 1997a), later reinforced by *The NHS Plan* in 2000, and the best value regime in local government (Department of the Environment, Transport and the Regions 1998) call for continuous improvement in both the quality and cost of provision.

Quality is set within national targets or service frameworks and local public service agreements. Labour continues to rely heavily upon external audits and performance management introduced by the Conservatives, alongside 'evidence-based' practice, as core tools in the monitoring process (Department of Health 1998b). Its political future is related to the attainment of such targets. The Health Minister has spoken of plans to create an independent regime of regulation, audit and inspection, and extending local accountability by requiring each PCT to produce an annual 'patient prospectus' delivered to each household.

The Modernization Agency

The Modernization Agency, established following publication of *The NHS Plan*, is to oversee the expected improvements by acting as a 'centre of excellence' and a 'leadership centre'. Not only will its board operate at a national level, helping to oversee the Plan's implementation, but local boards will also be created as 'a forum in which local stakeholders, including hospital consultants and patients groups, contribute to the health improvement programme' (Secretary of State for Health 2000: 6.52). Overall, the Agency's role is to 'redesign local services around the needs and convenience of patients' (Secretary of State for Health 2000: 6.15) by identifying, disseminating and 'celebrating' good practice, alongside the health observatories, while strengthening the service's leadership capacity at all levels. It also offers the carrot of greater 'earned autonomy' for good performance and has begun to promote diversity in provision alongside greater user choice.

Of particular importance for public health is its specific brief to support a 'healthy communities' collaborative, focused on disadvantaged neighbourhoods (Secretary of State for Health 2000: 6.18). Much is made within the Plan of the concept of 'earned autonomy'. However, it remains to be seen how this might work in relation to public health where outcomes are dependent upon high levels of collaboration with other agencies and improvements are only likely to show in the long term.

Conclusion

Labour's modernization agenda contains many opportunities for those concerned with public health to raise its profile and ensure that public health matters figure as a central feature in the work of other agencies and professionals. It offers the possibility of building on existing strengths, such as partnership working, and in so doing offering its expertise to others now required to develop new ways of working. By having something valuable to offer public health, professionals can quickly gain influence.

Nevertheless, a number of cautionary notes should be sounded. With so many agencies, many yet to fully materialize, having some responsibility for public health the situation may become so diffuse that nobody takes responsibility and drives the agenda. Public health might be part of every discussion but there may be much less certainty about how to move it forward. Unless strong and influential bodies emerge quickly a lack of confidence in making progress may come to stifle discussion and dissipate energy. At present there is a sense that there is no coherent point of leadership for public health.

Similarly, it is difficult to see exactly how the connections between different agencies will be developed and sustained. The time required to engage with the new structures could feel disproportionate to the outcomes and drift would then set in. The simultaneous engagement of different stakeholder groups, each with their own capacities, expectations and priorities may prove to be too overwhelming. Collaboration might be expected but in circumstances of complexity and confusion professional or agency specific service requirements may take priority over joint public health ventures. Since improvements in public health are so dependent upon the work of a number of agencies this could be a major stumbling block.

Successful collaboration, and local communities and civic organizations becoming engaged in deliberative and potentially influential forums, might depend upon the commitment, energy and strategic interventions of front line public health professionals. As a body, public health workers may lack the coherence to take this forward while setbacks may sap energy and commitment. There will be resistance both internally from the professionals with a core public health responsibility, and from other sectors, to the role envisaged for public health and the direction it is to take. It will be difficult to bring a clearly enunciated set of priorities to any public health dialogue while these internal issues remain unresolved. Yet while such eventualities provide public health with huge challenges that it might not be able to meet, there remains still within the modernization agenda the potential for public health to emerge as a powerful lever for change.

3

GABRIEL SCALLY
Public health: a vision for the future

Editors' introduction

A new century is a time for reflecting on the past and thinking about the future. For public health, the start of the 21st century also marks an era characterized by a broadening scope and an increasingly multidisciplinary workforce. This makes developing a concise vision for the future a challenging task.

In this chapter, the author helps public health workers to think about the future by focusing on several core themes. These include learning from historical public health, the need to function in a shared power world, the importance of public health management and leadership, the prospect of dedicated public health services, the importance of health protection and the impact of regionalism and internationalism.

Reflecting on the history of public health is identified as an important exercise that should be undertaken by public health professionals, not just academic historians, because important lessons can be learnt from the past. Learning can also be gained from looking at contemporary progress, paying attention to both failures and successes.

The author discusses the development of management and leadership within multidisciplinary public health teams. He argues that to achieve progress in a shared power world will require leadership skills of a different order to those exhibited in recent decades.

Consideration is then given to the continued and renewed concern about the communicable disease problem which is further complicated by the increasingly frequent engagement of public health with chemical and general environmental hazards. The implications for skill development in health protection within the public health workforce are considered.

The final section of the chapter demonstrates how regionalism in England aligns with the development within the European Union of the concept of a 'Europe of the Regions'. The EU strategy for public health is examined. It focuses on first, improving health information and knowledge; second, enhancing the capacity to respond to health threats, particularly communicable diseases; and third, addressing health determinants.

The author concludes by reiterating that the public health function in the UK is well established and its importance recognized, but a concern is the collective ability to support the breadth of skill development required within an increasing public health workforce.

> Convinced as we all are of the high ideal and real value of the health of all, we must stop being indifferent toward questions of hygiene and public health, and each one of us must make it his duty, so far as in him it lies, to promote this object in the future.
>
> (Max Von Pettenkofer 1873)

Attempts to write about the future of public health are blessed with certain advantages as well as disadvantages. Among the advantages are both the indisputable importance of the public health function and the certainty that a collective response to ill health will be a core requirement of whatever civil and political structures are in place in the future. The nature of threats to health and well being may alter, sometimes decisively, over time but nonetheless the principles of public health responses will undoubtedly remain reasonably consistent.

However, speculation about the future is handicapped by the ability of changes in civil society, which are generally not predicated by public health concerns, to radically change the organizational structures and climate within which public health practice is conducted. The major changes in United Kingdom public sector structures in 1974 (1973 in Northern Ireland), which saw the division of public health into its medical and environmental health components, created barriers which are only now, almost 30 years later, being gradually overcome.

Similarly the incorporation of major parts of the public health function within the structures of the NHS has meant that successive reorganizations, based, as is almost inevitable, on the needs of personal health services have posed major difficulties for the management of public health services. A continued drive to modernize public services inevitably means that a continuing theme of public health practice will be coping with, and indeed taking advantage of, organizational change.

Learning for the future from the past

In 1998 the anniversaries were celebrated of several important events in the history of health in the UK. While most attention was focused on the creation of the NHS in 1948 there was also a renewal of interest in the events that took place 100 years before that. In 1848 the first public health acts were passed by the Westminster Parliament. Their genesis was in the combination of squalor, overcrowding and disease created by the unregulated growth of the urban population combined with the threat of cholera spreading steadily from the East.

This important 150th anniversary generated a great deal of interest in the history of this part of the 19th century sanitary revolution. Many commentators noted the continuities between the determinants of health in the 19th century and the end of the 20th century. Issues such as poverty, housing and diet remain as major areas for public health concern and action.

Unfortunately, an appreciation of the history of public health remains a minority interest and is a topic of study by academic historians rather than by public health professionals. Partly this can be attributed to the historical discontinuity in the issues with which the public health community in the UK has been engaged. From 1974 until the end of the 20th century the major engagement was with issues of personal health service provision within the NHS. This role of aiding improvement in personal health service provision is undoubtedly important and is identified as one of the essential public health functions by the World Health Organisation. Nonetheless, the narrow basis for public health practice led to the neglect of the basic determinants of health and thus a historical discontinuity. The re-engagement of the public health system with the whole of the health agenda has, accompanied by the anniversary of the public health acts, increased interest in the history of public health. In future decades we may well see a steady growth in interest in public health history and an increased desire to learn from and use the lessons of the past.

Accompanying an increased interest in the retrospective analysis of public health successes and failures should be the paying of attention to the contemporary history of public health so as to facilitate study. For example, the important changes that have taken place in the public health workforce with the opening of leadership positions to those without medical qualifications has come about as the result of quite complicated pressures and processes involving a wide range of individuals and organizations. The accurate recording of these contemporary events will enable the learning to be extracted in an easier and more useful fashion. Thus the future practice of public health will be aided by our contemporary attention to analysis and recording of events that may, at that time, appear of limited significance.

The task of learning from contemporary events also needs to be extended to the analysis and recording of failures. The inability to learn from failures has been a major theme in the personal health services field. The adoption of root cause analysis as a means of learning from errors is in its early days in the health field in the UK. There are of course dangers in simply importing what are seen as good ideas from the personal health care arena. The adoption of clinical audit in public health practice is a good example of how processes do not necessarily adapt well to the different environment in public health. Nonetheless, as public health becomes more action orientated the ability to learn from failure as well as success would improve overall effectiveness of public health systems.

A shared power world

One of the immense advantages possessed by our predecessors in public health was the simplicity of the organizational structures with which they had to deal. The sanitary revolution of the 19th century was closely linked to the full flowering of municipal power. The role of central government was much more limited than today and the range of powers and responsibilities exercised by the corporations and councils that ran civil society at the local level was truly enormous. Their responsibilities literally ranged from the cradle to the grave and their full control of housing and utilities meant that their influence over the conditions under which people lived was all pervasive. When harnessed for the improvement of health this range of powers placed local authorities in a position of enormous strength. They were of course also responsible for the employment of the public health workforce including medical officers of health and sanitary inspectors. The role of the public health officials was largely to convince their employers, and important colleagues such as the borough engineer, that action to improve health needed to be taken.

The organizational situation has, however, changed out of all recognition. Not only is a substantial part of the public health function located with NHS bodies but also the powers of local authorities have been dissipated as utilities and transport have been privatized and responsibilities such as housing dispersed. There is little sign of this trend diminishing: rather the opposite. Continued dispersal of powers over factors important to public health seems set to continue.

Although there has been influential support for the return of public health functions to the local authorities, notably by a commission established by the Chartered Institute of Environmental Health (Commission on Environmental Health 1997), the nature of civil society in the future will undoubtedly mean that public health practitioners will need different skills if they are to fulfil the essential public health functions in an effective fashion. The ability to operate in a 'shared power world' will require an enhanced level of political and influencing skills as well as the ability to gain and maintain the confidence of the population served.

Public health management and leadership

The development of management in the realm of health services has proceeded apace in the UK since the early 1980s. Prior to then, the NHS was seen as an 'administered' rather than a 'managed' organization. In some ways the public health system in the UK remains in the realm of 'administration'. There is still a tendency for consensus methods to operate and the role to be seen as a professional advisory task rather than direct engagement in the production of change. Public health departments tend to be staffed with high level professionals and low status administrative and secretarial staff. This situation is changing as a growing skill mix is seen as appropriate but there is an urgent need to develop the management of public health operations.

As the tasks falling on public health increase there is also a need to invest time and energy in the performance management of public health functions. The growth of performance indicators in the personal health services field with the use of 'traffic lights' and 'star ratings' has left most of public health untouched. While good reasons can be produced for why this should be, such as long timescales and multi-partnership working, the absence of clear contemporary indicators of performance leaves public health at a distinct disadvantage. Over the next decade a key task will be the development of methods of 'keeping the score' in public health work.

In America the National Public Health Performance Standards Program has been developed to measure public health practice both at state and local level (National Association of County and City Health Officials 2002). The work has been in progress since 1998 and has lead to the creation of a local public health system performance surveillance and assessment tool. While many of the judgements required in the completion of the instrument are subjective the approach has merit and similar tools are needed in the UK.

The ability to display public health progress over short timescales will enhance the ability to attract resources and convince both the public and politicians of the benefits of taking public health action. Hunter (1997) has argued that the term 'public health management' seeks 'to clarify and give a sharper focus to the public health challenge and to the means of meeting it'. We need to invest resources in the production of approaches to public health practice that emphasize public health management as a core part of the discipline and to increase the opportunity for those with a professional management rather than a public health background to contribute to multidisciplinary public health teams. If senior public health practitioners are not good managers then they should at least work with good managers in their teams.

To achieve progress in the shared power world, as mentioned above, will require leadership skills of a different order to those exhibited in recent decades. In the NHS context public health leaders have become accustomed to an 'in charge' organization where all, or nearly all, that is needed to solve a problem lies within the direct control of the organization. The move towards integrated responses to complex social and economic problems with health consequences such as drug abuse or non-accidental injury poses different and more complex problems. No one body is in charge of the problem and many diverse and sometimes competitive organizations have partial responsibility. Bryson and Crosby, in their important work on public sector leadership, defined some of the skills that leaders must demonstrate:

> To be effective in this work, public leaders must understand the larger context, which often includes the economy, the polity, and even the society as a whole. They must attend to the people involved and to different levels of social organization from small groups to interorganizational networks. They must understand the policy change cycle and be skilful in designing and using forums, arenas, and courts.
>
> (Bryson and Crosby 1992: 31)

With the creation of a large number of director of public health posts in the primary care trusts in England and the local health boards in Wales there has never been a greater opportunity or need for high levels of leadership in public health. The first decade of the 21st century will demand that public health practitioners come out from behind closed doors and adopt new methods of working. In addition they will be required to relate to the public in much more direct ways. The view that directors of public health will be partly judged by the degree to which they are known and respected by their local communities means the adoption of new ways of communicating. The creation of programmes to develop public health leadership is at an early stage and will need to be speeded up and expanded.

(Public health management and leadership are also discussed in Chapters 1 and 2.)

Public health services

The organizational location of public health with NHS organizations has not only left the public health function vulnerable to organizational change but has also distorted priorities and resource initialization within public health. The House of Commons Health Select Committee, in its report on public health (House of Commons Health Select Committee 2001a), identified an overengagement with hospital services issues as being a major diversion from engagement on public health issues.

The centrality of targets for reduction in health inequalities to government policy seems fixed for the foreseeable future. The achievement of these inequalities targets, and the other important targets for reductions in cancer and cardiovascular disease, requires public health action across a wide range of organization and sectors. If the focus of public health activity should be within the realm of personal health services then these targets are unlikely to be achieved. An alternative, and increasingly accepted, approach is to think, talk and act in terms of essential public health services.

The development of the concept of essential public health services has been taken on board in some quarters internationally. The most cogent list of essential public health services is that developed and adopted by the American Public Health Organization. They have identified 11 essential public health functions and this provides a useful checklist against which the performance of the public health systems can be judged. More than this they provide an opportunity to change the language of discourse. In the future we should be thinking about how the functions can be carried out and talk in terms of bodies that host these functions. These organizational homes may change, merge or even be abolished but the focus of public health professionals should be on the functions that need to be carried out.

There is a strand of thought that there should be created, at some time in the future, a separate public health service. Those who support this approach see the advantage as the ability to pursue public health goals without the disadvantage of being dispersed minor players in much bigger organizations with more diverse agendas. In 2003 the Welsh Public Health Service came into being and this innovation represents an important experiment in structures. Although it remains within the NHS, the staff all being employed by one NHS trust, the gathering together of the bulk of Welsh public health resources in one organizational structure for the management of public health services in Wales is a major opportunity.

Health protection

Communicable disease

In the second half of the 20th century there was a feeling among some public health professionals that the burden of infectious disease was no longer a major problem in Western Europe. If it had been true this was clearly a major alteration in the purpose of public health systems, since they had been created and developed in response to communicable disease problems. Such a notion now appears fanciful, as a resurgence of the communicable disease problem has occurred.

There appear to be three major factors that lie behind the increased prominence of infectious diseases:

1   The resurgence of long established disease due to an alteration in the conditions that previously limited their occurrence and spread. Examples of this would be

malaria and tuberculosis. The collapse of malaria control programmes due to economic decline along with the development of drug resistance have facilitated the spread of malaria to areas from which it had previously been eradicated. Steadily increasing international travel and a growth in displaced peoples, along with drug resistance, have aided the spread of tuberculosis. Global warming has already led to shifting patterns of disease as climate change facilitates spread beyond traditional areas.

2   The identification of previously unidentified infectious diseases such as Legionnaires Disease and listeriosis. There has also been the discovery of the association between microbes and diseases that were not suspected to have had a microbiological origin. The best known example of this is the discovery of the association between E. pylori and peptic ulceration of the gastrointestinal tract.

3   The emergence of new communicable diseases. Pre-eminent among emergent organisms must be HIV. The global burden of HIV is enormous and unevenly distributed with devastation of the population taking place in many African countries and predicted for the future in many Asian countries.

These trends in communicable disease seem unlikely to diminish in the foreseeable future. The growth of antibiotic resistance is in itself a major threat to the control of communicable disease and this is compounded by the failure of the international pharmaceutical industry to develop new and effective antimicrobial therapies.

There is little public understanding of the threat represented by new or novel forms of existing diseases. The greatest threat in this regard would seem to be a significant degree of antigenac shift in the influenza virus. It is unlikely that the world's population would be devastated in the same way as happened in the world pandemic of influenza in 1918, if only because the general level of human health is better than it was at that time. However, given the high proportion of frail elderly people in developed countries and the large numbers of people with HIV infection in developing countries, worldwide mass mortality could easily occur. The 1997 outbreak of influenza in Hong Kong, which was associated with chicken flocks, is regarded as having been a close shave in this regard.

Environmental hazards

Adding to continued and renewed concern about communicable disease is increasingly frequent engagement of public health with chemical and general environmental hazards. Over the next decade the engagement of the public health system with environmental hazards is set to increase. The Integrated Pollution Prevention and Control regulations recognize health issues as an important ingredient in decision making. The inclusion of health bodies as statutory consultees, for example in applications for consent to discharge chemicals into watercourses, will impose a steadily increasing workload on public health professionals. It will also mean that the level of public engagement will increase since it is health concerns about pollution that are top of public concerns.

To this must also be added the possibility of deliberate action to cause mass casualties through the use of radiological, chemical or biological agents. The response to this will require a substantial development in the public health workforce to ensure that the skills are available to respond effectively to threats and incidents endangering the health of the population. Traditionally these skills have been well developed in the communicable disease field. It seems clear that the skill base will have to widen to ensure that all hazards can be dealt with.

Planning for emergencies

While response is vital, so too is the task of planning for emergencies. Prior to the end of the Cold War there was considerable reluctance on the part of many public health professionals to engage in emergency planning for nuclear warfare. The argument was that preparing for nuclear war increased the likelihood of it occurring and that it was unrealistic to contemplate survival. The reduction in international tension has lead to a broadening in the concept of and participation in planning. The continued development of this area, increasingly known as civil contingency planning, seems to be assured. The creation of the Health Protection Agency in 2003 brought together the previously disparate elements, whether it be planning, communicable disease or chemical and radiological hazards. The importance of the decision to construct a world class public health body of this nature cannot be underestimated and is likely to influence public health structures in other countries.

(See also Chapter 7 for more on health protection.)

Regionalism and internationalism

Regionalism in England

The growth of regionalism in England allied to the devolution to elected bodies in Scotland and Wales has changed, probably for ever, the political, organizational and policy context within which public health is developed and practised. Already there is considerable diversity among these three countries in Britain and should elected regional assemblies come into being one can expect the spectrum of variation to grow. The growth of regionalism in England has enabled public health to make major steps forward in creating solid working relationships across sectors. Although regional public health groups have only officially been linked to government offices of the regions since early 2002 there is already evidence of the benefits to be gained. In some ways this is a regaining of the ground that was lost with abolition of the regional health authorities in the 1990s. What is different, however, is that the focus has shifted, significantly if not completely, from concerns about the provision and planning of NHS services towards the broad determinants of health and the partnership working across sectors that is required if improvements are to be achieved.

As elected regional assemblies develop in England, albeit at a variable pace, public health is expected to be among their concerns and responsibilities. The regional director of public health is to be appointed by the elected regional assembly as their public health advisor with the task of ensuring that public health concerns are taken into account across the wide range of economic, planning and social functions that will be devolved to elected regional assemblies by central government.

(See also Chapters 1 and 2 for discussion on regionalism.)

'Europe of the Regions'

The growth of regionalism in England chimes with the development within the European Union of the concept of a 'Europe of the Regions'. Within the structures of the European Union this has been given an administrative form. The Committee of the Regions is the most recently created of the institutions, in 1991, as a result of the Maastricht Treaty. It was created to address the worrying gap that was opening up between the institutions of the EU and the population over whose lives it was having steadily increasing influence.

The Committee of the Regions is made up of 222 members appointed by the Council on the proposal of the individual member states. The United Kingdom has 24 members on the Committee. The Commission and the Council are obliged to consult the Committee of the Regions whenever they are making new proposals in defined areas and when these proposals will have an effect at regional or local level. Among the ten areas specifically identified is public health. There is, however, little evidence yet of attempts by the public health community in the UK to influence their members on the Committee even though they are considering important issues such as tobacco control and prevention and reduction of risks associated with drug dependence.

European Union health strategy

The EU has determined a direction for the future of public health that seems set to steadily increase the importance of the European dimension to all those concerned with the public health function. The EU's health strategy has been developed over a number of years and has been structured to take into account the lessons of the bovine spongiform encephalitis (BSE) crisis. The BSE crisis caused an enormous upheaval in the Commission and has shown that public health issues cannot be ignored in the future or regarded as subservient to economic or agricultural policies.

The EU strategy for public health focuses on three strands of action.

The first strand is about improving health information and knowledge. The development of pan-European surveillance mechanisms to collect, analyse and evaluate compatible health information will enable the health of the populations of Europe to be compared. Although this is done at the present time the data sources are diverse and timeliness is variable. A European Health Observatory has been proposed to lead this work. This will mirror the development of regional public health observatories in England and opens up the possibility of the English observatories making a substantial international contribution in the future. The information function is also seen as having the obligation of promoting the right of individuals to information, not only about public health but also about treatment of illnesses.

The second strand is aimed at enhancing the capacity to respond to health threats, particularly communicable diseases. The enlargement of the EU and the principle of free movement of people are seen as increasing the need for integrated approaches on important issues such as immunization. A challenge in this area will be the diversity of immunization schedules as practised in the EU countries at present. This work is also seen as extending into the safety of blood supplies and organs. Beyond the traditional communicable disease areas it is to be expected that the EU will continue to extend into the broader area of health protection with consideration of common issues such as electromagnetic and other forms of radiation.

The third and final strand is aimed at addressing health determinants. There is a history of the EU tackling some lifestyle issues in the past notably with the important and landmark campaign known as 'Europe Against Cancer'. The future direction seems set to encompass a wider range of lifestyle related health determinants but also sets the scene for involvement of public health with a wider range of social and economic determinants. It will be interesting to see how the strengthened concern with health determinants interacts with other higher profile EU programmes notably the Common Agricultural Policy.

The expansion of the EU to encompass countries with considerable problems of economic development, pollution and health status will pose a considerable challenge to the public health systems of the existing member countries. This, combined with the growing competence of the structures of the EU in public health issues, will increase the importance of an international perspective to those working in public health in the UK. The opportunity to learn from and contribute to public health on an international basis will be increasingly available to those working not just at national level but also to those engaged at a regional and local level.

(See also Chapter 1 for discussion about Europe in the future of public health.)

Conclusion

There have been many occasions when the public health community has viewed its future with something akin to concern and anxiety. Almost inevitably the pessimists have been proved wrong and despite organizational change things have in due course reached the stage where self-confidence returns. There is of course a cost to be borne. Many practitioners have had to change jobs and some have taken early retirement.

There are, however, no grounds for pessimism in the first decade of the 21st century. The public health function in the UK is well established and its importance recognized. The major concern is our collective ability to provide enough trained and experienced public health professionals to undertake the tasks that are flowing from the wide sweep of public health priorities. (Chapter 5 discusses capacity and capability in public health.)

The Irish born military leader, the Duke of Wellington, once remarked 'All of the business of war, and indeed all of the business of life, is to endeavour to find out what you don't know by what you do; that's what I called guessing what was on the other side of the hill' (Longford 2001). One of the delights of working in public health is that while one can speculate on what is on the other side of the hill, the range of possible scenarios is so great that there is always something challenging and new coming along.

PART 2

Participation and partnerships in 21st century public health

Editors' overview

Who plays a part in making public health action happen? Is there a large enough workforce with the necessary skills? How do people and organizations work together to take public health action forward? How are the public involved?

These are some of the questions addressed in Part 2. Participating in public health action, and working in partnership to achieve better health for the population, are central themes in multidisciplinary public health. This part of the book examines different conceptual frameworks, dimensions and processes involved in participation and partnership, setting them in their policy context and in the real world of practical experience.

Partnership working is now a major theme in all government policy. It is not new; indeed, it has been included in government policy for 30 years. But what *is* new is the recognition by policy makers that joint working does not just happen by goodwill and common sense. It needs attention to the structures and processes that underpin partnerships – issues which are explored in these chapters.

Multidisciplinary public health involves a wider range of professional groups than ever before, both within and outside the NHS; this wide range is explored in these chapters. There are challenges for health professionals to move out of their discrete professional specialisms and to work with other health professionals. Public health action also requires the public to be accepted as equal contributors in working for better health. The need to engage with non-health workers and lay people pushes health professionals' thinking towards even greater shifts.

In Chapter 4 Stephen Peckham asks the question, 'Who are the partners in public health?' He examines conceptual frameworks for partnerships between agencies, groups, communities and individuals, looks at interagency and interprofessional working and notions of 'joined up' policy, the dimensions of partnership and different levels of collaboration. Peckham identifies who should be involved in partnerships for public health and assesses whether there is a mismatch between the ideal and the reality of current partnership development.

Recent government policy emphasizes strengthening the public health function by expanding capacity and capability. In Chapter 5 this issue is examined by Jennie Naidoo, Judy Orme and Gill Barrett. They question government notions of 'capacity and capability' in public health, their application in practice and discuss issues about professional identity in public health. They examine which professional groups are involved in the current expansion of public health and why. They critically examine recent interrelated initiatives to support policy implementation. They discuss what is meant by 'public health professionals' and whether they always see themselves as contributing to public health.

In Chapter 6 Stephen Peckham and Pat Taylor discuss the current location of public health in primary care practice. They pose questions about how practice will need to change if primary care is to be an effective location for public health action. This chapter explores the devolution of the public health function to primary care trusts, the extent to which primary care trusts are managing this change, and the implications for wider public health development.

The traditional public health function of health protection, including disease surveillance and control, remain of central importance in contemporary public health. In Chapter 7 Melanie Grey and Joyshri Sarangi examine new challenges, policy frameworks and organizational arrangements for health protection. They discuss underpinning guiding principles to inform judgements and decision taking, and engaging the public in understanding decisions about health risks. Grey and Sarangi also map the wide range of resources for protecting health, and analyse key issues for multidisciplinary working practice.

In Chapter 8 Pat Taylor examines the lay contribution to public health. The 'public' is seen as a key partner in contemporary public health, and lay involvement is expected at all levels of public health activity. Taylor outlines the policy context for lay involvement before discussing some of the inherent problems, contradictions and conceptual and practical barriers. She discusses the reality as well as the potential for lay involvement in public health. Key questions are posed about expectations for lay involvement by different partners in current public health practice.

In Chapter 9 Alison Gilchrist examines the role of networking for health gain. She demonstrates the importance of social relationships in promoting general health and interagency working, arguing that robust and diverse networks provide useful mechanisms for emotional support, critical advice, communal learning and collective organizing. She links this with the concept of social capital, and discusses three aspects of networking: partnership approaches, personal networks and networking practice. The skills and strategies of effective and inclusive networking are identified as a vital dimension of public health.

4

STEPHEN PECKHAM
Who are the partners in public health?

Editors' introduction

An overarching theme in contemporary public health is the need for people to work together. The notion of collaboration and partnerships between agencies, professionals, communities and individuals is fundamental to policy for multidisciplinary public health.

Who needs to work together and how can they do it? This chapter examines the way that concepts for collaboration and partnership are embedded within public health policy and goes on to examine the nature of these partnerships. It considers the development of partnerships in the UK context and the different forms they take.

All public health workers – who by the very nature of their work are likely to find themselves working in partnerships with other people, organizations and the public – will find this chapter useful. It will help them to think critically about what 'partnership' and 'collaboration' actually mean in theory and practice, and why and how partnerships are successful. It also helps readers to find their way around the plethora of local, national and international partnerships.

The author starts by discussing definitions of partnership in current practice. A broad understanding of partnerships is identified and discussed, with a continuum of degrees of collaboration from isolation to integration. The discussion goes on to link the degrees of collaboration to the purpose of collaborations, the nature of the organizations involved and the influence of the wider context on them.

The next section discusses why partnership working is relevant and important for public health to achieve its objectives, with different contributions coming together to maximize resources for health improvement and addressing health inequalities. It acknowledges potential pitfalls and identifies opportunities for partnership working.

In the final section, the author takes an in-depth look at who are the partners in public health, basing discussion on national and international activity. He particularly concentrates on local relationships, where recent development has mostly focused. He concludes by summarizing key benefits and problems within current partnership developments in public health.

Introduction

This book has stressed throughout that 21st century public health is viewed as a collaborative endeavour – a shared responsibility. However, it has also been described as everyone's business but no one's specific responsibility. Recent government policy on public health has, more than before, explicitly recognized the need for a more multidisciplinary and multisectoral approach to public health with an emphasis on collaboration between agencies and individuals. (See Chapters 1 and 3 for an overview of recent and current public health policy.)

This chapter examines how concepts of collaboration and partnership (as a mode of organization) are embedded within current public health policy. It explores what form such collaborations take, how public health collaborations have developed in the UK and identifies partnership as a pragmatic endeavour – an incremental response to getting things done. The aim of the chapter is to provide frameworks for thinking about public health partnerships and to explore the inter-relationship between policy and practice. Thus this chapter will explore the patterns of intra- and interorganizational relationships as they relate to public health policy and action.

The chapter starts, however, by discussing what partnerships are, examining the concept of partnership and how it can be defined. The chapter then moves on to explore why partnership is of relevance to public health. Four broad approaches are discussed relating to the nature of public health, government policy, organizational approaches and working with the public and local communities. Finally the chapter examines a range of public health partnerships, drawing on the frameworks set out in the first two sections of the chapter.

What are partnerships?

The terms partnership and collaboration are often used interchangeably to explain ways of coordinating activity – whether between individuals or organizations. Warren *et al.* (1974) define 'coordination' as: 'A structure or process of concerted decision making wherein the decisions or action of two or more organizations [or individuals] are made simultaneously in part or in whole with some deliberate degree of adjustment to each other' (p. 16). In common usage, partnership conjures a picture of some formal or informal relationship – such as a GP or solicitor partnership, marriage or perhaps 'partners in crime'. However, the notion of partnership is not without problems.

The Audit Commission (1998) has suggested that partnership is a slippery concept and difficult to define precisely. Writing in the 1980s, before new Labour's attachment to the concept, Challis *et al.* (1988) argued that partnership is a word in search of a way of giving it effective meaning in practice. As Powell and Glendinning (2002) argue the key problem is that it is difficult to distinguish partnership from 'other forms of inter-organizational relationships (such as bureaucratic command or contracts) . . . Nor does it seem to map neatly onto network (as opposed to hierarchical or market) approaches to governance' (p. 3). Against such a background identifying public health partnerships becomes very complex.

Partnerships are formal structures of relationships among individuals or groups, all of which are banded together for a common purpose. It is the commitment to a common cause – frequently purposive change – that characterizes these partnerships, whether the partners are organizations or individuals, voluntary confederations of independent agencies or community assemblies developing multipurpose and long-term alliances (El Ansari *et al.* 2001). Embedded in such a definition is, however, the notion that partners are equal. This is rarely the case in reality and different professions and organizations come to partnerships with different values, levels of power, levels of commitment and resources. It is also true that partnerships do not have to be formal structures and many local partnerships, particularly between professionals or lay and professional people are informal but characterized by common purpose. For some commentators it is precisely this lack of a specific definition of 'partnership' which is seen as an advantage providing 'a form of organizational governance whose flexibility, responsiveness and adaptability is ideally suited to the demands of contemporary society [thus] collaborative activities can reflect local circumstances, needs and agreed joint objectives and remain appropriate to the expertise and levels of trust of local partners' (Glendinning 2002: 117).

The collaborative dimension

However, it would be simplistic to view partnerships as either existing or not existing for in reality we would expect to find different degrees of partnership. This collaborative dimension (Hudson *et al.* 1997, 1999) can be analysed using a framework which distinguishes between isolation, encounter, communication, collaboration and integration (see Box 4.1). Each of these represents points on a collaborative continuum

---

Box 4.1   The collaborative dimension – a framework

Isolation	No partnership exists and agencies or individuals work in isolation from each other.
Encounter	Some interagency and interprofessional contact, but this is informal, ad hoc and marginal to the goals of the separate organizations.
Communication	Separate organizations or professionals do engage in joint working of a formal and structured nature, but this still tends to be marginal to separate organizational goals or individual roles, and needs to be able to demonstrate how such activity will help achieve these respective goals or fulfil individual work roles.
Collaboration	Separate agencies recognize that joint working is central to their mainstream activities; this implies a trusting relationship in which organizations are seen to be reliable partners.
Integration	A situation where the degree of collaboration is so high that the separate organizations no longer see their separate identity as significant and may be willing to contemplate the creation of a unitary organization.

ranging from weak to strong. In fact the first and last points are not strictly collaborative measures, since isolation involves *no* interagency activity, while integration is strictly an *alternative* to collaboration.

In those interorganizational or professional relationships characterized by *isolation* and *encounter* we would expect to find:

- loose knit and lowly connected networks;
- infrequent and ad hoc interaction;
- divergently perceived organizational goals and interests; and
- interprofessional rivalry and stereotyping.

An example here would be the historically low level of interaction between general practice and public health in the UK, where they have been organizationally isolated but also premised upon different values, with general practice focusing on individual, reactive patient care and public health on population-based proactive preventive care (Taylor *et al.* 1998).

Where relationships are characterized by *communication* we would expect to find:

- more frequent interactions;
- a willingness to share information about mutual roles, responsibilities and availability;
- a willingness to share some information: some commitment to joint training;
- nominated persons who have some responsibility for liaison;
- relatively loose knit and lowly connected networks;
- limited acceptance of the notion of membership of a team;
- prime loyalty to the employing organization; and
- a high degree of expectation of reciprocation.

This situation would occur where public health professionals feel that they could achieve their own objectives better by working with others, such as when a health promotion worker makes contact with youth workers to achieve greater access to young people to promote sexual health. In such circumstances both the health promotion worker and the youth worker work together but guided by their own goals. Another example would be the new public health networks in England which will draw together professionals in local areas based upon the premise that individual primary care trusts will be able to fulfil all public health tasks on their own (Faculty of Public Health Medicine and Health Development Agency 2001).

Where *collaboration* develops we would expect to find:

- a willingness to participate in some formal and structured pattern of joint working;
- an acknowledgement of the value and existence of a team and agreement on the membership;
- relatively close knit and highly connected networks;

- a high degree of mutual trust and respect;
- a low degree of expectation of immediate reciprocation;
- a high degree of recognition of common interests, goals and interdependency;
- mutual secondments and other forms of cross-boundary deployment;
- clustering or co-location of personnel joint planning;
- joint service delivery; and
- joint commissioning.

Such characteristics are often demonstrated in joint projects. These are generally local and small scale but also include more ambitious projects such as healthy living centres (see Box 4.2).

Finally, with *integration* we should see very close knit and highly connected networks, little regard for reciprocation in relationships, a mutual and diffuse sense of long-term obligation, very high degrees of trust and respect, joint arrangements which are mainstream rather than marginal, joint arrangements, which encompass both strategic and operational issues, some shared or single management arrangements and the establishment of separate, unified organizations.

Levels of partnership

It would also be wrong to characterize the relationship between different agencies as being unidimensional – simply a linear continuum between isolation of one agency to

---

Box 4.2 Healthy living centres

The healthy living centre initiative is a government programme managed by the New Opportunities Fund and was launched on 29 January 1999. Healthy living centres are expected to seek to influence the wider determinants of health, such as social exclusion, poor access to services, and social and economic aspects of deprivation which can contribute to inequalities in health.

There is no blueprint for projects. The initiative is supposed to be flexible enough to allow for innovative proposals based on local needs, supporting national and local health strategies. Local communities and users are expected to be involved in all aspects of design and delivery of a project. Projects are likely to cover a range of activities including, for example, smoking cessation, dietary advice, physical activity, health screening programmes, training and skills schemes, arts programmes and complementary therapy.

The initiative supports *The NHS Plan*, the national strategy for health in England *Saving Lives: Our Healthier Nation* and the health strategies in Northern Ireland, Scotland and Wales. In England, proposals are expected to be part of health improvement programmes.

A range of projects have been established covering an enormous variety of topics and population groups.

integration with other agencies. In practice partnership occurs at a number of levels (Hudson 1987; Rummery and Glendinning 1997; Exworthy and Powell 2000). These include:

- internationally between governments and international agencies, as in UNESCO or the World Health Organisation;
- at a national level, regionally or, for example, in the UK between devolved areas/regions within national government;
- between key local agencies (such as local government, health, voluntary agencies) – as in health action zones or local strategic partnerships;
- locality or area based such as community partnerships, Sure Start, healthy living centres, Neighbourhood Renewal;
- between individuals – joint working.

Types of partnership

Additionally, Hudson and Hardy (2001) identify six key types of partnerships: governing partnerships; accountability partnerships; purchaser–provider partnerships; NHS–local authority partnerships; partnerships with patients/publics; and central–local partnerships. Yet these perhaps simplify the multiplex nature of inter-professional partnerships and partnerships between professionals and patients and the public. Importantly Powell and Exworthy (2002) have argued that partnerships do not just exist horizontally within these levels but that they can also be vertical, between levels (see Figure 4.1).

Stewart (2002) has suggested that partnerships can be categorized as being strategic (or coordinating), facilitative or implementing partnerships. However, like

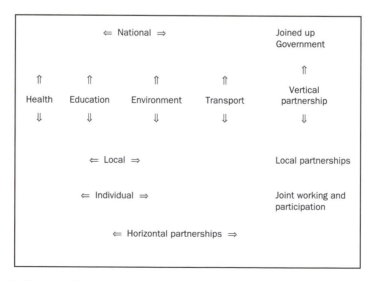

Figure 4.1 Vertical and horizontal partnerships

most frameworks for partnership this categorization suffers problems from the fact that some formalized partnerships have more than one of these roles and often the members are not clear what their role is. In order to assist in discussion and analysis Ling (2000) has suggested that partnerships can be described by four key dimensions:

- their membership;
- the links between members;
- the scale and boundaries of the partnership; and
- the wider context within which the partnership operates.

In practice the dimensions described by Ling are defined by, for example, the context and purpose of the partnership – such as could be found in a partnership approach to stopping smoking, a healthy schools project or in child protection committees. Similarly the membership of a partnership will be directly related to the availability of partners so that two healthy living centres in different areas focusing on say young people are likely to have different members depending on local agency structure, local community profile, number and range of community and voluntary organizations, levels of coterminosity between statutory agencies and so on. While accepting the problems surrounding the definition of 'partnership' it is this term which will be used for the remainder of the chapter to denote arrangements developed in relation to public health.

Why partnerships for public health?

This section explores why partnerships are relevant to public health. Since 1997 there has been an increasing concern to develop joined up processes at national, regional and local levels, as well as increasing vertical partnership between levels. The Labour government has pursued a 'collaborative discourse' (Clarence and Painter 1998) that has included 'joined-up government at the centre and joined-up governance at local levels' (Powell and Exworthy 2001: 21). Many attempts to promote greater collaboration (possibly including the current policy drive) have been 'largely rhetorical invocations of a vague ideal' but collaboration has become the *zeitgeist* of the Labour government (Hudson 1999) as a result of its 'third way' philosophy (Powell 1998). However, in public health as elsewhere in government policy, various mechanisms have been introduced which cannot be considered simply rhetorical. Three broad strategies have been employed in developing partnerships:

- cooperation based on agreement between different organizations/individuals;
- incentives such as funding; more flexibility over resource allocation such as given to areas with health action zones who were able to use health and local authority resources more flexibly than authorities outside these zones (Matka *et al.* 2002); and
- authoritarian approaches setting out specific organizational forms or other 'must do' requirements; these include local strategic partnerships, membership of

primary care group/trust boards, range of partners for healthy living centres, Sure Start or health action zones.

These have been applied at both national and local levels and have been variously called joint working, partnership and collaboration. From a public health policy perspective it is important to recognize the role of national government and the need for partnerships at national and local levels as well as between these levels. The need for national collaboration was clearly recognized in *The Health of the Nation* White Paper (Secretary of State for Health 1992). In fact government policy on public health partnerships has traditionally operated at both national and local levels addressing (to some degree at least) partnership on public health policy, organizational partnerships and joint working between professionals.

The relative emphasis on these aspects of partnership have been changing over the past ten years reflecting the general shift in public health policy from the Conservative government of the 1980s and 1990s to the new Labour government elected in 1997. The next sections explore the context of these developments outlining five broad themes for partnership relating to the nature of public health, organizational issues, government policy working with the public and the need to address health inequalities.

The nature of public health

The need for partnership can be seen to arise from the recognition that there are many factors which contribute towards public health. In fact this was an explicit element of the Alma Ata (WHO/UNICEF 1978) declaration where collaboration is one of the key pillars of primary health care (the others being participation and equity – see Macdonald 1992). Collaboration was also a key element of the Health for All approach promoted by the World Health Organisation during the 1980s (WHO 1991).

The history of public health in the UK has been characterized by the gradual domination of the medical model and public health medicine promulgated by medical practitioners (Macdonald 1992; Baggott 2000). This has led to an emphasis on disease control and monitoring, epidemiological studies, individual health promotion and support to medical practitioners – most recently in relation to evidence-based medicine. (See Chapter 7 on disease control; Chapter 15 on epidemiology; and Chapter 14 on evidence-based public health.)

Yet it is widely recognized that most advances in health are the result of improvements in people's economic and social status – better housing, higher incomes, better education and so on. These improvements are not just the consequences of government intervention but derive from the actions of individuals, communities, organizations and international circumstances. Moreover, as suggested in Chapter 9, social and community ties have been identified as important protective elements which promote health. Recognition of the importance of healthy communities would appear to be reflected in current health policy with, for example, the creation of health action zones, healthy living centres, health improvement programmes and the development of primary care organizations (see Chapter 6 and Peckham and Exworthy 2003 for a fuller discussion). All these organizations have a broad and ambitious brief to employ both individual and community approaches for addressing local health problems.

Clearly this encompasses a range of activities undertaken by a wide range of actors (different government departments and agencies, professionals, private organizations, community groups, families and so on, and hence gives rise to the notion that public health is everyone's business (Secretary of State for Health 1999). Current policy and practice are framed by government policies on public health in England that aim to develop a three way partnership between individuals, communities (and local agencies) and government to achieve better public health. Similar emphasis can be found in government proposals in Scotland, Northern Ireland and Wales (Scottish Executive 1998; Secretary of State for Northern Ireland 1998; Secretary of State for Wales 1998).

While the need for involving a range of agencies, and individuals, in public health has long been acknowledged (in both policy and practice) the current government has perhaps more fully embraced action which sits more firmly in the wider social model of health with its emphasis on intersectoral action and participation as advocated by WHO. The government has fully endorsed the need for multidisciplinary approaches to public health and in England has supported new approaches to tackling public health issues such as health action zones, healthy living centres and local strategic partnerships. In Scotland local authorities are required to develop community planning to provide a strategic framework for joint planning, partnership working, and to address fragmented public policy and service provision (Fernie and McCarthy 2001). As Barnes and Sullivan argue 'Partnership was understood to be the key vehicle that would enable the resources of government to be brought to bear on improving health, reducing inequalities and improving services in a coordinated and cohesive manner' (Barnes and Sullivan 2002: 81). (See Chapters 1 and 2 for further discussion of government policy in public health.)

Addressing health inequalities

Tackling health inequalities is a major focus of government policy. One of the first acts of the 1997 Labour government was to set up an inquiry on health inequalities chaired by Sir Donald Acheson. The report makes a number of recommendations for action ranging across the whole scope of government. Central to the report's approach to tackling health inequalities is the need for government to act across all departments to tackle the causes of ill health including poverty, transport, education, housing, health and so on. Echoing the findings of earlier studies (Townsend 1988) the Acheson enquiry emphasized the need for coordinated action to address the causes of health inequality. The government has established key targets for tackling health inequalities to reduce geographical and socio-economic differences in mortality. There are also additional targets related to smoking and teenage pregnancy. (See Chapter 10 for in-depth discussion of tackling inequalities in health.)

Policies to tackle health inequalities can be identified across government (Department of Health 2001c) including tax and benefit reform, welfare to work, interventions in the early years of life and across the life course, diet and nutrition programmes, among many others. The government's approach to health inequalities also emphasizes the need to tackle these at national, regional and local levels (Secretary of State for Health 1999; Bull and Hamer 2002). These policies have been pursued at a local level using primary care and partnership working as the main local vehicles for policy implementation. At a regional level there is greater strategic coordination bringing regional public health directors into the existing government regional offices. These approaches have been reinforced by the issues emerging from the Department of Health consultation (on a plan for delivery) (Department of Health 2002a) and the Treasury cross-cutting review on health inequalities (HM Treasury and Department of Health 2002). Thus the very nature of health inequalities calls for a partnership approach placing this at the centre of public health policy and developments.

Organizational issues

The growing emphasis upon partnership also arises in part from the acknowledged limits of organizational individualism where agencies work in isolation from each other. Huxham and Macdonald ([1882] 1999), for example, identify four 'pitfalls of individualism' which all have direct relevance to public health:

- *repetition:* where two or more organizations carry out an action or task which need only be done by one;
- *omission:* where activities which are important to the objectives of more than one organization are not carried out because they have not been identified as important, because they come into no organization's remit, or because each organization assumes the other is performing the activity;
- *divergence:* the actions of the various organizations may become diluted across a range of activities rather than being used towards common goals;
- *counterproduction:* organizations working in isolation may take actions which conflict with those taken by others.

Pratt *et al.* (1998) have also argued that partnerships need to be related to whether the goals being pursued are collective or individual and the predicted gains are high or low. This can be shown diagrammatically as in Figure 4.2. Public health goals are collective, although health is also an individual goal. The framework developed by

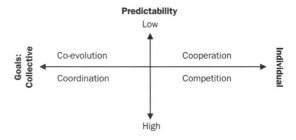

Figure 4.2 Strategies for partnership

Pratt *et al.* shows that in addressing collective public health goals if the gains are uncertain or low we would expect to see co-evolution – the gradual development in separate agencies towards the collective goal. However, where it is clear gains are high – such as with accident prevention – we would expect to see coordination through partnership. Even where the focus is on individual agency goals Pratt *et al.* view the gains as generally low, as people may not control all the determinants of their health, a strategy of cooperation would be best to achieve the best individual outcomes. Clearly where individual gains are high but the context is uncertain agencies may compete for obtaining the best health. Public health strategy needs to balance these approaches but if the goals are to maximize population health then co-evolution or coordination are the best strategies for partnerships.

Government policy

The drive towards 'joined up' thinking, generating 'joined up' solutions are a response to the need to address what have been described as 'wicked issues' (Audit Commission 1998; Clarence and Painter 1998; Powell and Exworthy 2001; Glendinning *et al.* 2002). In other words, the issues facing local communities – such as tackling health inequalities, promoting health, tackling social exclusion and so on – are multifaceted and require multiagency and multidisciplinary attention. This new approach is embodied in government policy documents such as *Saving Lives: Our Healthier Nation* which emphasize the important role of integration and partnership 'working across Government to attack the breeding ground of poor health – poverty and social exclusion – and we believe in creating partnerships with local authorities, health authorities and other agencies to tackle the root causes of ill-health in places where people live' (Secretary of State of Health 1999: 3). The emphasis is also embodied in *The NHS Plan* identifying the NHS's role in helping to 'develop Local Strategic Partnerships, into which, in the medium term, health actions zones and other local action zones could be integrated to strengthen links between health, education, employment and other causes of social exclusion' (Secretary of State for Health 2000: 111). (These policy issues are also discussed in Chapters 1 and 2.)

Working with the public and communities

The increasing emphasis on community and public involvement is of particular relevance to public health. Recent research on health inequalities has identified the important connection between individual, relative inequality within any given geographical community, as well as inequality between communities (Wilkinson 1997). It is widely recognized that there are inequalities in health status, morbidity and mortality between deprived and affluent communities shaped by a range of individual, geographical and social factors. The relative effect of these will vary according to specific circumstances. At the same time early life factors and/or the cumulative effects on social cohesion of life events caused by deprivation play a significant role (Wilkinson 1996, 1997). Thus developing approaches to reduce health inequalities will require tailoring towards individual circumstances and addressing specific characteristics of local areas and communities. There has tended to be little recognition of the role of the community in promoting its own health through community-based action and community health initiatives (Petersen and Lupton 1996; Taylor *et al.* 1998). Yet, individuals, families and communities provide significant amounts of self-care and ill health prevention as illustrated in Figure 4.3 (WHO/UNICEF 1978; Zakus and Lysack 1998). (See Chapter 8 for discussion of the lay contribution to public health.)

Despite the domination of a medical approach to public health most advances in health are the result of improvements in people's economic and social status – better housing, higher incomes, better education and so on. These improvements are not just the consequences of government intervention but derive from the actions of individuals, communities, organizations and international circumstances. Recognition of the importance of healthy communities would appear to be reflected in current health policy. For example, the creation of health action zones, healthy living centres, health improvement programmes and the development of primary care organizations all have a broad and ambitious brief to employ both individual and community approaches for addressing local health problems.

Self-evidently, in adopting a more enlightened public health perspective, individuals and communities need to be seen as equal partners in promoting and producing health alongside many others. The medical and health professions are just one part of a range of individuals and organizations which have an impact on health including local authorities, voluntary organizations, and private companies and those that work within them.

So, partnership or collaboration is an essential ingredient of public health in four key ways:

- tackling the key determinants of health (as conceptualized in the social model of health) requires action by a range of international, national and local agencies;
- seeing public health as a shared responsibility;
- needing to avoid overlap and duplication; and
- recognizing the important role individuals and communities play in promoting their own health.

But this still raises the question of what a partnership is and what sort of partnerships are needed to deliver public health. While accepting the need to address international aspects and the important role of cross-national partnership arrangements this chapter will focus on the UK context.

Who are the partners in public health?

Partnership can be seen to exist between individual workers in the context of interprofessional partnership. There are important and ongoing relationships between NHS public health specialists, environmental health officers, nurses, doctors, community workers and so on, that operate within, but independently of, organizational and institutional arrangements – although it is presumably hoped that such arrangements support rather than hinder such joint working. In recent years there has been

Who		Act as	How	Who with	Comments
Individuals		Patients, health providers, health educators	Self care, shared care, user involvement, complaints, preventive care	Themselves, health professionals, other users	Individuals undertake a range of self-directed and motivated preventive health measures and have contact with professionals on an individual basis
Families		Patients, health providers, carers/parents, supporters, advocates	Direct care, shared care, user involvement, complaints, preventive care	Themselves, health professionals	Contact with individual health care practitioners and professionals providing support and information (e.g. health visitors)
Communities of interest	**Informal networks**	Supporters, health providers, information providers	Friend and kinship networks, self-help groups	Themselves, health professionals	May work collaboratively with specific health professionals but main emphasis is on mutual support (e.g. self-help groups)
	Formal networks	Health providers, supporters, advocates, information providers	Community associations, patient groups	Members	May provide a range of information and support services to members. This may involve specialist and professional health providers (e.g. patient participation group, food cooperative)
	Community/ voluntary organizations	Providers of services, supporters, advocates	Campaigning, delivering services, participating in working groups	Members, users, health professionals, health agencies	More formalized than networks and may have specific aims to provide services as well as support users (e.g. MIND, SCOPE, Royal National Institute for the Deaf)
Geographical communities		Polity, electors, providers, advocates	Voting, campaigning, developing networks between other groups	Health agencies, local authorities, government	E.g. neighbourhood health action group, environmental groups

Figure 4.3 Individuals, communities, the public and health

an increase in joint educational approaches through multidisciplinary public health training (for example, at the University of the West of England, Bristol). However, professional networks still tend to be uniprofessional although the Faculty of Public Health has begun to broaden itself into a more multidisciplinary profession in line with government policy.

Partnership can be contextualized in both formal and informal ways. Formal partnerships include organizational arrangements such as cross-representation and joint budgets; informal arrangements are those such as professionals working alongside each other, and local networking. Generally, formalization occurs at all levels with policy gradually increasing institutional and organizational structures to support this. Informal approaches have tended to be seen as less important but have also occurred predominantly at senior management levels and between professionals working in the community.

International partnerships

International collaboration is an expanding feature of public health. Increasingly it is recognized that public health issues transcend national boundaries and action between countries (such as in the European Union or WHO) is becoming important. Mobility between countries, international trade (particularly in foodstuffs) and common health problems mean that countries can no longer be isolated in their approaches to public health. The need for global responses to diseases like HIV/AIDS and, increasingly, the transfer of other diseases through global travel means dealing with poverty and health issues in many developing countries requires cooperation at an international level (McKee et al. 2001). (Chapter 13 discusses globalization and its impact on health.)

National partnerships – joined up government

At the national level, joined up government has been promoted in policy making and service delivery through cross-departmental programmes and initiatives such as Sure Start, the Teenage Pregnancy Unit and the rough sleepers initiative. These seek to overcome the long recognized problem of departmentalism, that is, the strong tradition and culture that civil servants and ministers seek to defend and, if possible, augment their own sphere of responsibility; ministers thus become 'barons'. Issues that cut across more than one department (such as health inequalities) might suffer from a lack of departmental ownership or sufficient accountability. This has led Kavanagh and Richards to conclude that 'It is questionable to what extent joined-up government can be properly established when departments remain crucial holders of resources and continue to dominate policy-making and policy delivery' (Kavanagh and Richards, 2001: 17).

Since 1997 there has been an increasing attempt to link up government departments. When the Labour government published its Green Paper on public health (Department of Health 1998c) it was only signed by the Secretary of State for Health. This was criticized for a lack of joint government commitment, a position rectified in the White Paper which carried the signatures of ministers from other key departments

(Secretary of State for Health 1999). In addition, initiatives in local government and urban policy have increasingly been linked to health. In England, for example, single regeneration bids now explicitly including health targets, joint health and social care targets have been set for the NHS and local government, and the Neighbourhood Renewal Unit has a presence in both the Department of Health and the Office for the Deputy Prime Minister. The Cabinet Office has also provided a focus for coordinated approaches such as the Social Exclusion Unit and more recently the Treasury has undertaken a number of cross-cutting spending reviews including one into tackling the causes of health inequalities (HM Treasury and Department of Health 2002). These approaches are a clear attempt to join up policy and government action and have more recently been reflected in changes to regional structures bringing the NHS more closely aligned with regional government offices and regional public health forums bringing together local authorities, the NHS and regional agencies.

With devolution, cross-national relationships are developing between England, Wales, Scotland and Northern Ireland. In the case of Northern Ireland the recently established Joint Irish Institute for Public Health with Eire has been formed. Importantly, while there are distinct differences in approaches to public health, particularly between Wales, Scotland and England, policy consistencies such as an emphasis on partnerships between health and other divisions of government such as the environment, transport and so on are more evident across the UK. In Scotland and Wales the focus for much of this approach lies within the Scottish Parliament and the Welsh Assembly, providing a political coordination at national level. In contracts in England responsibility for developing a partnership approach lies within the government regions with newly appointed directors of public health. As Powell and Exworthy (2002) have demonstrated in their study on health inequalities policy, such national approaches to partnership are becoming more common and important, and are likely to continue to provide both an attempt at joined up policy and to join up the mechanisms of central government. However, they and others (Davies *et al.* 2000) argue that this is not yet by any means perfect. (Perspectives on 'joined up' government are also discussed in Chapters 1 and 2.)

Local partnerships

For most public health workers and activists it is at the local level that partnerships are more likely to be developed or experienced. Local partnerships now constitute a wide range of activity encouraged by central government policy initiatives but also developed through local action.

Since 1997 the government has tried to develop a new framework for addressing public health, introducing a number of new mechanisms. These include a statutory duty of partnership upon health agencies and local authorities with provisions for local strategic partnerships, the development of joint investment plans, health improvement and modernization plans and partnership structures such as health action zones, healthy living centres and Sure Start projects which have sought to widen partnerships beyond health and local authorities with a wider public health remit. In addition, local approaches to tackling teenage pregnancy are predicated on local partnerships and there exist a wide range of formal and informal groupings at local level which may constitute partnerships, such as action on stopping smoking, healthy schools initiatives, child protection committees, community safety groups, drug action teams and so on. The nature and range of such groups will vary from area to area, and some have a long history, some have developed for one off reasons and others are highly informal, based on ad hoc groupings of individual workers. Drawing on Stewart's (2002) framework of strategic (or coordinating), facilitative and implementing partnerships it is useful to examine local partnerships in more detail.

Strategic or coordinating partnerships would include health action zones (HAZs) and local strategic partnerships. HAZs were established from 1998 onwards to develop partnership approaches to tackling health inequalities. They were given additional funding and developed a core staff with partnership, both horizontally across major local agencies, but also vertically with other local agencies. The evaluation of health action zones has suggested that collaboration is an important ingredient in success but that having a long history of partnership is helpful and that a commitment to partnership does not address imbalances in power between different members. These are well recognized problems (Gillies 1998a; Department of Transport, Local Government and the Regions 2002; Stewart 2002).

However, the evidence from the HAZ evaluation is that there have been successes partly due to the changing national context, with new policies supporting a partnership approach – providing local freedoms, for example, flexibilities through new approaches to funding (Secretary of State for Health 2000; Barnes and Sullivan 2002). Initially these were in the 88 neighbourhood renewal areas but now they are being set up across England. While initially seen as being established for single local authority areas, a fifth cover more than one district – the largest being 12 local authority districts. More recently local strategic partnerships have begun to form across the country bringing together the public, private, voluntary and community sectors to action the local community strategy. Such changes are located within the broader framework of the modernization of local government and democratic renewal. Local strategic partnerships are a key element of intersectoral partnerships in England (DETR 2000; DETR 2001) and have key roles in engaging communities in partnership arrangements and provide rationalization of other strategic planning processes. Tackling health inequalities is central to the process 'ensuring committed NHS participation in local strategic partnerships by bringing knowledge, expertise and resources to the partnership' (Department of Health 2001c). (Public health initiatives at neighbourhood level, such as HAZs, are also discussed in Chapter 11.)

There are fears that they are being dominated by local authorities with little community input (Biles et al. 2001). Health improvement and modernization plans currently remain separate from the community plans being developed by local authorities. There does not appear, at present, to be any significant dovetailing of NHS planning with these new local strategic partnerships. Yet public health – and specifically health inequalities – is clearly expected to be a prominent issue for the local strategic partnerships.

Local strategic partnerships have only gradually been established in the past two years and do not have the structures and funding which underpinned the development of HAZs. Currently there is an evaluation underway but at the moment these partnership arrangements are still developing. Whether they can fulfil the coordination role envisaged by government to tackle complex issues such as deprivation and poor health, only time will tell as most have only started since the year 2000, although nearly half of these developed from existing formal or informal partnership arrangements (Stewart 2002). One problem may be that they are too large to really provide a coordination role. The average membership is 41 with some having over 50 members. Such large memberships potentially demonstrate a desire to address governance issues and draw together representatives from all the local agencies – stressing everyone's responsibility.

It is perhaps in the layer just below these strategic approaches to partnership where there has been most activity and development. Clearly primary care organizations would fit here as would healthy living centres, community partnerships, Neighbourhood Renewal, Sure Start and so on. As discussed in Chapter 6, primary care has become a focus for public health partnerships. In England, following the publication of *The NHS Plan* (Secretary of State for Health 2000) and *Shifting the Balance* (Department of Health 2001a, 2002b) primary care trusts are seen as central to developing local public health action and collaboration. In Wales these institutional and organizational arrangements are extended to include further local authority and voluntary agency representation on local health boards which will also be co-terminous with local authorities. While these arrangements have focused on planning and strategy they have also included approaches to joint commissioning. Similarly in Scotland, Scottish PCTs and, in particular, their constituent local health care cooperatives are expected to address public health issues. There is significant emphasis placed, both in policy and in practice, on public health partnerships. This means that for primary care organizations, partnerships will include local authority departments – such as housing, education, leisure and environmental health as well as local voluntary agencies and private organizations. There is also an increased emphasis on partnership within the NHS, between practices, with hospitals and potentially with other primary care organizations. This is a potentially complex set of relationships and shifts the focus to seeing partnerships as a network – explicitly so in England (Department of Health 2002b).

The evidence suggests, however, that partnership working is slow to develop. In 2000–01 telephone interviews were undertaken with chief executives and chairs of the majority of the 72 PCGs/PCTs in the Tracker Survey in England. The survey found that 44 PCGs had worked with departments of urban regeneration, 38 with leisure services, 31 with housing services and 29 with education (Gillam *et al.* 2001). However, while such links were described as rudimentary consisting of membership of multiagency groups, Gillam *et al.* argued that such links are a prerequisite of developing working relationships and they back this argument with evidence showing that primary care organizations are beginning to allocate funding to health improvement activities.

In Scotland there is a strong emphasis on public health. This may relate to the fact that the Scottish population has a worse health status than in England. Historically both Scotland and Wales have been closely identified with health inequalities. During the interwar period many of the most extreme examples of ill health and social deprivation were found in the South Wales valleys and in the industrial belt of central Scotland (Levitt 1988). Some areas of Glasgow have among the highest rates of infant mortality in Europe, and in the UK, 52 percent of the 'worst off million people in terms of health live in Scotland' (Shaw *et al.* 1999). At a policy level Scotland has followed the model of *Saving Lives: Our Healthier Nation* with a similarly focused White Paper *Working Together for a Healthier Scotland* (Scottish Executive 1998). In Scotland there has been a more specific emphasis on developing strategies and action to address public health issues with a Health Improvement Fund, increasing public health intelligence but with the public health function retained by the Scottish health boards who remain the key commissioning agencies.

In 2000 the Secretary of State for Health, Alan Milburn, highlighted Sure Start as making one of the most important contributions to health improvement in the UK (Milburn 2000). Sure Start is one of many community partnership approaches being developed in many areas around the country which seeks to address individual problems through community-based responses but by working with the local communities involved. Sure Start is based on a similar approach pioneered in the USA and has a strong neighbourhood focus, with each programme serving the local community 'within pram pushing distance'. The programme is targeted on children and families in deprived circumstances. It is being delivered through local partnerships with the aim of providing a range of support services, including childcare, early learning and play opportunities, and support with parenting skills, as well as improved access to primary health care (see Box 4.3).

Partnerships with communities

Increasingly, community-based approaches to health have been incorporated into a range of government policy objectives at a local level emphasizing partnerships between local communities and statutory agencies within programmes such as

---

Box 4.3   Rose Hill – Littlemore Sure Start

The Sure Start project started in 1999 in an area of Oxford with the second largest 0–16-year-old population. The area also had the highest number of people reporting a limited long-term illness and high levels of unemployment. Rose Hill had a high proportion (25 percent) on the school roll of children from Asian families and a high number of children on the special education needs register. There were no locally based health services in the area and few resources for under-4s and their families.

The project has worked with local parents to establish a centre based at the First School for 0–3-year-olds providing a community café, health clinics, crèche, playroom and so on. The project has also worked with the local early education project.

The project is a partnership between statutory and voluntary services and local families. There are parent representatives on the project group, and a research group is conducting a local evaluation of the project.

The focus of work is on prevention rather than crisis intervention and thus should be seen as playing an important role in addressing local health and welfare issues from a public health perspective.

Standard Regeneration Budget, New Deal for Communities and the Neighbourhood Renewal programme. The emphasis is on the need for local regeneration activity which engages local communities as citizens, service users and neighbours (Audit Commission 2002). The focus is on deprived neighbourhoods and the Neighbourhood Renewal programme aims to build on the experiences of previous programmes to improve local neighbourhoods so that 'within 10–20 years no one should be seriously disadvantaged by where they live' and to 'narrow the gap on [worklessness, crime, health, skills, housing and physical environment] measures between the most deprived neighbourhoods and the rest of the country' (Social Exclusion Unit 2001a: 8). More importantly neighbourhood renewal is a cross-departmental approach and there is an attempt to join up policy initiatives across government – especially between local government and health. Such partnerships can be seen as both facilitation and implementation partnerships but they face many difficulties in relation to community engagement, imbalances in power, problems of governance as new ways of working challenge traditional local authority and health service models of bureaucracy, management and budgetary control.

Finally, at a more individual level joint working has traditionally developed health promotion (both in local authorities and the NHS) and public health departments around specific issues to meet individual patient/client needs (for example, diet and smoking) or targeted at specific population groups (such as young people and pregnant women). However, some general practices have also developed joint working arrangements for public health. While these have involved interprofessional working the emphasis has been predominantly intraorganizational within the NHS. Notable examples include the West End Health Centre in Newcastle and the Bromley by Bow Centre.

More rarely wider collaborative approaches have been pioneered such as the Arts for Health Movement and Local Exchange Schemes or Time Banks (Cowe 2000) (see Box 4.4).

Local partnerships can, therefore, be seen to have a range of agencies involved, an organizational context, an individual context and a range of purposes. These are shown in Chapter 17, Figure 17.3. What all the local partnerships share is an attempt to draw together local agencies and professionals to avoid overlap, improve coordination and bring a range of approaches, professionalisms, perspectives and resources to bear on local problems. In some cases this approach is defined and set by

---

Box 4.4 Rushey Green Time Bank

The time bank is closely related to the local exchange trading schemes where community members trade skills. In the time bank people trade hours of activity.

There are a dozen or more time banks in the UK. One of these pioneering schemes was led by a GP who saw the potential for time banks to have a health impact. He instigated a scheme in Rushey Green in 1999 which encourages local people to offer time to other local residents. Tasks on offer include story telling, fishing, odd jobs, baby sitting and visiting elderly and house bound people.

central government or is at least reliant on a context which has been set centrally. However, it is also true that many initiatives derive from local circumstances, personal agendas and endeavours despite continuing problems of traditional management approaches and poor interagency coordination.

Conclusion

The discussion in this chapter has demonstrated that partnership is a fundamental concept which underpins public health policy and action. This is both a strength and a weakness. Clearly the nature of public health and the need to address inequalities in health requires multisectoral action which, if it is be effective, requires some level of coordination. The multisectoral approach requiring action by all those agencies and individuals which have an impact on health, strengthens approaches to address health problems and inequalities. However, it is their coordination which creates problems both in terms of 'joining up' policy and action and ensuring accountability. Thus public health may be everyone's responsibility but how do we ensure that responsibility is taken up and also held to account?

Partnerships are also generally based on ideas of voluntarism and current policy; emphasizing the development of formal partnerships raises questions about whether such enforcement of collaborative working is possible. Public health policy continually emphasizes new forms of partnership through PCTs, healthy living centres and local strategic partnerships. However, research on partnership has identified the need for partnerships to develop through the establishment of relationships between different agencies and individuals. Such partnerships are more likely to be successful and be sustained. Yet, in the very policy push towards establishing partnerships many traditional partnerships are being reorganized dismantling the very relationships which support sustained collaboration. Many areas are currently in the process of dismantling health action zone structures devolving aspects of their work to PCTs, local strategic partnerships and other local agencies and in other areas long standing community and joint planning forums are being superseded by new structures. In formalizing partnerships the government has also attempted to establish who partners should be, and there is a danger that insufficient coordination will be achieved between different partnerships such as public health networks and other local health partnerships in the community. In England local strategic partnerships have been given the task of overall coordination but as discussed above these are only just beginning to develop. It may be some time, if at all, before they can act as local coordinating bodies.

Despite this there is still a strong sense of support for partnership and many policy makers, workers and representatives from community and voluntary agencies are committed to developing partnership approaches. Recent policy changes do provide some new frameworks and a new context which make partnerships easier through changes in funding regulations, structures and the ability to experiment with new organizational forms. Ultimately the success of public health partnerships is likely to rest upon the flexibility for actors at all levels to develop real and appropriate partnerships within a policy framework that recognizes variation and flexibility but which provides clarity on purpose and accountability.

5

JENNIE NAIDOO, JUDY ORME AND GILL BARRETT

Capacity and capability in public health

Editors' introduction

Public health work in the 21st century needs people with a wide range of knowledge and skills. What are the competencies – the combination of knowledge, attitudes and skills – which we need to develop in the public health workforce? Are there enough people being trained? Do we have the right range of expertise?

In this chapter, the authors address the question of capacity and capability in the public health workforce. The chapter aims to help public health workers and trainers from all disciplines and professional backgrounds to see themselves as part of a wider workforce, with responsibilities to continuously develop their skills and knowledge, and to apply them in new situations, often in multidisciplinary teams.

The authors first review the scope of the public health workforce, identifying different levels of skills and expertise, and some barriers to collaborative working within and across these levels. They discuss the range of public health skills and competencies and highlight the issue of multidisciplinary practice. They argue that a mapping exercise, matching the National Standards skills and competencies with existing professional skills and expertise, would provide a useful baseline from which to assess the existing public health workforce and future training needs.

The chapter moves on to review the concept of the 'professional project' in public health. Particular challenges are identified and discussed, including issues of multi-disciplinary working, challenging the dominance of health professions, using the evidence base for public health, and issues about integrating and financing training in public health.

The authors argue that the important progression to make is to a true multi-disciplinary public health where contributions from the range of professional groups are recognized and valued.

The chapter concludes with a case study focused on asylum seekers to illustrate the range of professional groups who can potentially contribute to the health and well being of this marginalized group of people with complex needs.

Introduction

Public health depends on the capacity and capability of a large workforce, employed in a variety of roles and organizations, to protect and promote the public health in a range of contexts and environments and throughout the life cycle. The potential workforce for public health is huge, spanning not just health but also education, social care, environmental health, housing, transport and voluntary sector staff. This leads to many complexities when trying to develop capacity and capability in public health.

This chapter first reviews the scope of the public health workforce, identifying different levels of skills and expertise, and some of the barriers to collaborative working within and across these levels. The range of public health skills and competencies is then discussed, and the issue of multidisciplinary practice is highlighted. The concept of the professional project is then reviewed and related to developments in public health practice. Particular challenges are identified and discussed, and the potential for developing capacity and capability in different ways is illustrated using examples of good practice.

The public health workforce

The government clearly recognizes that people from a range of backgrounds and at all levels of seniority contribute to the public health workforce (Department of Health 2001b). The Chief Medical Officer's project to strengthen the public health function identifies three different levels of involvement in public health:

- Specialists from a variety of professional backgrounds, with the ability to manage strategic change and lead public health initiatives. These include consultants in public health medicine, directors of public health, leads in public health and environmental health officers.
- Practitioners who spend a substantial part of their working time furthering health by working with communities and groups. These include public health nurses, community nurses, community and youth workers, and health promotion specialists.
- Professionals whose work includes elements of public health and who would benefit from a better understanding of public health. These would include social workers, teachers and police officers.

This framework is important because it acknowledges theoretical views of the broad determinants of public health, for example, the importance of social capital for public health (Popay 2001; Duggan 2002), and hence the potential of a wide variety of professionals to promote the public health.

Challenges

However, this 'three levels' framework also presents many practical challenges. Not all these players necessarily see themselves as having a public health function, and the range of professional and disciplinary backgrounds is immense. Whether the multi-disciplinary public health banner is sufficient to weld a commonality of purpose among these diverse groups is questionable. Adequate funding for public health training and accreditation, and a supportive policy context which recognizes the multidisciplinary roots of public health are key prerequisites if a unifying public health purpose and function is to evolve.

A separate challenge is the historical dominance of public health medicine in the field of public health, and the problems this poses for true multidisciplinary practice (McPherson and Fox 1997). The picture is complicated due to the relative weakness of public health medicine within medical specialties, which leads to a defensiveness and policing of the boundaries of public health medicine in an effort to assert identity and retain autonomy (Lewis 1991). Sociologists term this process 'professional closure' – an attempt to close ranks, limit the number of people admitted to the profession and thus retain a protected monopoly provider position which is more likely to be well rewarded both financially and in terms of power and kudos (Freidson 1986; Annandale 1998). Recent developments such as the lower ranking and pay scale of recently appointed non-medical directors of public health in England compared to medical directors of public health illustrate this point. The introduction of the voluntary register for public health practitioners which follows closely the traditional curriculum of medical public health specialists (Faculty of Public Health Medicine 2002) also demonstrates an attempt at professional closure, as predicted by sociologists.

Public health and a range of other professions are associated with a specific and broad-ranging skills mix which includes considerable areas of overlap. Investigation of a range of professions reveals the full range of skills, capabilities and competencies, which overlap and encompass many public health competencies and skills. For example, teachers have educational skills, community workers have community development skills, public health nurses have needs assessment skills, environmental health officers have risk assessment and management skills and so on. Rather than re-inventing these skills, public health should draw upon existing expertise, including professional training and accreditation schemes as well as accredited specialists, for instance in health promotion or environmental health. This is not only desirable but essential given the lack of specialist public health capacity and capability on the ground (Singleton and Aird 2002).

Commentators have also identified the crucial need for developing a more flexible skills mix among existing NHS staff in order to deliver quality care and the targets for staffing (Buchan 2002). The introduction of new roles and skill mix will pose the most challenging test for the human resources agenda, and the priority should be on developing the skills of existing staff rather than introducing new types of workers (Buchan 2002).

Public health skills and competencies

Important developments in the mapping of public health practice are the recently published *National Standards for Specialist Practice in Public Health* (Healthwork UK 2001) and the functional map of public health practice under discussion (Skills for

Health 2002a). *Key purposes* for public health identified during this process of developing standards are to:

- improve health and well being in the population;
- prevent disease and minimize its consequences;
- prolong valued life; and
- reduce inequalities in health.

The key purposes are broken down into ten smaller constituent parts, termed *key areas*, which are:

- surveillance and assessment of the population's health and well being;
- promoting and protecting the population's health and well being;
- developing quality and risk management within an evaluative culture;
- collaborative working for health and well being;
- developing health programmes and services and reducing inequalities;
- policy and strategy development and implementation to improve health and well being;
- working with and for communities to improve health and well being;
- strategic leadership for health and well being;
- research and development to improve health and well being;
- ethically managing self, people and resources to improve health and well being.

Scrutiny of these key areas and their sub-areas demonstrates the breadth and sub-stance of public health but does not effectively convey the level of competence required in each of these areas. They are therefore open to a significant amount of interpretation.

Public health training needs

A mapping exercise, matching the National Standards skills and competencies with existing professional skills and expertise, would provide a useful baseline from which to assess the existing public health workforce and future training needs. Training needs may be 'top up' programmes re-enforcing potential public health roles and expertise of existing professionals as well as initial training programmes for new staff. For example, this process of targeted educational enhancement may be particularly important for those professionals who have applied unsuccessfully for director of public health posts in primary care trusts. The important progression to make is to a true multidisciplinary public health, where contributions from the range of pro-fessional groups are recognized and valued. If this does not happen in a proactive and productive way, it is unlikely that we will come near developing the capacity and capability in public health that the Chief Medical Officer drew attention to in his report (Department of Health 2001b).

The emphasis on and commitment to 'joined up' working is analysed in other parts of this book (see especially Chapters 1 and 2). The assumption, however, that groups can and will work across professional and organizational boundaries is not necessarily borne out in practice. Interprofessional education and training can help to instigate and facilitate partnership working (Centre for the Advancement of Inter-professional Education 1997). Skilful management and expertise in multidisciplinary education in public health is needed to ensure that the needs of professionals who are anxious to forge their own identity and not keen to be assimilated in one agenda are addressed appropriately. It could be argued that there are certain areas of focus within public health which act as real vehicles to enable professions to work together and to cross boundaries, for example, social capital, neighbourhood renewal and building healthy communities.

The public health professional project

Larson (1977) discusses the concept of the 'professional project', which is useful when thinking about public health practice. Key aspects of the professional project are about acquiring a monopoly in valued areas of expertise. This monopoly is supported by specific training that restricts the number of practitioners and certifies a certain level of competence; this in turn is recognized and supported by the state. Foucault (1979) uses the concept of 'governmentality' to encompass all those pro-cedures, techniques, mechanisms, institutions and areas of knowledge – including professions – that empower political programmes. Foucault therefore emphasizes the fluidity of the professional project, which is constantly being renegotiated within a political and technological context.

The professional project is a fairly accurate description of public health specialists. For capacity and capability in public health to develop in an effective multidisciplinary manner, some aspects of the professional project, such as state recognition and support, and certified training and education, need also to apply to practitioners and the wider workforce. Without a widening of the public health professional project, public health will remain a beleaguered medical specialty. Its potential as a multidisciplinary resource and activity enhancing the public health in its broadest sense will remain unfulfilled. A key question for practitioners and the wider workforce is whether the identity of being a public health professional, or engaging in the public health professional project, will complement or challenge existing professional identities. This in turn will impact on the ability to generate genuine multidisciplinary working in the interests of the public health.

Issues of multidisciplinary working

The Department of Health (2001f) in their *A Research and Development Strategy for Public Health* recognize the central importance of partnership, participation of all stakeholders and the plurality of approach in public health. While the policy context appears to be supportive, practical difficulties abound. These include developing effective communication, establishing genuine teams and teamwork, escaping the dominance of public health medicine, practising evidence-based public health, and the provision of appropriate training and education.

Communication across professional groups and different sectors can be problematic. There is a range of different jargon with no unifying means of communication. There is a need for a communication which understands and respects contributors' unique positions and strengths and builds on these. To facilitate this process, interprofessional education and training in public health is essential, as well as multidisciplinary forums on public health where practitioners can learn together and develop a common means of communicating.

Genuine teamwork seeks to develop and utilize partners' specific skills and expertise, recognizing the value of practitioners at different levels, in different organizations and agencies, with different remits and priorities. This requires practitioners to be confident in their identity and expertise, and to feel supported by their own employing organization. One practical way of demonstrating confidence and commitment is for employers to support staff training in public health.

Teamwork is essential because public health skills and competencies cover such a broad area that it is unrealistic to expect any one person to be expert in all fields – indeed, it would be quite a challenge to have a team which encompassed all these skills within its membership. Arguably, the key public health skills are those of facilitation, leadership and partnership – skills that serve to combine expertise and resources for public health goals. Innovative ways of spreading expertise and resource are needed. One example of this is the development of public health networks spanning several primary care trusts which 'By pooling resource, particularly specialist skills . . . could help to provide the capacity needed for effective public health, which a single Primary Care Trust could not' (Shaw and Abbot 2002: 29).

Challenging the dominance of health professions

The traditional dominance of public health medicine and the visibility of health professions is problematic because it marginalizes those who should be key or lead players in public health. These include local authorities' staff such as environmental health officers, neighbourhood renewal workers and staff of voluntary organizations such as carers' organizations. However, the appointment of non-medical directors of public health within primary care trusts is a step in the right direction, demonstrating that public health has a broad disciplinary and professional base which goes beyond medicine. The decision of the Faculty of Public Health Medicine in 2001 to open up membership to non-medical candidates is another indication of positive change and progress.

Using the evidence base for public health

There is now an extensive database of research and evidence about sound public health interventions (NHS Centre for Reviews and Dissemination 2000a). This evidence base can effectively guide the work of a wide range of practitioners, not only those whose work directly impacts on health, such as doctors, nurses, health visitors and environmental health officers, but also those who make an indirect impact, such as housing officers, architects, environmental engineers, teachers, the police, probation, fire and prison officers (Department of Health 2001b). However, as

Nutbeam (2002) points out, the ability to mobilize this evidence to improve health is much less well developed than the ability to collect good quality evidence in the UK. While research and evaluation skills are important to determine whether evidence exists and how sound it is, what is needed now is action to protect and promote the public health.

Effective action depends on an understanding of the socio-economic and political context of policy, and an overt and transparent ethical and value base. It is important to recognize the catalytic work of the Health Development Agency here, both at a national policy level and at a regional and local level. Some of its key functions are:

- maintaining an up-to-date map of the evidence base for public health and health improvement;

- advising on setting of standards in the light of that evidence for public health and health promotion practice; and

- effective and authoritative dissemination to practitioners.

Alongside this work of actively exploring and developing the evidence base for public health theory and practice, there is a productive facilitation of collaborative working between different professional groups focused on a range of cross-cutting public health themes such as inequalities in health, social exclusion and public health evidence base. (See Chapter 14 for a detailed discussion about evidence-based public health.)

Integrating and financing training in public health

The provision of appropriate training and education requires not just the provision of relevant curricula and programmes, but also financing and resourcing so that relevant personnel are able to undertake opportunities for further training and education in public health.

On the point of training provision, public health does not currently fit into the existing curricula of most professions. There is an urgent need for training needs analysis to be undertaken for all professionals who contribute to public health. The potential for integration of at least certain aspects of their training can then be explored so that common ground can be secured in relevant areas of their work. This could involve environmental health officers, health promotion specialists, community nurses, community development workers and general practitioners. The provision of recently developed postgraduate programmes in public health that are underpinned by interprofessional educational approaches means that these students are more likely to establish important common ground.

With regard to financing and resourcing, there are gaps in all areas nationally, although there are also examples of good practice demonstrating the way forward. Funding streams for public health education and training are not clearly identified at present. However, there is evidence of regional funding structures for public health education and training being developed involving the lead for public health being taken by one workforce development confederation in a region. The role of managed public health networks could be to undertake a skills audit and subsequently work with workforce development confederations to coordinate and ensure appropriate access to training opportunities and to ensure these opportunities meet identified needs. This would need to be supported by a funded development programme, agreed with workforce development confederations and linked with academic institutions, to fill gaps in capability and capacity in public health (Faculty of Public Health Medicine 2002). The government's commitment to building capacity and capability in the field is welcomed; the funding of this construction does, however, need to be supported.

Primary care trusts are starting to respond to the need for continuing professional development in public health by linking with relevant education providers. Funding streams for local authority professionals such as environmental health officers are not clearly identified, and continuing professional development is supported on an individual basis with no coordination in the field.

It is necessary to look at the ability of providers to provide the range of education and training to facilitate necessary capacity and capability. It is also necessary to decide at what level to assess training needs – locality or primary care trust or regional – in order to 'skill up' the workforce. The process needs to operate at all levels in a synergistic way without duplication.

The way forward?

Dilemmas emerge in terms of appropriate ways forward for public health education and training. Consideration needs to be given to whether public health is managed by leads with vision, or whether practitioners should be skilled up to have the broad vision and competencies, or should it be a combination of both, which may be confusing. For instance, public health nurses could move forward with both the first and second model, but the question would need to be asked about what is meant by the first option in terms of tasks and necessary infrastructures.

Conclusion

If the full potential of public health is to be achieved, capacity and capability in public health needs to extend beyond its current narrow medical and health boundaries to embrace a wide range of different professionals and activities. This broadening out process depends on several different, mutually supportive factors, including a diverse workforce which recognizes and embraces its public health role, appropriate training and education opportunities, and a supportive political and policy context which encourages a broad perspective on public health.

The central task is to recognize existing competencies and expertise as public health skills, not to attempt to build up capacity and capability from nothing. Abundant public health skills and competencies exist already, ranging from community development workers and social workers to public health and community nurses to voluntary sector workers and beyond. What is needed is a vision and purpose which binds such diverse workers together in a common public health agenda.

To some extent this is being provided by the policy context, which recognizes varying levels of public health skills and competencies, a broad public health workforce and the need to go beyond public health medicine. However, this public recognition needs to be backed up by practical support for multidisciplinary training and education in order to deliver a broad public health identity and commitment, and mechanisms to encourage collaborative working for public health.

The concept of the professional project enables identification of key aspects of this process – effective communication to facilitate collaboration and team-work, evidence-based practice to inspire trust and confidence in the public health enterprise, and appropriate recognized training and education opportunities for public health staff at all levels and in different roles. It is possible to chart progress in all these areas, although much scope for development and progress still exists.

People and action skills are high on different professional agendas, and health promoters in particular are skilled at bringing people and agencies together to work collaboratively. This range of contributory skills and specialisms are vital to the furtherance of public health; this needs to be acknowledged instead of being ignored. Thus it is only by recognizing the vision and skills encompassed by this range of different contributory professions that public health can become an effective force for change and positive health.

Case study: asylum seekers

The needs of asylum seekers

The following case study, focused on asylum seekers, has been developed to illustrate the range of professional groups who can potentially contribute to the health and well being of this marginalized group of people with complex needs.

Although asylum seekers are not a homogeneous group, they are likely to share a range of public health needs associated with their experiences of migration. Being a marginalized group they may be exposed to a range of health problems associated with social deprivation and social exclusion.

However, they may also experience the following problems specific to their asylum seeker status. They may suffer a number of physical health problems associated with their exposure to atrocities in their country of origin and during their journey to the UK. This may include physical injury from the effects of war or trauma associated with torture and rape. In addition, asylum seekers experience high levels of stress and depression associated with the experience of uncertainty, separation from family members and cultural bereavement. For some, these mental health problems will be compounded by psychological trauma associated with witnessing the destruction of their homes, the ill treatment of family members or the psychological after effects of torture and rape.

Asylum seekers include families, single adults (predominantly young single males) and unaccompanied children; their health needs are likely to be affected by their age, gender and family composition. Some of the complex range of public health needs likely to be experienced by asylum seekers are identified below.

The need for security, shelter and safety

Asylum seekers are required to accept the accommodation offered to them or lose their benefits. Coker (2001) reports that asylum seekers are often housed in sub-standard accommodation in deprived areas. Leifler (1999) refers to two male asylum seekers who were 'living on the ninth floor of a building in which the running water only reached the eighth floor and the electricity meters did not work' and the Campaign against Racism and Facism (2000) cite the case of asylum seekers living in high-rise apartments with no central heating, broken lifts, infestations and stairs littered with rubbish.

An additional potential problem associated with housing is that of asylum seekers being housed in inappropriate areas, for example, Leifler (1999) cites a case where a local council had planned to house a group of Kosovars near to a group of Serbian refugees.

Asylum seekers experience hostility and abuse from some members of the public and racially motivated attacks have been reported in a number of areas within the UK (Wong and Butler 2000). Asylum seekers need information on areas and situations that may expose them to increased risk, in addition to advice on how to optimize their personal safety.

Mechanisms to enable asylum seekers to report the experience of crime are also required because of language barriers, lack of familiarity with UK procedures and 'concern that their involvement with police may affect their claim for asylum' (Wong and Butler 2000).

Current legislation restricts asylum seekers from accessing employment within the UK (Refugee Council 2002). Asylum seekers who were granted a work permit under previous legislation can work but difficulties arise through lack of recognition of professional qualifications (Lynch and Cuninghame 2000) or barriers to obtaining verification from an asylum seeker's home country (D'Cruze 2000). Employment restrictions mean that many asylum seekers are dependent upon the state for financial support. Although children are eligible for benefits at the full income support rate, adults receive only 70 percent of income support benefit.

The need for community and social support

The practice of dispersal means that asylum seekers may not have access to the support of friends and family members resident in the UK or community groups who share a similar culture.

The need for access to a range of services

Asylum seekers need access to a range of primary and secondary health care services because of their complex physical and mental health needs. They need an empathetic response with services provided by staff who have received adequate training to enable them to understand the perspective of the asylum seeker and the traumatic experiences that they may have encountered.

Although asylum seekers are entitled to the full range of NHS services in the same way as any other UK resident, in reality they experience a number of barriers to access. Within the UK general practitioners are gatekeepers to most NHS services and therefore entitlement is dependent upon registration with a GP practice. General practitioners are free to decide which patients they will accept onto their lists and, according to Fassil (2000) and Coker (2001), many asylum seekers experience difficulty in registering with a general practitioner.

Possible reasons for this are identified as language difficulties resulting in lengthy consultations (Jones and Gill 1998); a reputation for high mobility (Jones and Gill 1998); and the potential for asylum seekers to affect practice payments if they refuse vaccinations or cervical cytology screening (Department of Health 2000b).

Many asylum seekers have no option but to accept temporary registration which limits their access to routine preventive health services and means that the general practitioner has no access to past records.

When they do negotiate access to a general practitioner, although they are entitled to access NHS services, they are not automatically entitled to free NHS prescriptions, dental or eye care. In order to receive these services they need to complete an HC1 form which is only available in English.

An additional barrier relates to lack of information on the part of asylum seekers and professionals regarding entitlement to NHS and other services. Many asylum seekers are not familiar with the UK model of health service provision. Martell and Murray (2001) and Hampshire (2001) highlight the problem that asylum seekers may have no concept of a general practitioner or practice nurse because for many primary care does not exist in their country of origin.

Language barriers mean that asylum seekers need access to quality interpreting services. This may be provided through 'hands free' technology or through face to face interpreters. Family or community members are sometimes used as interpreters but this may be inappropriate and can create problems in respect of confidentiality.

All children, whether unaccompanied or part of an asylum seeking family, have the right to access education but evidence suggests that not all children receive an immediate school place (Lynch and Cuninghame 2000). In addition, schools may not have adequate resources to meet the language needs of children for whom English is a second language (Lynch and Cuninghame 2000).

An additional difficulty that may be experienced by asylum seeking children is that of integration within UK schools. Difficulty can arise as a result of language barriers, racial hostility, bullying (Hampshire 2001) and unresolved stress associated with the experience of trauma, loss and grief (Wong and Butler 2000).

Strategies to meet the needs of asylum seekers

The needs of asylum seekers are diverse and broad ranging, and a comprehensive range of strategies is required to address these needs. The role of public health specialists, practitioners and the wider public health workforce in meeting asylum seekers' needs is set out in Figure 5.1.

Next, the applicability of the national standards for specialist public health in helping to develop an integrated strategy is considered. The ten key areas identified in the National Standards for specialist public health practice (discussed earlier in this chapter) are all applicable to meeting the needs of asylum seekers. An example is presented for each of the ten standards to illustrate their relevance in practice.

It is also possible to map the ten standards across the three levels of involvement

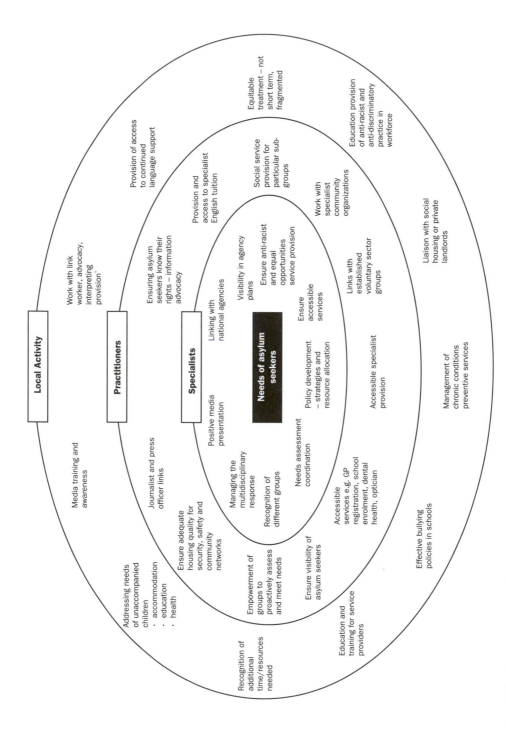

Figure 5.1 The role of public health specialists, practitioners and the wider public health workforce in meeting the needs of asylum seekers

in public health; this may be a helpful exercise in assessing public health educational and training needs.

Surveillance and assessment of the population's health and well being
In addition to visible and easily recognized health needs such as respiratory or gastro-intestinal illnesses, asylum seekers may have hidden health problems. For example, they may have experienced torture leading to enduring mental health problems and/or ongoing depression due to loss of family, home, work and community. Health needs assessment in these cases would need to be sensitive and may well require specialist input, a longer time scale and additional resources.

Promoting and protecting the public health and well being
Asylum seekers, especially children, may not be up-to-date with UK immunization programmes. The fact that they are often registered as temporary residents with general practices may result in fragmented service provision, and lack of continuity in record keeping may mean future immunizations and preventative programmes are missed.

Developing quality and risk management within an evaluative culture
Research documenting health needs of asylum seekers exists in a variety of formats including academic journals and anecdotal accounts. National agencies such as the Health Development Agency and the Audit Commission, and voluntary organiza-tions such as The Refugee Council or Asylum Aid, provide literature reviews and policy recommendations based on these accounts.

Collaborative working
Statutory services are often inaccessible to asylum seekers, and one of the main bar-riers is language. Working collaboratively with link worker, advocacy and interpreting providers is an essential component in ensuring that asylum seekers have access to the full range of health, education, housing and social services to which they are entitled. High quality face to face interpreting and advocacy services should be prioritized.

Developing services and programmes and reducing inequalities
Asylum seekers are likely to be a small group within the local population, but one with a high level of health needs. In developing public health programmes and services for this marginalized group, care needs to be taken to ensure the process is transparent and equitable. National guidelines and resources may provide useful additional support for developing specific services.

Policy and strategy development and implementation
To date, asylum seekers are entitled to reduced levels of income support which will inevitably result in high levels of poverty. The links between poverty and ill health are well established. One proven avenue to improving health is to reduce poverty, which can be tackled at local and national levels. In addition to lobbying for adequate income levels, supportive strategies such as benefits advisors and interpreters are needed to ensure asylum seekers receive all the benefits they are entitled to.

Working with and for communities

Asylum seekers bring a wealth of skills and expertise to their newly established communities. Facilitating and empowering these communities to work in partnership with statutory agencies to address community needs brings benefits to everyone. User involvement in agencies helps to ensure appropriate service provision and maximum uptake.

Strategic leadership

Strategic leadership includes working towards positive media representation of asylum seekers and their contribution to the community. Asylum seekers should not be represented as a specific isolated group who make demands on services but rather as a marginalized group who share features with other excluded groups. By meeting their needs, services are improved for everyone. Proactive press releases and fostering a good working relationship with the local media are important strategies.

Research and development

Asylum seekers are subject to many social factors which will impact negatively on their health, for example, poor housing, discrimination, low income and poor access to services. Research can help to identify which strategies are most effective in tackling these factors and promoting health. Research needs to be sensitive, ethical and take into account the possible risk of over-researching this vulnerable group.

Ethically managing self, people and resources (including education and continuing professional development)

Good communication is central to effective management. This is particularly important within a multidisciplinary team where different agencies and professions use different terminologies within their areas of expertise. It is therefore vital to ensure that all forms of written and verbal communication have minimum jargon and are understood by all. Good communication with user representatives is also essential. This is especially relevant for asylum seekers who may not speak English, for whom interpreting and translation services need to be provided and costed.

6

STEPHEN PECKHAM AND PAT TAYLOR
Public health and primary care

Editors' Introduction

Primary care workers have a key role in 21st century public health; primary care is now central to the government's agenda for health and health improvement. The government's policy is to move from an emphasis on secondary care towards placing primary care at the centre of health care development, commissioning and public health.

The chapter examines the current role and understanding of primary care. The authors identify the common definition of primary care as care delivered through medical practice. More accurately, this is primary *medical* care, which is at odds with the definition of primary care promoted by the World Health Organisation, which includes addressing wider community health needs, with primary medical care as one component. This wider concept of primary health care underpins the contribution of primary care to multidisciplinary public health.

The authors examine policy changes which have affected primary care, culminating in setting up primary care trusts with responsibility for leading public health development. They contrast the position for primary care in England with developments in the rest of the UK where primary care is not expected to lead public health development.

The authors acknowledge that recently public health practice has been separated from its historical roots within local communities. However, initiatives such as Health for All and the Healthy Cities movement developed alternative local public health approaches in parallel to mainstream NHS developments. Current policy seeks to reconnect these initiatives with mainstream primary (medical) care.

The chapter presents research that has identified key factors which promote and hinder the development of public health in primary care. Equity, collaboration and participation are identified as key drivers in the process.

The chapter goes on to identify tensions and obstacles which may affect the ability of primary care to embrace the new agenda of promoting public health. They include the emphasis on performance management and achieving capacity targets; the need for financial balance; and the integration of the health and social care agenda. The authors conclude by raising some questions about the capacity of primary care to succeed in leading public health in the face of so many competing priorities.

Introduction

Primary care is now recognized as playing a central role in the UK National Health Service and has become a major focus of health policy (Peckham and Exworthy 2002). The changes introduced by the Labour government from 1997 have significantly shifted health care policy from an emphasis on secondary care – which has dominated health policy since before the Second World War – to placing primary care at the centre of health care development, commissioning and public health. These changes to the health care system in the UK came at the end of a sustained period of health care reform in the 1990s in the UK and also many other developed countries. (Health policy changes from the 1990s onwards are discussed fully in Chapters 1 and 2.)

This chapter examines the public health role of primary care and explores the issues arising from recent developments in policy in the UK.

Re-evaluating primary care

Primary care has long been acknowledged to be one of the major strengths of British health and social care arrangements with its focus on universality of access, emphasis on continuity of family and individual care, and its role as a gateway to other services (Starfield 1998). However, the theory and practice of primary care has been undergoing re-evaluation and change (WHO/UNICEF 1978; Macdonald 1992; Starfield 1998), a situation reflected in the re-examination of primary care in the UK (Fry and Hodder 1994; Meads *et al.* 1999; Peckham and Exworthy 2003).

This re-evaluation from within primary care services has been accompanied by impetus for change coming from national policy (DHSS 1986; DHSS 1987; Department of Health 1997a, 2001a, 2002b; Secretary of State for Health 2000). Initially, the main thrust for change was on quality and then, with the introduction of the internal market and fund holding, on the purchasing role of primary care which was intended to lead to greater efficiency and responsiveness (Le Grand *et al.* 1998). At the same time, there has been a re-assessment of the role of general practice and, latterly, more radical solutions have been sought, with a range of new developments from the mid-1990s onwards. These have included:

- primary care act pilots which explore new organizational arrangements for general practice;
- total purchasing – where groups of practice held the whole purchasing budget for their population;

- GP commissioning which brought together GPs and health authorities on commissioning.

The latter two were the forerunners of the primary care groups (PCGs), primary care trusts (PCTs) and care trusts in England and Northern Ireland, primary care trusts in Scotland, and local health groups in Wales. (These organizations are sometimes collectively referred to as primary care organizations.)

Current government policy emphasizes the promotion and integration of primary and community care. The intention is to ensure a more efficient response to the needs of vulnerable groups, by managing the care of these groups as much as possible in the community and by developing interagency work. However, in England the policy emphasis for primary care organizations on developing services and commissioning health care is secondary to promoting the health of the local community, creating a new key emphasis on public health (Department of Health 1997a; NHS Executive 1998a; Secretary of State for Health 1999). This contrasts with the situation in Scotland and Wales, for example, where the Scottish Parliament and Welsh Regional Assembly retain a significant interest and role in public health.

Defining primary care

One key obstacle to this re-evaluation of primary care remains the 'taken for granted' meaning of the term itself. Primary care in the UK context is generally used as a form of shorthand for primary medical care (Macdonald 1992; Pratt 1995). Summerton (1999) has described primary care as a portmanteau concept 'a favourite of politicians and can be viewed variously as a set of activities, a process, a level of care or even a strategy for organizing the health care system as a whole' (Summerton 1999: 63).

Use of the term primary care in the UK often appears synonymous with the assumption that primary care operates mainly through medical practice. This approach epitomizes the 'medical model' of primary care which concentrates on illness and medically defined solutions to health needs. This is at odds with broader definitions of primary care which may be more accurately labelled primary health care 'a reorientation of all health services towards the health needs of communities, both local and national' (Macdonald 1992: 14). Such debates have mainly been relevant to non-industrialized countries as it was assumed that medical care would provide answers to all health problems in industrialized countries and, eventually, in the 'third world' (Walsh and Warren 1979). It is now apparent in the 'developed' world that health care is being revaluated because medical advances escalate health care costs and evidence is emerging to question how far medical interventions are able to substantially influence the health status of populations. There is a rediscovery of the importance of public health perspectives in tackling inequalities and promoting healthier lifestyles.

Re-evaluating public health: developing a primary care perspective

From local authorities to the NHS and partnerships

Organizationally, the history of public health is complex (Lewis 1991; Baggott 2000) with responsibility being split between the NHS and local authorities. Until 1974, public health services (community medicine, health visiting and so on) were located within local authorities. In 1974 medical public health and nursing was transferred to the NHS health authorities and community health services, while environmental health services remained in local authorities alongside housing, social services, leisure, education and other local authority services.

As discussed in earlier chapters (see especially Chapters 1 and 2) public health is now undergoing another transition with a greater role for primary care and an emphasis on partnerships between local authorities and health care services through health action zones, local strategic partnerships, healthy living centres, urban and neighbourhood renewal and, in England, the development of a public health function within PCTs. (See Chapters 11, 12 and 13 for more about these partnership initiatives and urban renewal.)

Yet this transition of public health to primary care has occurred over a long period. For example, throughout the 1980s and 1990s moves were made to link community nurses into general practice to form the primary health care teams. However, for many community nurses, particularly health visitors, this closer relationship with general practice has actually meant a diminution of their public health role as they were drawn into the agenda of primary medical care. Although individual health visitors have worked hard to preserve their public health roles, the overall impact of this move has been for them to prioritize individual health promotion work with families and to be drawn into child protection work. They have also been increasingly drawn into the medical agenda and targets for general practice such as immunization, and to have less time to concentrate on the population aspect of health issues or to work with local authority colleagues (Craig and Lindsay 2000). This is making many health visitors feel frustrated at being forced to follow a general practice agenda thus wasting much of their training.

The emergence of community health movements

It is relevant to chart another aspect of public health development which has run alongside the 'official' history of primary care, but in the 21st century public health is arguably as important in current developments. The Health for All and Healthy City initiatives emerged in the 1980s as a result of the Alma Ata declaration (WHO/UNICEF 1978) and embraced the key dimensions of equity, collaboration and participation. Five UK cities became involved in the European Healthy City initiative and many other areas embraced a Health for All approach as an umbrella for joint working between local authorities, health authorities and voluntary and community organizations (Ottewill and Wall 1990; Smithies and Webster 1998).

This movement also stimulated many community health development projects with a focus on addressing underlying social, environmental and physical causes of ill health contributing to health inequalities. It also involved many non-medical staff in developing public health perspectives. While there were local examples of close collaboration between community health projects within the Health for All movement and mainstream health services, the experience overall was one of parallel existence. When the NHS was being driven towards more market-based approaches to health care provision focused on competition rather than collaboration (Klein 1998) this was particularly the case. The community health movement produced important information and research but this was not officially recognized by government or the NHS (Ashton and Seymour 1988; Townsend *et al.* 1992).

Public health and primary care: making new connections

Until the early 1990s, public health developments in primary care were peripheral, focusing on the role of community nurses and developing health promotion in general practice. The growth of primary care commissioning required more emphasis on health needs assessment (Harris 1995) and this stimulated the debates about the need to rediscover the relationship between the two. Historically, individual GPs have played an important role in raising public health concerns of their local area and, with their close and continuous knowledge of local populations, have always been well placed to raise wider issues of concern to the health of their local communities. Many individual GPs have attempted to retain this part of their role (Tudor-Hart 1988; Widgery 1991) and have played significant roles in health campaigns in their local communities. However, the profession as a whole has failed to embrace this role in any significant way, seeing their focus as one of developing medical specialties within general practice rather than health promotion and 'lifestyle advice' (Fitzpatrick 2001).

The first real policy attempt to develop public health as a key priority for the NHS as a whole began in 1992 with the first national strategy for health in England, *The Health of the Nation* (Secretary of State for Health 1992). This was welcomed as the first time in its history that the NHS had had an explicit policy for health promotion, albeit one which largely emphasized the individual's responsibility for leading healthier lifestyles (Ranade 1998). Health authorities were to promote and facilitate individuals' responsibility for their own health and within this, GP practices were given extra funding to offer advice and information to patients to develop healthier lifestyles. The success of this approach was very variable across the country and was dependent on the commitment and enthusiasm of individual practitioners to make it more than an add-on to mainstream medical advice (Hunter 1998).

The Health of the Nation also brought in the key ideas of working in partnership with other organizations to improve health in settings such as schools and workplaces. This partnership working approach was mainly led by health promotion specialists working within health authorities but many initiatives drew in individual primary care professionals.

A model of public health in primary care

Research was commissioned by the Public Health Alliance (now the UK Public Health Association) between 1996–98 to develop a model of public health in primary care (Taylor *et al.* 1998). It came as a response to concerns from primary care practitioners in the Public Health Alliance who highlighted practical difficulties in undertaking public health work within primary care settings. The research began by developing a conceptual model of a public health approach in primary care based on the WHO definition of primary care: 'primary health care is essential health care based on practical, scientifically sound and socially acceptable methods and technology made universally accessible to individuals and families in the community through their full participation' (WHO/UNICEF 1978).

Using this underpinning definition it identified three sets of interests: primary care, public health professionals and the communities served by them (see Figure 6.1). It represented them as three circles which needed to overlap to create a public health model of primary care. The model also identified three motivational drivers for each group most likely to bring them together. Primary care professionals needed to accept that they could not deliver a holistic level of care alone and needed to collaborate with others.

Equity was the key factor for public health professionals requiring them to refocus their practice at a community level. The community needed to actively contribute to health and to participate in the services and resources to promote health and well being. The research tested the model with representatives of these three groups in four different case study sites just prior to the reforms implemented by the Labour government after 1997. It found that the model was useful for identifying evidence of public health activity in primary care as well as providing a framework to develop an understanding of how it might be developed in the future. Crucially, the research identified key themes which adversely affected the development of public health activity in primary care; these are set out in Box 6.1.

The research also identified a series of facilitating factors which appeared to assist the development of a public health approach in primary care; see Box 6.2.

Crucially the report concluded with the recommendation that any strategy to develop effective public health action within primary care needed to be developed

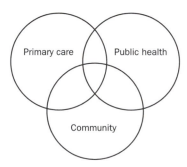

Figure 6.1 A public health model of primary care

Box 6.1   Factors which inhibit the promotion of public health in primary care

- There were no easily agreed definitions of primary care, public health or community participation and without this agreement initiatives tended to remain at a project level outside the mainstream of core activity.

- The dominance of the medical model in both primary care and public health inhibited the development or acceptance of community perspectives on health. In primary care the predominant focus on individuals made it difficult to take a population-based approach to health or to respond to community-based health initiatives which did not offer services to individuals. Public health specialists in health authorities were predominately focused on providing evidence in relation to commissioning and resource issues and had little time to work within the community.

- There was a recognition by all the participants that inequity contributed to ill health, but much less confidence at any level that it could be tackled by public health or within primary care.

- Existing organizational structures reflect the predominant medical model and the contract culture, both of which have militated against successful collaboration.

- Participation by local people in health related activities was perceived as helpful but difficult to achieve and maintain.

Source: Taylor *et al*. (1998)

Box 6.2   Factors promoting the development of public health in primary care

- The commitment and enthusiasm of individuals prepared to innovate and work on the 'edges of their brief'. Primary care professionals who lived in the community or who were themselves active in the community in non-health roles helped to establish bridges with the wider community.

- The mediating role of community-based projects able to play a bridging role between primary care professionals and other agencies and community groups. A neutral geographical base was also useful for joint working. Jointly funded posts and collaborative mechanisms also helped.

- Access to and control over resources and funding was essential for innovative initiatives to be established.

- A history of collaboration was important to establish effective community participation – it was unlikely to be achieved through short-term funded projects.

Source: Taylor *et al*. (1998)

---

within the three drivers of equity, collaboration and participation; and at the three levels of macro (national) level, meso (regional, county) level and micro (community and neighbourhood) level.

Current developments in primary care and public health

The change in government in 1997 brought a significant shift in policy away from seeing health as largely an individual responsibility to accepting a social responsibility for health inequalities. The use of public, private and voluntary sector providers in health and welfare was to be retained but the emphasis on competition within health and welfare provision was to be replaced by a commitment to collaboration and working in partnerships. (This is discussed in more detail in Chapter 1.) Public health and primary care became key components in the new government's reforms of the NHS. The new NHS (Department of Health 1997a) introduced changes to both sectors which gave a rationale to their interdependence.

The advent of primary care groups and primary care trusts

The experimental changes in primary care discussed at the beginning of this chapter were used as the basis for full reform of primary care. All general practices and community nurses in England were required to become part of new geographically based primary care groups (PCGs) acting as sub-committees of the health authority to give guidance on commissioning, health improvement and to plan developments in primary care.

PCGs had their own boards made up of a majority of GPs with two community nursing representatives, a lay member, social services representative and a non-executive director of the health authority. This represented a radical change for primary care, creating, for the first time, a formal mechanism for general practices to both work together and work with their nursing colleagues, other agencies and with their local communities; it also charged them with wider responsibilities in primary care. It brought the requirements to work in partnership and to be involved in the realities of planning and commissioning down to the grassroots level, drawing in practitioners responsible for 'hands on' services.

One director of public health commented: 'primary care groups are a fundamental "mindset" change for individuals as well as organization. The biggest obstacles are attitudinal not structural' (Director of Public Health quoted in Meads *et al.* 1999: 47)

The government's policy for primary care established PCGs and PCTs (in England) as the vehicles for commissioning, primary care development and health improvement (including tackling health inequalities) (Department of Health 1997a; Secretary of State for Health 2000). They have three main functions (NHS Executive 1998a):

- to improve the health of, and address health inequalities, in their community;
- to develop primary care and community health services across their area (including improved integration of services); and
- to advise (PCGs) or take on (PCTs) the commissioning of hospital services for patients within their area to appropriately meet patient needs.

Primary care trusts

The framework for primary care reform laid out in *The New NHS* in 1997 identified four increasing levels of responsibility for these new primary care organizations such that they would eventually become primary care trusts, independent of the health authority and with separate executive committees and boards with a lay majority. Ultimately the government envisaged the establishment of integrated health and social care services in care trusts; the first care trust started during 2002. Initially the move towards primary care trust status had been seen as a progression under the control of individual PCGs and health authorities, but *The NHS Plan* in 2000 accelerated the process and required all primary care groups to become PCTs by 2003.

In *Shifting the Balance of Power: Next Steps* (Department of Health 2002b) the government abolished existing English health authorities and transferred most of their functions to PCTs who were then responsible for spending 75 percent of the overall NHS budget in England. Strategic and performance management responsibilities including clinical quality, targets and incentives and penalties were taken on by 28 new strategic health authorities. In 2002 the government also indicated that social services departments will be disbanded; all adult care will be delivered by care trusts, and children's services (currently in social services, education and health) will be organized by new children's trusts (Alan Millburn's speech to Social Services Conference, October 2002). This programme of change represents a massive challenge for primary care at all levels.

Research undertaken in England (Starkey *et al.* 2001; Wilkin *et al.* 2001) indicated that the development of PCGs was variable and there was much criticism about the continuing dominance of GPs in the new structures. However, there were indications that changes in the mindsets of the individuals were beginning to take place particularly because of the mixture of stakeholders on the PCG boards. More recent research (Wilkin *et al.* 2002) suggests that the change to PCTs has led to greater management control and less practitioner involvement in the management of primary care. In addition, studies have also found that the move to PCT status has shifted the focus of attention in primary care from looking 'inwards and downwards' to their local communities, responding to local needs and demands, to looking 'outwards and upwards', being more focused on national targets, priorities and central government directives (Abbott *et al.* 2001; Heller 2002).

The public health function in health improvement

Public health has also experienced large scale change. In *The New NHS* (Department of Health 1997a) and *Saving Lives: Our Healthier Nation* (Secretary of State for Health 1999) the government laid out its plans for health improvement. Each health authority was required to produce a health improvement plan (HIMP) for its population, leading a partnership with other local agencies. Community interests, general practices and primary health care teams were encouraged to engage in this process.

The *Independent Inquiry into Inequalities in Health* chaired by Sir Donald Acheson was established and reported in 1998 (Acheson 1998). Among its 36 recommendations it identified inequities in access to primary care and differential consultation rates between population groups and geographical areas. Importantly the link was made between deprivation and lower levels of access to preventative services and health promotion. It also consolidated much of the recent thinking on developing public health as a multisectoral and multidisciplinary programme (Acheson 1998). (See Chapter 10 for more about tackling inequalities in health.)

The PCT role in public health

More recent policy proposed in *Shifting the Balance of Power* (Department of Health 2001a, 2002b) places PCTs at the heart of the government's plans for modernizing and developing the NHS. This includes the transfer of the public health function and the majority of the NHS budget to PCTs. PCTs will thus become the main vehicles for policy implementation including the NHS's contribution to public health.

The evidence suggests that most PCGs/PCTs have strengthened strategic planning capacity in support of health improvement, a process required specifically in the metamorphosis from PCG to PCT. PCGs/PCTs have identified local priorities and some can point to evidence of implementation in addressing health inequalities. For example, the most recent National Tracker Survey of PCGs/PCTs for 2001/02 (Wilkin *et al.* 2002) found a substantial increase in local health needs assessment activity and 82 percent of PCGs/PCTs have their own health improvement plan (compared to 73 percent in 2000/01). Nearly all (92 percent) of PCGs/PCTs have designated a health improvement lead and there is a clear trend towards appointing public health specialists (from 14 percent in 2000/01 to 43 percent in 2001/02) but also, interestingly, an increase in nurse leads (from 9 percent to 20 percent) suggesting that some PCGs/PCTs do not universally see public health doctors as being the natural leads (Gillam and Smith 2002). In addition, 67 percent of PCGs/PCTs had set health improvement targets and just over half had targets for reducing smoking, 43 percent for reducing teenage conception rates, and 33 percent to reducing differences in life expectancy (Gillam and Smith 2002). The extent of health inequality targets contrasted with the previous years when it was found that the uptake on addressing broader health inequalities was still low and that the strategies in use needed to be expanded.

The importance of the role of PCTs in England was further emphasized by the abolition of English health authorities and the National Health Service executive regions in 2002 (Department of Health 2002b). Larger strategic health authorities are taking a more strategic role through the development of regional public health networks that draw together the NHS and local authorities. Such developments see an expansion of multiprofessional public health practice with new public health specialists including those with nursing and community backgrounds (Department of Health 2001b). It is at the regional level of interorganizational collaboration that the shape of public health will be formed in the future.

The role of the PCT director of public health

Each PCT in England is required to appoint a director of public health and to develop clear inequalities strategies which focus on local neighbourhoods and communities. The director of public health should have a public health support team, who are the health representatives on local authorities' local strategic partnerships and other joint working arrangements.

At the time of writing (2003) PCTs are only just developing their public health staff groups. The director of public health role is now open for the first time to suitably trained individuals from any background. Directors do not need to be medically qualified but in fact the majority are public health doctors who have moved from the old health authority public health departments. In September 2002, of the 300 PCTs in existence 260 had made director appointments of which 211 (83.7 percent) were medics and 42 (16.3 percent) were non-medics (personal communication from M. Tagney, Department of Health).

Middleton (2002) debates the issues involved in the contribution of medicine to 21st century public health. He believes that part of the skill of directors of public health is to harness the wide range of expertise needed within their public health team, highlighting that it is unlikely that most medical directors of public health would possess all the necessary skills. Measuring health problems, recommending the appropriate interventions to deal with those problems and monitoring the effectiveness of interventions are considered to be central to their work (Middleton 2002: 84).

While the appointment of directors of public health and support teams with an explicit focus on the broad health improvement agenda is to be warmly welcomed, there are some real challenges around delivery. Directors of public health need adequately resourced public health teams and much work remains to build and develop these teams; currently (2003) single handed directors of public health are the reality in some areas. The creation of the new PCTs in large numbers has highlighted the shortage of fully trained specialists in public health. Although this is being addressed by the extension of training schemes to those from non-medical backgrounds, much remains to be done.

The separation of the health protection function into the Health Protection Agency also poses significant challenges to PCTs in delivering and coordinating the health protection function, and there are risks of fragmentation in this area. (The role of the Health Protection Agency is discussed more fully in Chapter 7.)

Partnership working

The New NHS introduced the 'duty of partnership' between local authorities and NHS organizations and the National Health Service Act 1998 introduced new budget flexibilities to allow more joint working between health and local authority services. This was a significant change as financial constraints had long been used as a reason for a lack of cooperation and joint working. The contribution of non-NHS organizations to the new agenda for public health in primary care has also been taken forward in the requirement for local authorities to take responsibility for health and well being and to develop local strategic partnerships across their areas of responsibility. Health improvement programmes, now the responsibility of PCTs, must link into the newer local strategic partnerships and areas of overlap must be identified and accommodated through joint working and collaboration.

The Labour government's commitment to tackling inequalities and its policy initiatives to address those in communities experiencing poor health has led to multiple initiatives led by a range of government departments. New Deal, Sure Start, Neighbourhood Renewal, health action zones and healthy living centres all build on and recognize this early work on community health development and *Health for All*.

Primary care trusts are required to work with these wider health initiatives. They are required to work closely with these initiatives and to make connections with their mainstream work

Public health in PCTs: tensions in practice

While there is some sense in charging PCTs with health improvement responsibilities, doubts have been expressed about their capacity to fulfil these tasks and also the relative priority accorded to the tasks compared with their other roles of commissioning and primary care development. Gillam *et al.* (2001) argue that the development of the new primary care organizations provides an opportunity to develop partnerships and take a population approach which was not possible from an individual practice approach. This will require dealing with substantial complexity and involve developing new skills. In a survey of key local public health stakeholders Woodhead *et al.* (2002) found that respondents felt that devolution of the public health function to PCTs would avail expertise to the community. Also, while there was more potential for effective utilization of public health expertise at local level, the inadequate availability of staff was a potential drawback. (See Chapter 5 for a detailed look at capacity and capability in public health.)

These points were echoed by public health professionals participating in a joint NHS Leadership Centre and Faculty of Public Health Medicine meeting exploring leadership issues. Moving public health to PCTs was seen as beneficial as it was felt that this would enhance local sensitivity, improve working with local government, harness front line workers, focus more on the wider determinants of health and bring new skills and a non-medical perspective. However, concern was also expressed about isolation, replication of functions across many agencies, a large and varied agenda, PCTs being too small a unit and a loss of corporate memory through disrupting public health departments built up in health authorities (Scott 2002).

One key weakness of national policy is the apparent lack of coordination between NHS organizational policy and public health. PCTs have an equally significant, and some would argue more pressing, role in developing the integration of primary and social care services at a local level. The performance management framework emphasizes these requirements in much more specific and tangible targets. This agenda is challenging in requiring two organizations, PCTs and local authority social services, to work together, but in many respects it fits more easily within the current medical paradigm. This balance may change in the future with the government's stated intention to include performance management targets for tackling inequalities (Milburn 2002).

These issues were identified by the Health Committee's inquiry into public health (2001) and were acknowledged to some extent with the publication of *The NHS Plan* (Secretary of State for Health 2000) which noted that 'the wider inability to forge effective partnerships with local government, business and community organizations has inhibited the NHS's ability to prevent ill-health and tackle health inequalities' (p. 29). Thus we have seen a renewed emphasis on the development of partnerships, although the effectiveness of these (and other) strategies to tackle health inequality are not yet known since many of the mechanisms proposed in these documents have only been established since the turn of the century. Empirical evidence (at the local level) suggests that there is widespread support for such policies but their implementation is being hampered by competing priorities from central government and local partnership difficulties (Exworthy and Powell 2000).

Developments in Northern Ireland, Scotland and Wales

The policy for primary care development has been taken forward in Northern Ireland, Scotland and Wales in slightly different ways, driven respectively by the existing patterns of health and social services boards in Northern Ireland, and the Scottish Parliament and Welsh Assembly who have both retained significant responsibility for the strategic direction of health development and resource allocation.

In Scotland health boards have been retained with strategic responsibility and community trusts still employ community health staff. GPs are required to work together in local health care cooperatives. These cooperatives have responsibility for working with other local providers to tackle health improvement and reduce health inequalities. The cooperatives are local partnerships between health care and local authority services and form constituent parts of Scottish PCTs (Scottish Executive Health Department 2001).

Local health groups in Wales bring together community and primary care professionals with representatives from the local voluntary sector and their boards have a broader membership than in either England or Scotland. Also in Wales local government and the health service have been reorganized to create coterminous boundaries and local health boards will gradually replace health groups taking on wider responsibilities for public health in partnership with local authorities (Welsh Assembly Government 2002). The emphasis on partnership reflects developments in Scotland and England but extends beyond a focus on health and social care partnerships which are dominant in England and, to a lesser extent, in Scotland.

Details of the approach to be adopted in Northern Ireland are only just emerging with the establishment of local health and social care groups. These groups will have an increased responsibility for promoting the health of their local populations. The emphasis in the consultation document is on the unique position of primary care professionals to develop local partnership working to address wider health issues (Northern Ireland Executive 2002).

The level of change outside England appears to be slower and more incremental with a greater level of responsibility for strategic change kept at the national level – particularly in Wales where the Assembly sees itself playing a key role in public health issues. While divergence between the different countries within the UK is currently predominantly structural in nature, devolution and its effect on health policy is becoming increasingly important and is likely to lead to distinct differences in both the object and substance of public health policy, particularly as it relates to primary care (Exworthy and Powell 2000). Yet we can also see some distinct similarities in relation to public health with all the home countries identifying an increasing public health role for primary care. Only England has gone as far as establishing public health directors within PCTs but all models share a renewed emphasis on the public health role of primary care. There is little development of these ideas and emphases vary, with Scotland, for example, placing public health nursing at the forefront of primary care, Wales and Northern Ireland emphasizing local partnerships and England developing a public health function within the PCTs.

Current realities influencing the development of public health in primary care

Even if the connections between public health and primary care are clearly set out in policy and accepted as positive by many practitioners in primary care, it is clear from the above discussions that the relationship between primary care and public health will have a number of problems in the implementation stages. Primary care organizations are establishing themselves as new organizations and will inevitably be struggling with the realities of organizational and cultural change. Primary care trusts are required to achieve financial balance and are struggling with the complexities of commissioning and acute sector overspending. Initiatives around public health action and inequalities are likely to require radical changes in practice for primary care professionals. This will require training to be in place and resources to fund new ways of working, which may not be easy in a tight financial climate already crowded by other pressing agendas.

It will be some time before the reality (or, more accurately, the various realities) of public health practice in primary care will emerge. While there appears to be a strong policy focus towards establishing public health practice within primary care and some significant organizational moves to enable this to happen, there would seem to be other initiatives and drivers operating against these developments.

7

MELANIE GREY AND JOYSHRI SARANGI
Protecting the public's health

Editors' introduction

Threats to public health are not new; for as long as human kind has existed there has been a constant interface with the dangers of the surrounding environment. Since the 1800s, protection from threats to health in people's environment – such as air pollution, lack of adequate sanitation, poor housing, disease transmitted by people or animals – have been an essential and fundamental part of public health action.

But what is new about health protection in the 21st century? Who plays a part? What partnerships and agencies are involved? These questions are addressed in this chapter. It will be of interest to any public health worker who wants a contemporary overview of public health action to protect the population's health.

This chapter is concerned with threats to health from the physical and biological environment, which are moderated by global, national and local, socio-economic and political circumstances. It takes a wide view of protecting the public health, beyond that of protection for basic human needs, to providing human environments which make a positive contribution to health.

The authors start with an overview of current threats to health and emerging health protection policy. Global, technological, population and societal changes are resulting in new threats, such as climate change and terrorism, as well as the re-emergence of existing threats, such as infectious diseases common in the 19th century. They discuss underpinning guiding principles to inform judgements and decision taking, including the precautionary principle, principles around uncertainty of hazard and risk assessment, and engagement of society in understanding risk decisions.

Driving forward organizational and structural change in health protection is the need for informed, transparent, integrated and effective systems for prevention and rapid emergency health response. The chapter maps the wide range of resources for protecting health in different sectors and organizations, and analyses key issues for multidisciplinary working practice. The authors conclude that protecting the public's health in the 21st century requires collaborative partnerships at local and regional level, supported and informed by an integrated national and regional expertise, and an explicit, well driven policy framework.

Health threats and emerging health protection policy

The scope of health protection

Health protection has its origins and organizational arrangements based on the prevention and control of communicable disease, non-infectious environmental hazards and health related emergency planning (Regan 1999). Acute responses as well as proactive interventions are required to deal with the diverse nature of risks to a particular population. The Department of Health and the Welsh Office consultation document on health protection (Department of Health/Welsh Office 2002) distinguishes hazards to health as *involuntary* hazards. Although very different in nature they have the following characteristics in common (Department of Health/Welsh Office 2002):

- they can affect large groups of the population in a relatively short space of time, for example, epidemics;
- when a problem arises it may not be clear initially which hazard has caused it – infectious agent, chemical or radiological hazard;
- speedy and coordinated action to trace the source and deal with it is of the essence to ensure infection and contamination do not spread;
- management of these hazards requires collaboration between the NHS and other agencies such as emergency services and local authorities.

The emergence and re-emergence of significant public health threats, assessment of risk, development of policies and organizational systems and aspects related to practice for the preventative and emergency health response provide the focus for protecting the public's health.

Contemporary health threats

The scale and nature of health threats from infectious diseases or environmental hazards are very wide ranging, including:

- an acute major incident (such as a radioactive leak from a nuclear installation site);
- a major food poisoning outbreak or food contamination;
- a public accident (such as a major rail crash);
- longer term and chronic health threats (such as exposure to hazardous materials from a landfill site or the effects of air pollution);

- the uncertain hazards of new technologies (such as genetic modification of foods or mobile telecommunication technology);
- newly emerging infectious diseases including zoonotic (of animal origin).

A health impact can be small and limited to the local population, or widespread extending to whole populations. An effect on the public's health can be acute and immediate and/or chronic and delayed over a period of many years.

The risks to health increasingly include those of global origin and have international and national as well as local implications. Over the past decade these threats have included:

- climate change and consequential health impacts (for example, flooding) (Department of Health 2001a);

- bioterrorism risks (anthrax, smallpox) post-11 September 2001 (House of Commons Defence Committee 2001/02);

- continuing communicable diseases such as HIV and AIDS (Department of Health 2002c: 39);

- food implicated health threats such as new variant Creutzfeldt-Jacob Disease (vCJD) from bovine spongiform encephalopathy (BSE) in cattle (Patterson and Painter 1999; Phillips Report 2000);

- animal disease outbreaks such as the foot and mouth disease outbreak of 2001, where control procedures resulted in potential health risks from environmental hazards (Environment Agency 2000; Department of Health 2002d).

- newly emergent communicable diseases such as Severe Acute Respiratory Syndrome (SARS), thought to be caused by a coronavirus of animal origin and newly manifest in humans, which originated in China in November 2002 (WHO 2003).

As well as the direct health impacts, these health threats have also resulted in indirect effects such as the impact on national economies and the destabilizing effect on populations and communities.

Global and local environmental changes resulting from the impact of resource over-utilization and ecosystem degradation are now presenting themselves and are being linked to newly emerging diseases (Lee 2000a). The scale is illustrated by the emergence of at least 30 previously unknown infectious diseases since the 1970s (Department of Health 2002d). In policy terms this places emphasis on the importance of surveillance systems and networks for early warning and preventative action. This includes animal health surveillance to detect species drift of infectious agents of potential risk to human health, a successful example of which is the virulent strain of the influenza virus, 'Avian Flu', which was prevalent in the early 1990s in chickens in Hong Kong and began to infect people in 1997. Early action involved destruction of infected chickens, thus preventing a potential worldwide (pandemic) influenza outbreak (Chief Medical Officer 1997). Similarly effective surveillance and rapid alert networks have assisted the response to SARS, although lack of transparency in China, the country of origin, delayed the control measures nationally and globally.

Emerging health protection policy and organization

The policy and public communication disasters of the BSE crisis and the lessons to be learnt from this (O'Brien 2000), undoubtedly have informed a number of changes in European and British policies for protecting health. Openness and transparency in relation to health hazards and risk uncertainty are key changes, as well as development of precautionary and preventative policies which are integrated into all policies (European Community 1999). Political and economic constraints including the influences of the World Trade Organisation and free trade agreements, coupled with challenges to the strength of the scientific evidence and risk, make implementing these policies a slow process. (Globalization and health is discussed in depth in Chapter 13.)

The Food Standards Agency (FSA) was created in 1998 in response to the number of food safety issues including the BSE crisis (MAFF 1998). The setting up of the FSA went some way to addressing the criticism of government departments regarding the interests of commercial producers, agri-business and the food industry over that of consumer and public health. Public concern and heightened risk perception regarding food safety issues in the UK continues to have a significant influence, for example, on policies in relation to genetically modified food controversies and the government response.

European Union policy, and implicitly that of the member states, requires a high level of health protection to be adopted (European Community 1999). Since 1996 public health has become a European policy objective and protecting public health has a focus within the European Commission Directorate for Health and Consumer Protection. Transparency and public engagement are important themes for EU policy and include policy mechanisms for better information and for support of non-governmental organizations and consumer and public health organizations, such as the European Public Health Alliance. (For further reading, see Randall 2001: Chapter 5.)

The EU Public Health Action programme 2003–08 includes the need for and the direction of improvements in health information and rapid response to health threats (European Community 2001). This requires comparability and coordination Europe-wide, as well as greater cooperation with international organizations such as the World Health Organisation, Organisation for Economic Cooperation and Development (OECD), Food and Agriculture Organisation and the World Trade Organisation (WTO). (See Table 7.1 for a list of organizations and their functions in health protection.) The communicable disease network of the EC set up in 1999 (Giesecke and Weinberg 1998; European Community 1999; *Eurosurveillance Weekly*) was enhanced to provide a telematic early warning response system (EWRS) in 2000, alerting public health authorities to health threats. Since 2002 this also provides for a coordinated response to biological, chemical and nuclear threats.

Table 7.1 Organizations and their functions in health protection

Organization/Abbreviation	Function
Cabinet Office (CO)	Government office – coordinating/cross-cutting: includes the UK Resilience Unit and Contingency Planning Secretariat.
Centre for Applied Microbiological Research (CAMR)	National centre for microbiological research (under HPA).
Chemical Incident Response Service (CIRS)	Expert advisory unit for chemical incident response (under HPA). (One of five regional service provider units.)
Committee on Medical Effects of Air Pollution (COMEAP)	Department of Health, a committee on air pollution and health.
Consultants in Communicable Disease Control (CCDC)	Specialists in surveillance and control of communicable disease (within regional/local HPA).
Department of Environment, Food and Rural Affairs (DEFRA)	Government department for environment, food and rural affairs.
Department for Transport (DfT)	Government department for transport.
Drinking Water Inspectorate (DWI)	Regulation of drinking water quality (under DEFRA).
Environment Agency (EA)	National agency for environmental protection.
Emergency Planning Coordination Unit (EPCU)	Department of Health unit for health services emergency planning coordination.
European Public Health Alliance (EPHA)	Alliance of non-governmental public health organizations in Europe.
Expert Panel on Air Quality Standards (EPAQ)	Government standing expert panel.
Food and Agricultural Organisation (FAO)	United Nations international body for food policy, food security and agricultural development and standards.
Food Standards Agency (FSA)	National body monitoring food safety and health.
Health and Safety Executive (HSE)	Executive arm of the HSC for implementation of health and safety of the workplace.
Health and Safety Commission (HSC)	National commission for health and safety.
Health Protection Agency (HPA)	National coordinating body for health protection (April 2003).
Home Office (HO)	Government office for internal affairs.
Interdepartmental Group on Geographic Information Systems (IGGC)	Government group (Ordinance Survey) developing the application of geographic information systems (GIS).
Local Authorities Coordination of Regulatory Services (LACORS)	Coordinates local government regulatory services such as food and consumer safety.

Table 7.1 Contd.

Organization/Abbreviation	Function
National Focus for Chemical Incidents (NFCI)	National expert advisory body for chemical incidents (under HPA).
National Radiological Protection Board (NRPB)	National body providing expertise on radiological protection.
Office of Deputy Prime Minister (ODPM)	Government office – for regional and local government. Regional Coordination Unit.
Organisation for Economic Cooperation and Development (OECD)	International organization on social and economic development.
Public Health Laboratory Service (PHLS) and Communicable Disease Surveillance Centre (CDSC)	National/regional microbiological services and national centre for communicable disease surveillance (under HPA).
Public Health Observatories (PHO)	Regional NHS organizations for health and disease monitoring and coordinating information and health trends.
Regional Health Emergency Planning Advisors (RHEPA)	Advisors for emergency planning and response (under regional HPA).
Regional Service Provider Units (RSPU)	Toxicological expert units (under regional HPA).
World Trade Organisation (WTO)	International organization for trade tariffs and agreements.

The precautionary principle

European Community policy makes it clear that the precautionary principle must be applied having regard to the size of the risk (proportionality), analysis of costs and benefits and consistency of application. Conditions under which the precautionary principle would apply are defined in the *Rio Declaration on Environment and Development* (UNCED 1992b). These are:

- when there are threats of serious or irreversible damage;
- when there is lack of scientific certainty; and
- when cost-effective measures are possible to prevent environmental degradation.

'When in doubt about the impact of a development it will be managed according to the worst case scenario of its impact on the environment and human health' (UNCED 1992b).

Towards prevention

'Polluter pays' policy mechanisms involving punitive fines and environmental remediation are now moving towards the inclusion of other policy mechanisms such as fiscal measures, for example, a carbon tax as an energy and greenhouse gas reduction measure and a landfill tax as a waste reduction measure. This is shifting policy away from control and clean-up, towards prevention of activities involving adverse environmental and health impacts. The European Union Sixth Environment Action Programme commencing in 2001 is a ten year programme which furthers action on environment and human health threats as well as on quality of life issues through integrated approaches (European Community 2002). The developing policy debate on food and farming methods is also relevant as regards public health and the protection of natural resources and the environment (DEFRA 2002).

These policies widen the responsibility for protection and conservation of natural resources beyond governments and the private sector to society as a whole. In wider health impact terms this raises issues such as pricing of goods and services, for example, food, fuel and energy costs related to fiscal environmental measures and the differential impact on low income households. Such developments in policy aimed at reducing global environmental effects and achieving a more sustainable approach to resource utilization, need to be considered in terms of their wider health impacts on specific population groups, such as fuel poverty and the cost of essential goods such as food. (Sustainability and health is discussed in depth in Chapter 12.)

Responding to new threats

The spectre of deliberate releases of biological and chemical agents and terrorist activities has heightened public and government awareness of the potential impacts on health and on economic and social stability. These new and re-emerging health threats have shown that despite developments in international and national surveillance, there are limitations within current organizational frameworks for the management of risk. The Chief Medical Officer's report *Getting Ahead of the Curve* (Department of Health 2002c) and the consultation document *Creating a Health Protection Agency* (Department of Health/Welsh Office 2002) set out the strategies to integrate policies and programmes under the umbrella of health protection. The broad strategy aims cover:

- scoping of health threats;
- establishing priorities; and
- integrating infectious disease challenges within wider health protection needs.

Overall, in policy terms, there is the need to move forward with preventative and proactive programmes based on surveillance and assessment of risks and integration of environment and health impacts, together with public engagement on these issues. This must take account of evidential uncertainty regarding risk, and public anxiety regarding health threats.

Organizations and structures for health protection

Historical development of health protection in UK

In the UK, policy roots for environmental and health protection exist within the public health regulations of the 19th century. The piecemeal and separate development of policies that followed has resulted in lack of integration of both policies and administrative arrangements to implement them. It was not until the mid-1990s that moves to integrate policies to protect the environment and health began to develop (Department of the Environment/Welsh Office 1993) with the creation of the Environment Agency in England and Wales, and the Scottish Environmental Protection Agency. Policy mechanisms such as, for example, Integrated Pollution Prevention and Control has enabled the integrated assessment of the environment and health impacts of industrial processes (CHMRC 2002).

The policies for protection from workplace hazards have developed through a complex set of regulatory requirements that were integrated, after 1974, under the national Health and Safety Commission and its executive arm, the Health and Safety Executive. A more proactive approach to implementing workplace health promotion has been strengthened through policies such as *Revitalising Health and Safety* (HSC/DETR 1999). Special hazards posing national risks, such as nuclear installation sites, have a well developed regulatory system and interagency working supported by the National Radiological Protection Board expert body.

Infectious disease surveillance and control of outbreaks of infection since 1974 has been split between the health service and local authorities, supported by the Public Health Laboratory Services. Collaboration between local authorities and the health authority was weak following the loss of the medical officer of health from local authorities in 1974. This loss of public health expertise was cited as a key factor in the failures of public health services during the infectious disease outbreaks in the 1980s (Acheson 1988). Specialist consultants in communicable disease control and their infection control teams subsequently have provided health and epidemiological expertise to health and local authority environmental health services.

Since the introduction of regulation of food adulteration and unsafe food in the 19th century, environmental health services of local authorities together with trading standard services, has continued to have responsibility for food and consumer protection issues at a local level. These services were separate at county and district levels, until the advent of unitary local authority areas, although in non-unitary local government areas this separation remains. Local protection from hazards to the public and the working population, including emergency planning arrangements, have continued to be the focus of local authority services for protecting public health.

The health protection agency

The increasing range and complexity of health threats has focused attention on the need for coordinated national expert advice and information to support improved coordination at all levels of surveillance and response. The national Health Protection Agency, set up in April 2003 as an expert coordinating body, reduces the number of separate national bodies. In developing the strategy the report *Creating a Health Protection Agency* (Department of Health/Welsh Office 2002) identified that planning for or dealing with any health threat event, where causation may very well be unknown in the early stages, required broadly similar emergency response and investigation.

The Health Protection Authority is a special health authority within the NHS at the outset and it is anticipated that it will have responsibility for providing, supporting or collaborating with the following national, regional and local agencies and services:

At national level (these organizations are integrated within the Health Protection Authority):

- Centre of Applied Microbiological Research;
- National Focus for Chemical Incidents; and
- Public Health Laboratory Services including the Communicable Disease Surveillance Centre.

The National Radiological Protection Board is to operate together with the above organizations under the Health Protection Authority to provide the national expertise base.

At regional level (these organizations are integrated within the Health Protection Authority):

- regional service provider units;
- public health laboratories;
- regional health emergency planning advisors; and
- health protection staff from central or local services.

At local level:

- consultants in communicable disease control and other health protection staff in local health protection units for the primary care trusts.

There are no immediate plans in the Health Protection Authority consultation document supporting interface working between the Health Protection Authority and other national organizations such as the Environment Agency, the Health and Safety Executive, the Food Standards Agency or with local authority services at local level. However, in some regions, emergency and contingency planning needs have enabled such arrangements to be established ahead of the establishment of the Health Protection Authority.

UK-wide coordination on major national emergencies, for example, terrorism threats, the foot and mouth outbreak or widespread flooding, requires government cross-cutting approaches. This is now the focus for the Contingency Planning for Emergencies Secretariat and the UK Resilience Unit of the Cabinet Office (www.ukresilience.info/home.htm), as well as the regional coordination function of the Office for the Deputy Prime Minister, Regional Coordination Unit (www.rcu.gov.uk).

The emerging organizational structure for protecting health in England is set out in Figure 7.1. (As mentioned above, Table 7.1 lists organizations, their abbreviations and their functions in health protection.)

NATIONAL

Government departments

Health
Cabinet Office
Home Office
Transport
Environment, Food and Rural Affairs
Office of Deputy Prime Minister
Trade and Industry

Health Protection Agency

Coordination

| National Focus for Chemical Incidents | Centre for Applied Microbiological Research | Public Health Laboratory Service |
| Food Standards Agency | Environment Agency | Health and Safety Executive |

Other agencies and organizations

| National Radiological Protection Board | Drinking Water Inspectorate | Other |

REGIONAL

Government Office for the Regions

Regional director of public health
Regional Public Health Observatories

Regional health protection

Regional health emergency planning advisors
Regional service provider units
Chemical Incident Response Service
Regional epidemiologist
Public Health Laboratory Service

Sub-regional

Strategic Health Authority

Regional offices

Environment Agency
Health and Safety Executive

LOCAL

Health services

Primary care trusts
Directors of public health
Local health protection units

NHS trust
Acute trusts
Ambulance trust

Local authority

Environmental health
Trading standards
Emergency planning
Transport and planning

Emergency and essential services

Fire, police, ambulance
Utilities: water, sewerage, communication, power

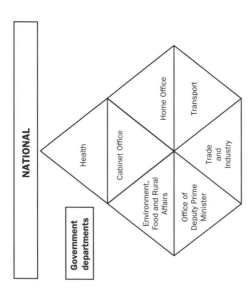

Figure 7.1 The emerging structure for protecting public health (England)

Regional and local organizations and structures

Emergency planning and response

Local NHS bodies have been responsible for many years for ensuring that they have plans for responding to major incidents and mass casualties, together with local stakeholders – the emergency services and local authority emergency planning teams. Following the health services structural changes in April 2002, the National Audit Office has conducted a review of emergency planning service provision by the NHS. The report identifies key requirements and best practice already in place, which needed to be systematically spread to address deficiencies in the way that the NHS plans and prepares for major incidents (National Audit Office 2002).

The Department of Health Emergency Planning Coordination Unit has also reviewed the organizational arrangements for the NHS which are set out in the guidance document *Emergency Planning and Response to Major Incidents: Summary of Roles and Responsibilities* (Department of Health EPCU 2002a). This guidance document sets the framework within which individual NHS organizations are required to meet the requirements of controls assurance for emergency planning (refer to the document Annex – summary diagram at www.doh.gov.uk/epcu/pdf/eprolesandresponsibilitiesv5.doc). Guidance from the NHS Executive on major incident planning, covers aspects of integration and coordination of the health services, together with local authorities and other emergency services (NHS Executive 1998b; Department of Health EPCU 2002b).

Regional health emergency planning advisors have been established since 1980 to assist and provide regional coordination, together with additional toxicological expertise provided since 1993, through the five regional service provider units, including the Chemical Incident Response Service.

In anticipation of the establishment of the Health Protection Authority in April 2003 and in response to terrorism contingency planning, a number of regions are establishing regional health protection units, employing existing experts and advisory staff from the regional and local organizations. The establishment of regional coordination for contingency planning for health protection has already shown that multiagency working can impact on the effectiveness of response to a major Legionnaires disease outbreak in 2002, whereby a significant reduction in the fatality rate for this disease was achieved (Spear 2003). In some regions the intention is also to integrate a wider skills mix including environmental health officers from local authorities (Spear 2003).

Environmental and infectious disease monitoring

The Public Health Laboratory Service (PHLS) provides services to local authorities and public health authorities for routine and incident environmental and infectious disease monitoring. While the new Health Protection Authority will support a Public Health Laboratory Service laboratory in each region, the transfer of some Public Health Laboratory Service laboratories and staff to mainstream NHS services may impact on the availability of these services, which are a vital part of surveillance.

The health service role

The expertise-based national Health Protection Authority is being set up at a time when there has also been radical restructuring of the health sector (Department of Health 2001c). At regional level the overall accountability for health protection, including coordinating the government's response to emergencies and disasters, rests with the regional director of public health, with the public health function co-located within the regional offices of government for England.

In recent years the requirement to provide environment and health impact assessment for management of major incidents has resulted in the role of public health staff being extended, for example, during the foot and mouth outbreak (Department of Health 2002d: 125). There is also the statutory public health consultee role required for pollution prevention, under the Integrated Pollution Prevention and Control regulatory regime (Kibble and Saunders 2001; CHMRC 2002).

In England at local level, responsibility for the health of the population within primary care trusts rests with the director of public health for the PCT, and includes the responsibility for health protection of that population, supported by specialist health protection units under the overall responsibility of the regional director for public health. This function is supported by the public health observatories located in each NHS region, tasked with monitoring health and disease trends, identifying gaps in health information and looking ahead to give early warning of future public health problems.

The local authority role

Local authorities have continued since the 19th century local boards of health under the medical officer for health, to have responsibility at local level for environmental health and public and environmental protection services – dealing with environmental conditions, infectious disease control, food safety, consumer safety and trading standards, housing and working conditions, and emergency planning and response.

Coordination and advice for the regulatory functions of these services is provided by the national local authorities coordinators of regulatory services, advising on food safety, consumer protection and animal health. Local authorities coordinators of regulatory services also support the local consumer support networks. National agencies such as the Environment Agency, Food Standards Agency and the Health and Safety Executive provide advice to local authorities and monitor provision for some function areas.

The Home Office report (Home Office 1999) reviewed civil protection and emergency planning for local authorities setting out standards of good practice and the Department of Health guidance also informs local authority services (NHS Executive 1998b: Appendix A). The central role at local level of local authorities for emergency planning is well established and although there are well developed practices, the new threats are posing particular challenges requiring multiagency training development and field rehearsal for incidents.

Protection of public health at the local level can be enhanced through reconnecting local authorities to the public health agenda together with health and other services. The link between local authorities and public health thus needs to be reforged with key drivers in health protection being the health challenges and risks which are emerging. Health protection must be explicit within local partnerships, including the secondment or transfer and joint development and training of staff in the health, local authority and emergency sectors, together with an important role for public health workers of engagement with the community regarding health threats and risks in their area.

The Commission on Environmental Health report *Agendas for Change* (CIEH 1997) identified the need for environmental health practitioners in local authorities to link up organizations at local level and to be a major part of an integrated multidisciplinary public health programme. The impact on local services of centralization and direction, for example, best value and performance regimes of the late 1990s, tended to mitigate against local authority services contributing to the multidisciplinary public health agenda, although the willingness of professionals to contribute is clear and the climate of engagement around key health issues is driving forward change. The contribution and widening role of environment health practitioners in public health development is considered by the joint Health Development Agency and Chartered Institute of Environmental Health report (HDA/CIEH 2002).

Health protection: principles and practice

Hazards, risk and health impact assessment

The first principle in establishing an effective system for protecting health is the identification of hazards and their potential to cause harm – the risk. While hazard is the intrinsic ability of an agent to cause a specific adverse consequence in terms of population health and/or environmental impact, the risk can be described as the potential of a hazard to cause harm depending on specific circumstances. This can be considered in terms of:

- the host (human exposure, susceptibility, response);
- the harmful agent (infectious, chemical, physical, biological);
- the environment, the pathway or mechanism for the agent to cause harm.

Risk assessment is the process of estimating the potential impact of a chemical, physical, microbiological or psychosocial hazard on a specified human population or ecological system under a specific set of conditions for exposure and for a certain time frame (Pencheon *et al.* 2001: 208). For certain hazardous agents dose response relationships and toxicological and epidemiological data exist and risk assessment can be quantified in terms of a specified human population exposure under a specific set of conditions and over a specific time frame.

However, in many situations, especially for complex and long-term patterns of exposure, the assessment of the acceptable risk level is uncertain, due to weaknesses in the evidence arising from:

- incomplete data (lack of exposure data, unreliable health data or low statistical power);

- variability inherent in the data (difficulties in measuring human exposure and dose response studies, which are often retrospective or opportunistic, and of extrapolating high dose acute exposure studies to low dose exposure);

- confounding factors (other factors which affect health status which cannot be removed).

(Developed from SWPHO 2002: 25)

Where evidence exists and is strong, exposure indices can be developed and applied in order to reduce exposure and prevent harm. Developed exposure indices for hazards include:

- ambient (background) environmental exposure for all individuals;

- individualized exposure (for example, for occupational exposure or high risk groups);

- exposure through combined exposure pathways (for example, through inhalation, ingestion and contact).

An example of ambient exposure indices is air quality standards for individual pollutants such as ozone and particulate matter, set by the government's Expert Panel on Air Quality Standards on advice from the Department of Health Committee on Medical Effects of Air Pollution. In 1995 the Committee, on reviewing the evidence base, concluded that 'air pollution is likely to be having a serious effect on health in the UK – more than 12,000 deaths are brought forward and between 14,000 and 24,000 admissions and readmissions to hospital are associated with short term exposure to air pollutants' (Department of Health COMEAP 1995, 1997). In Europe it is claimed that poor air quality, through causing premature death, claims as many lives as AIDS (European Commission 2002). In 1997 in England and Wales, the national air quality management strategy was adopted to secure improvements in local air quality, applying standards at local level for eight key air pollutants (Department of the Environment, Transport and the Regions 1997).

In relation to the broader public health implications of diverse and complex environmental hazards, the epidemiological and toxicological evidence is more often than not insufficient or inconclusive. A recent study evaluated the state of the evidence into waste management activities and health (SWPHO 2002). In the concluding summary the report states 'the nature of existing epidemiological research in this area is such that most studies are useful for generating hypotheses, but are unable to test the hypotheses or provide convincing evidence of association between exposure and health impacts' (SWPHO 2002: 40). Also studies which focus on physical health effects ignore the wider health impacts of waste facilities, such as psycho-social effects of living nearby.

Miller (1996) came to a similar conclusion for studies on the health impacts of hazardous waste. Fehr (1999) describes the use of integrated environmental and health impact assessment for the planned extension of a non-toxic waste disposal facility. Fehr argues that such an assessment should be used more often as a tool in health protection and promotion, but that consensus is needed on the concept and further development needed of the tool. The National Assembly for Wales has produced guidelines on health impact assessment, which stresses that it must do more than just indicate that a development may create pollution or a health hazard: it must assess options in relation to health outcomes (National Assembly for Wales 1999: 19).

(For further reading on health and environmental impact assessment, see British Medical Association 1998; European Community (1999). For methodological aspects of health impact assessment, see Department of Health (1999b). (Health impact assessment is also discussed in depth in Chapter 18.)

Making decisions about hazards and risks

Uncertainty and the lack of knowledge about risks from health threats need to be addressed within decision-making models. In these situations risk-based decisions tend to be intuitive and value based, influenced by individual perception, by society and by those empowered to make judgements.

When there is little knowledge and much uncertainty about risks, experts are prone to use the same mental strategies, known as heuristics, as the non-scientifically trained public (SWPHO 2002: 35). Thus scientists tend to underestimate the risk of technologies they are familiar with, while the public tend to overestimate the risk, as they unfamiliar with the technology.

Other aspects influence outcomes, such as outrage factors, which cover qualitative aspects of a judgement, including lack of choice, global catastrophic potential and affecting people personally (SWPHO 2002: 36). For example, involuntary manmade hazards such as pollution, especially if poorly understood by science, are perceived to be a higher risk than voluntary ones, such as dangerous sports or smoking. These perceptions of risks are not of necessity unpredictable and are not unreasonable. Thus there is recognition that communication strategies which inform, engage and empower the public, should be employed within decision-making processes for protecting against health threats. (For further reading see Royal Society 1992; Department of Health 1997b; Saffron 1993; Dickson 1997; Bennett and Calman 1999.)

Surveillance and prevention

The actions required to contain new and emerging infections are set out in the government's strategy document, *Getting Ahead of the Curve*, and include a surveillance system with comprehensive coverage to detect unusual disease presentations and changes in occurrence or profile of micro-organisms, and the use of data to predict outbreaks or epidemics and prevent them (Department of Health 2002c: 56). For example, the drop in uptake of MMR (Measles, Mumps and Rubella) triple vaccinations resulting from public scares over possible heath risks is a predicator of gaps in the immunity of populations and a future rise of this disease.

Primary and secondary prevention

Effective surveillance enables primary prevention, including health information, for specific infectious diseases. For example, in order to reduce lifestyle risk factors which predispose individuals to sexually transmitted infections, health education interventions can minimize the spread of infections by targeting particular risk groups (such as people with multiple sexual partners).

Secondary prevention of certain infectious diseases can be achieved through screening leading to the identification of these infections at a time when remedial action can be taken to prevent or alleviate the effects. Screening can enable estimation of trends in the population burden of disease and contributes to the estimation of future health impact. The longstanding specific antenatal screening programmes for rubella and syphilis have now been supplemented by the addition of universal antenatal screening for Hepatitis B and by offering an HIV test to women booking for antenatal care (Acheson 1998; Department of Health 1999c). These systems for early detection at an asymptomatic stage enable specific therapeutic steps to be taken, for example, the administration of Hepatitis B vaccine to the babies of mothers identified as Hepatitis B positive during their antenatal care (Department of Health 1998a).

Surveillance systems and their limitations

The Communicable Disease Surveillance Centre of the Public Health Laboratory Service is responsible for collection, collation and dissemination of information on communicable diseases in England and Wales. In Scotland, the Scottish Centre for Infection and Environmental Health and in Northern Ireland, the Department of Health and Social Services and Public Safety fulfil this function.

While established systems exist, including statutorily required disease notifications and special surveillance systems such as those for sexually transmitted disease surveillance, there are gaps in the reporting of many diseases with public health implications. For example, the current statutory notification system of specified diseases to the local authority 'Proper Officer' (Public Health Control of Infectious Diseases Act 1984) has discrepancies when compared with presentation of microbiology laboratory isolate data. Also reporting rates are variable, for example, the rise in cases of tuberculosis recorded nationwide masks underreporting of a disease considered to be yesterday's problem (British Thoracic Society 2000; Department of Health 2002c: 60).

Surveillance data from these sources in England and Wales are analysed for trends by the Communicable Disease Surveillance Centre (*Communicable Disease Reports Weekly* and *Journal of Communicable Diseases and Public Health*) and comprehensive surveillance data down to district level are available online through the Public Health Laboratory Service website. Other surveillance systems include food and hazardous product alert and information systems enabling rapid response and recall at the earliest point in the supply chain, for example, at the port of entry or recall from suppliers or consumers and hazardous product alert systems.

Routine and incident surveillance for environmental hazards include monitoring of air, water, food, soil and vegetation. This is the responsibility of several government departments and national agencies (see Table 7.1) including the Environment Agency, Food Standards Agency and the National Radiological Protection Board and at local level, the local authority. The Chemical Releases Inventory was introduced in 1991 in England and Wales to provide data on an annual basis of emissions from industrial processes under the regulatory Integrated Prevention and Pollution Control regime.

Despite the apparent transparency of this information, there are severe limitations through inconsistencies and lack of reporting. In addition, many industrial activities and sites are excluded from the Integrated Prevention and Pollution Control process and are separately regulated, such as landfill waste, mining and sewage treatment. Of over 100,000 chemicals catalogued as being in commercial use, many have not been fully assessed for toxicity, persistence and bioaccumulation (Murkerjee 1995; Santillo *et al.* 1999). Thus gaps in knowledge or lack of systematic methodologies mean delays in establishing routine monitoring; an example is chemicals which mimic human reproductive hormones and are suspected of decreasing sperm counts and increasing the incidence of cancers (IEH 1995; Colborn *et al.* 1997).

Where monitoring is undertaken, the analysis of population health impacts can be facilitated by data sets on health and environmental quality being coordinated on common geographical boundaries, so that links between health events, ambient environmental quality changes or pollution release incidents can be ascertained. Geographic Information Systems (GIS) enable geomapping of population and boundaries with other data sets and tools for analysis of the information. The Inter-Departmental Group on Geographic Information Systems was set up by the government in 1993 to develop the use and application of Ordinance Survey information. An example is the HAZMOD intranet web-based GIS service for the emergency planning community which is under development by the Civil Contingencies Secretariat of the Cabinet Office (Cabinet Office 2001c). The use of GIS systems is also relevant to, for example:

- mapping infectious disease outbreak and related environmental data;

- population data such as standardized deprivation indexes and environmental exposure;

- mapping ambient air quality monitoring data;

- mapping chemical release inventories, waste sites facilities or *Control of Major Accident Hazard Regulations 1999* (COMAH 1999) sites.

Modelling of routine, accidental or deliberate releases, together with GIS is developing as a powerful tool in mapping long-term trends of health impact and in predicting patterns of exposure for acute hazard incidents. The EU health informatics network is likewise being developed to include environmental information to provide reliable data for health impact assessment.

Health emergency planning and response

Tertiary prevention in terms of health protection consists of measures to reduce or eliminate the adverse health effects of particular incidents or outbreaks. In relation to the acute response the nature, degree and timing of specific health protection responses will vary depending on the circumstances and potential population health implications.

A major incident may be defined as:

> any occurrence which presents a serious threat to the health of the community, disruption to the service or causes (or is likely to cause) such numbers or types of casualties as to require special arrangements to be implemented by hospitals, ambulance services or health communities.
>
> (NHS Executive 1998b: glossary)

Thus an acute response is required for a major incident such as a fire in a chemical plant, as well as ongoing longer-term measures consisting of health impact assessment and health surveillance. In order to achieve a combined and coordinated response to a major incident, the capabilities of the emergency services must be closely linked with those of local authorities and other agencies. The management of the response can be divided into three levels: operational, tactical and strategic (NHS Executive 1998b):

- Operational (bronze): this is the front-line control at the scene of any incident.

- Tactical (silver): the tactical level of command is used to determine priority in allocating resources, to plan and coordinate tasks, and to obtain other resources as required.

- Strategic (gold): this senior tier of management would only be used in a large incident to make strategic decisions about deployment of resources, managing populations, providing information and restoring normality.

The requirement to implement one or more of these management levels will depend upon the nature of the incident.

Emergency planning

Following the fuel crisis and severe flooding in 2000, the Cabinet Office has undertaken an extensive emergency planning review and has set up the UK Resilience Unit and the Civil Contingencies Secretariat to support national and regional resilience to emergencies which in turn will support local services (Cabinet Office 2001d). This is to effectively coordinate communication between government and regional/local implementation and to enable 'horizon scanning' as regards risks, contingency planning and validation of the emergency response plans.

Individual emergency plans need to reflect the concept of integrated emergency management, where the aim is to achieve maximum effectiveness by integrating the contribution made by a number of different agencies and authorities, with the emphasis on planning the response to an incident regardless of cause. This can only be achieved through multiagency, multiprofessional and multidisciplinary collaboration under the auspices of a lead agency. While the lead agency is usually the police in the acute phase of a response and the local authority in terms of dealing with the aftermath, there are situations where the lead coordinating role is undertaken by another agency at a local or national level. For example, during the foot and mouth crisis the Cabinet Office provided the necessary lead for coordinated national action (Cabinet Office 2002).

Dealing with major incidents

> A major incident can have a huge impact on one part of the health service, while leaving others relatively unaffected. In a similar way, an NHS major incident is not necessarily a major incident for other emergency services, such as police, fire or local authority services – and vice versa ... When the number and type of casualties overwhelm or threaten to overwhelm normal services, special arrangements are needed to deal with them.
>
> (NHS Executive 1998b: 14)

The United States terrorist incident on 11 September 2001 indicated that extensive emergency planning arrangements would need to be consolidated in the UK in order to deal with the implications of a terrorist incident resulting in mass casualties. For major incidents involving chemical industries, arrangements exist which require on and off site planning and rehearsal involving local communities (COMAH 1999). For incidents involving radioactive nuclear installations, the National Radiological Protection Board provides expertise and coordination based on guidance contained in their handbook (McCol and Kruse 2002).

In practice a major health incident may start in a number of ways (NHS Executive 1998b: 6):

- Big bang: a health service major incident is classically triggered by a sudden major transport or industrial accident such as a chemical explosion.

- Rising tide: the problem creeps up gradually such as occurs in a developing infectious disease epidemic or a winter bed availability crisis.

- Cloud on the horizon: an incident in one place may affect others following the incident.

- Headline news: a wave of public or media alarm over a health issue as a reaction to a perceived threat may create a major incident for the health services even if fears are unfounded.

- Internal incidents: the service itself may be affected by its own internal major incident or by an external incident that impairs its ability to work normally.

- Deliberate release: a deliberate release of chemical, biological, radiological or nuclear materials requires specific action to be taken in terms of public health intervention.

The range of responses to incidents

Environmental incidents with less extensive population health implications also require coordinated action to be taken by relevant local agencies. For example, the evacuation of a household following kerosene contamination of the property from a leaking domestic fuel storage tank or pipeline may require thorough local authority environmental health investigation of the site, biological sampling for medical toxicology assessment of the individuals, as well as social services assistance for housing. Accurate toxicological analysis of environmental samples for kerosene contamination could determine the nature and extent of public health action necessary.

A low scale incident at local level may escalate into a situation which requires particular action to be taken by statutory agencies with health protection responsibilities, for example, the Health and Safety Executive regarding a Legionnaire's Disease outbreak which is usually associated with workplaces. While a limited health protection response is required in terms of contact tracing in relation to a case of, for example, non-infectious tuberculosis – a far more extensive response may be required for a case of infectious tuberculosis on a hospital ward catering for cancer patients whose immune system is already weakened.

The role of microbiology laboratories may determine the particular public health measures necessary. For example, the identification of a case of infectious multidrug resistant tuberculosis will necessitate the patient's urgent hospital admission and isolation in a special facility, as well as detailed investigation and screening of close contacts to minimize the spread of this potentially fatal infection.

The nature of crises which may require an incident response are thus diverse and require multiagency partnership in order to ensure that appropriate risk management-based decisions are made in the interests of health protection. The response must include the management of public anxiety as part of major incident management, such as the coordinated media response triggered by the BSE crisis (Department of Health 2002c: 129). The difficulty for decision takers is determining when, what, who and how to communicate issues involving public health risks. The threat of anthrax through the postal system in 2002 and subsequent incidents in 2003 indicate that preparation and training is needed at all levels to prepare in the event of a major incident.

Overview: the challenges

The diverse health threats of the past decade have undoubtedly moved health protection needs, particularly health and hazard surveillance and emergency response, up the political agenda, not least because of the economic and destabilizing effects of such threats nationally and globally.

Health protection policy and provision is implicitly about prevention and promotion of health, although it has been influenced by intervention and control models of health. While key successes have been made, for example, in European and national surveillance networks for communicable disease and in rapid hazard alert systems, there remains much to be done in providing integrated surveillance and prevention and an integrated response to incidents when they occur, across responsible agencies at local, regional and national level.

Health protection policy and practice must be related to the assessment of the risk and health outcomes, but the complexity and uncertainty in risk assessment must not hinder the implementation of preventative and precautionary policies. While integrated health and environmental information, modelling and health impact assessment tools together with geographic information systems are being refined, there needs to be consensus in policy development about their use in determining local and regional priorities for health protection.

Transparency, information and communication about health risks in decision making are key requirements, whether concerning acute incident response or in relation to planned hazard prevention. There is now undoubtedly a plethora of publicly available information about health and environmental risk. How much and in what way this influences the response in relation to risk perception, or facilitates contribution to decision making, is open to debate. There is an important role for public health specialists working with communities to inform and engage them in the process of understanding risk and the requirements to reduce risk. Ongoing research regarding the social amplification of risk should provide guidance on the way forward on engagement with the public about risk and facilitate a more involved public and community role.

'Think globally and act locally' is perhaps an overused phrase, but has some resonance here, not only in relation to the broad concept of sustainable development and natural resource utilization to which it usually refers, but also in relation to health risks and specific national and local responses. Collaborative partnerships focused on communities, local agencies and services are as relevant to health protection as they are to the broader context of health improvement. The new primary care structure coupled with a growing policy agenda for health and sustainability within local authorities, provides an opportunity for local health protection to be connected to the wider public health agenda for local populations, targeting risks and addressing health inequalities arising from these health challenges.

The Department of Health policies for health protection in England and Wales (Department of Health 2002c; Department of Health/Welsh Office 2002) are being implemented at a time of significant health sector organizational change. A key issue is maintaining existing provision through the process of change at a time when health threats are greater and have the potential for massive health impacts. This will require explicit policy drivers for health protection and adapting within new structures to integrate health protection through effective partnership arrangements having regard to the disciplines and expertise available at local level, and the coordination of expertise and support at the national and regional level.

8

PAT TAYLOR
The lay contribution to public health

Editors' introduction

The public are no longer seen as passive recipients of paternalistic professional efforts to improve their health. Rather, they are active participants in plans and programmes which aim to improve their health and well being, drawing on the resources of their own perspectives, experience and knowledge. The 'public' – lay people – are key partners in contemporary public health and lay involvement is expected at all levels of current public health activity.

This chapter will be useful for all public health workers as it examines the contribution of lay perspectives to public health, addressing questions of why and how lay people can and should be involved in public health practice.

The author starts by considering current policy for public involvement in the overall historical context of lay involvement in the NHS. She identifies that most of the policy for public involvement concentrates on patient involvement in health *services* rather than on the wider arena of public health. She then considers why lay perspectives are important to public health and shows the place of lay perspectives and lay action in the development of health services and public health action in the UK.

The chapter outlines the nature of lay perspectives on health and demonstrates that they are a different and unique contribution to multidisciplinary public health. But there are significant difficulties in accessing and articulating lay views in the face of the dominance of the biomedical model in any public discussion on health. Medical perspectives on lay involvement are examined and key obstacles in health professional approaches to public involvement are discussed.

The author concludes by looking at ways of promoting an effective lay contribution to public health. She identifies four approaches and four levels to lay involvement and shows that the connections between them need to be understood by those responsible for developing lay involvement. Public health particularly requires strong links to local and informal networks within communities and local populations, in order to establish the full contribution of lay involvement.

Introduction

> Today we need a new outlook. An approach that accepts that there are wide determinants of ill health – and a wide ranging programme of action is necessary and indeed is underway to deal with them . . . an approach which also understands that the NHS can make a specific contribution to improving health prospects by working with the communities it serves: making the task of tackling health inequality something done with local people not just done to them.
>
> (Milburn 2002)

The quote above highlights a significant change in the way the public are being perceived in government policy – no longer as passive receivers of expert health care but as active participants in the processes of health improvement. How realistic is this aspiration in practice? How has the rhetoric of policy actually opened up opportunities for lay people to articulate and influence the agendas for health improvement and health service development?

Structure of this chapter

The chapter starts by considering why lay involvement is important to public health and the changing nature of public involvement in public services. A brief consideration of the historical development of public health illustrates that lay perspectives have always underpinned the development of public health. The chapter then outlines lay perspectives in health and demonstrates that there is a different and unique contribution that lay perspectives bring to a multidisciplinary public health. A discussion of medical perspectives on lay involvement follows.

The chapter concludes with a section on promoting an effective lay contribution to public health. It identifies four approaches and four levels of public involvement and further shows that there are key practical, attitudinal and conceptual obstacles to promoting an effective lay contribution to multidisciplinary public health. It considers some of the conceptual leaps needed for public health to ensure that it accesses a vibrant and rich vein of lay input to inform its future development.

Why is lay involvement important to public health?

The lay perspective is a crucial area of knowledge for public health. Listening to, and understanding, lay people's experience of their health, ill health and how it is affected by their daily lives can:

- give insight into patterns of behaviour and lifestyles which can identify new areas for investigation in relation to mortality and disease;
- help us to understand factors which underpin and create health inequalities;
- suggest new factors which influence people's health and their ability to use existing resources;

- help us to understand how people live and manage their lives in different circumstances, which is crucial to understanding how information and support can be most effectively offered;

- encourage people's interest and achieve their active involvement in maintaining their health;

- create continuing mechanisms for dialogue and debate and for successfully implementing and monitoring programmes of health improvement with the ownership of the people they aim to help.

This can only be done by in-depth engagement and ongoing dialogue with people within the context of their everyday lives.

The concept of public health action

One way of understanding the dimensions of lay involvement in public health is to distinguish between public health *resource* and public health *action*. Public health resource refers to the range of expertise and services that can support and promote health, such as health promotion and disease surveillance. Public health action refers to the wider activities in society that can promote health and well being and can include the activities of organizations, groups, communities and individuals who may not necessarily perceive themselves as being primarily involved in health.

It is this concept of public health action that underpins the drive for partnership working and is the starting point for understanding the lay contribution to public health. The development of public health action may influence and alter the nature of public health resources. Lay perspectives may eventually be seen as a form of public health expertise; this has happened within health services where patients with long-term chronic illness have now better established their right to have their experience equally valued in the development of services (Department of Health 2001e).

The changing nature of public involvement in the NHS

Four eras of public involvement

Milewa *et al.* (2002) have reviewed the changing nature of public involvement in the NHS since the inception of the health service in 1948; they identify four distinct periods: pre-1974, 1974–90, 1990–97 and post-1997.

Up to 1974 – democratic accountability in local authorities
The first period was prior to 1974, when the NHS had public representatives throughout its structures. Some were the elected members from the municipal authorities in which local NHS services were provided and others were appointed as lay members on hospital boards and committees.

The medical officer of health and other public health specialists such as environmental health officers, health visitors and social workers were outside the

NHS structure, working with local politicians and the local democratic processes within the local authority to address the wider health needs of local populations.

1974–90: community health councils in health authorities
The year 1974 marked the start of the second period, when the medical officer of health and community nurses left their local authority colleagues to enter the NHS, fragmenting public health as a comprehensive set of locally focused activities. (This is discussed in the Introduction to this book.) The role of the medical officer of health as an influential, but independent figure within the local authority being able to identify key local health concerns was lost; the director of public health within health authorities did not have the same sphere of influence or independence.

After 1974 the roles of lay representatives were reduced. Community health councils were set up within the NHS in 1974 to represent the 'interests of the public' but this was essentially a token gesture to lay representation. The community health councils have retained a statutory responsibility for aspects of public consultation in relation to health service changes and have worked behind the scenes to promote patient interests. But throughout their nearly 30 year history (and now imminent demise) they have struggled to gain recognition for their work despite the resurgence of interest in patient and public involvement (Buckland *et al.* 1994).

In the 1980s the increasing interest in managing the NHS and in using market approaches within public services brought the 'needs' of the patient back into focus with an emphasis on responsiveness, accessibility and quality. The model of lay involvement in this period was the patient as consumer, but there was little interest in any other public representation within the wider processes of health care planning and service delivery. However, Milewa *et al.* (2002) assert that this did signal a change in policy from seeing patients as 'passive recipients' to seeing them as more active 'consumers' of health care. It also created an opportunity for groups of health service users to express their views within the different mechanisms created for 'consumer' feedback (McIver 1991; Barnes 1999).

1990–97: the Patient's Charter and *Local Voices*
In 1990 the Patient's Charter gave patients some procedural rights in their use of services and in 1992 *Local Voices* (National Health Services Management Executive 1992) was issued as an advisory document to encourage health authorities, who were purchasers of health care on behalf of their local communities, to consult their communities about their health needs. This stimulated a variety of initiatives and methods in local areas, from local community activities, user and self-help groups to more market research methods such as surveys, focus groups and patient panels.

Research undertaken at that time (Lupton and Taylor 1994) indicated significant differences in public involvement activity depending on which part of the health authority took responsibility for it. Managers developing quality assurance tended to favour market-based methods, public relations staff tended to prioritize information giving, and public health specialists were more inclined to work with local democratic networks and community-based groups. Some commentators (Harrison and Mort 1998) viewed public involvement activity as primarily concerned with legitimating managerial decisions or curbing professional autonomy, but others (Pickard 1998;

Barnes *et al.* 1999) also indicated that there had been an increasing degree of service user involvement and influence in service delivery.

1997: change of government

Public and service user involvement remained firmly on the policy agenda with the change of government in 1997 and has remained central within the reforms in primary care and in health improvement. This Labour government has built on the foundations developed over the past 12 years by funding national initiatives that give recognition to public and patient involvement, such as the national service frameworks and the Expert Patient (Department of Health 2000a) and in bodies such as Consumers in NHS Research. National initiatives such as health action zones and healthy living centres also provide opportunities for lay people to become involved in developing their own perspectives on health. (See Chapter 2 for more about the public health policy of the 1997 Labour government.)

Primary care groups were required to include a lay representative on their boards and then their successor bodies – primary care trusts – were required to develop explicit arrangements for public involvement to be integrated throughout their activities (Department of Health 2001e).

Policy changes in the early 2000s are being implemented to create new structures for patient involvement with the requirement to have patient advice and liaison services in each PCT and NHS trust, and a patient forum attached to each trust. The forum would be affiliated to the new National Commission for Patient and Public Involvement (Department of Health 2001e). These forums are intended to act as a coordinating mechanism for patient and public involvement activities in each local trust area, including those relating to wider initiatives on health within other agencies and in the community in general. In addition the local authority now has re-established a formal relationship with health and the NHS by being given responsibility to include health within its statutory powers of scrutiny.

This section has showed that most experience of public involvement in health is related to patients and health services rather than public health. But in the early 21st century, as well as policy relating specifically to health services, there are parallel policy initiatives relevant to the development of lay perspectives in public health. They include the Sure Start programme, Neighbourhood Renewal Strategy and the regeneration programmes. These all include very clear intentions to involve local communities in their programmes and are likely to offer opportunities for lay people to contribute to the health in their communities.

The next section looks specifically at the involvement of lay people in public health, as distinct from the development of health services.

Lay perspectives in the history of public health

A consideration of the place of lay perspectives within the history of public health may help to develop an understanding of the part they have played in establishing the modern public health knowledge base.

The history of public health identifies different historical periods in which public health consciousness was higher in society in general and viewed as a wider social responsibility. It is in these periods when there have been clear alliances forged between health professionals and lay people. Then there were other periods when public health activity has been confined to specific public health services such as disease surveillance and protection, and the responsibility of experts.

There are two clear traditions which have underpinned lay input into public health action. One is the voluntary and charitable tradition: much of the hospital provision in this country was provided through charitable and religious activity prior to 1948. The other tradition stems from the activities of the organized Labour movement.

Voluntary and charitable tradition and the Labour movement

The 19th century was characterized by a high level of public health activity with social concerns generated by the growth of cities and the fear of the spread of disease and social unrest. The charitable activities of the rich were not wholly altruistic but were underpinned by self-interest and moral superiority. Ashton and Seymour (1988) identify the Sanatarians, led by Chadwick, a doctor who worked to persuade municipal authorities and politicians and campaigned for widespread legislation to establish modern standards of clean water and sanitation. The Personal Preventors such as Eleanor Rathbone and Josephine Butler, the founders of modern health visiting, began from a starting point of being voluntary visitors to the poor, and went on to found the tradition of working with families to improve their own life circumstances as well as campaigning for better housing and social conditions. Immunization and child surveillance followed on from these actions. The Rowntree surveys on poverty contributed to this (Owen 1965). Social philanthropists such as Peabody, the Cadbury and Fry families established 'model' housing schemes to demonstrate the importance of decent housing to people's health and well being.

The Labour movement, with its concern for the working and living conditions of workers, also contributed to public health activity. Unions provided their own organizations for holidays, sports and convalescent homes. Organizations such as the Co-operative Societies, the Ramblers and Workers Educational Association were established by the trade unions. The Labour movement also supported mutual aid societies, forerunners of modern building societies, enabling working people to contribute to insurance for essential health care, sickness benefit, funeral costs and early unemployment support (Gladstone 1979; Richardson and Goodman 1983; Brenton 1985). For many older people, growing up before 1945, their first experiences of social and health support came from trade union and mutual aid organizations.

The welfare state and the NHS

The two world wars were also times of wide social concern for health and social needs. In the First World War there was widespread concern for the health status of recruits to the armed services prompting debates about adequate diet, housing and health services. This provided an opportunity for the trade union movement to be successful in their demands for better social provision for improvements in social conditions and welfare benefits. The social upheavals of the 1930s' mass unemployment and the Second World War consolidated these demands and led to the Beveridge Report (Beveridge 1942) and a political commitment to the establishment of the welfare state to tackle the 'five giants' of poverty, disease, ignorance, squalor and idleness.

The establishment of the NHS and other welfare services in 1948 was accompanied by a widespread expectation that many social problems would be solved. This and the success of earlier public health activists and the success of immunizations led to public complacency about the wider threats to the population's health. Confidence in the power of drugs grew in the public mind as the key solution to all aspects of health.

Lay action in the 1970s

It was not until the 1960s that it became clear that these expectations were not being fulfilled and a growing body of evidence demonstrated enduring poverty and disadvantage among different groups in the population and in particular geographical areas. During the 1970s there was a resurgence of lay action which took a variety of forms. The voluntary sector resumed its role in highlighting the problems for different groups of people suffering disadvantage and campaigning for improvements and recognition from the public services. New kinds of voluntary and community action grew alongside the traditional voluntary groups founded within the charitable tradition of 'noblesse oblige'. These groups drew their forms of organization more from the traditions of self-help and the Labour movement and were helped by state investment in community development projects (Brenton 1985; Smithies and Webster 1998).

This renewal of voluntary and community action in the 1970s contained within it the beginnings of social movements that would be sustained throughout the following two decades. New social movements such as Women's Rights, Disability Action, Action against Racism, provide some pertinent examples (Barnes and Sullivan 2002). These new forms of lay action had wide ranging influences. They often worked at the level of local authorities and health services, working to improve services and set up new forms of social support. They were influential in taking part in the early interest in service user consultations in the setting up of community care services in the early 1990s (Lindow 1993). They also worked to influence the larger and more well established voluntary organizations to become more responsive to the people they purported to represent and so built up a greater awareness of the need for interest groups to be in touch with their constituencies. Barnes and Sullivan (2002) note that these new lay movements wanted to go further than gaining improved services and support, they wanted to achieve a transformation in social attitudes and understanding towards their members and their experiences.

The early community health movement

The 1970s also saw the beginning of a community health movement with the first community health project being set up in 1977 in London (Smithies and Webster 1998). These projects were often connected to other community activities and developed health related activities in local communities using community development methods to help local people articulate and take action on health concerns. Food cooperatives, mental health support groups, antitranquillizer groups, community swimming sessions, environmental clean up campaigns, women's refuges and boys' football clubs were all examples of communities' perspectives on health.

Individual health professionals did get involved in these projects, but they were rarely given organizational backing for their involvement. Overall, community health work remained outside mainstream NHS consciousness. The community projects related instead to other community activities and to their local authorities, joining and being supported by the Health for All and Healthy Cities movements.

While the NHS and mainstream health services remained relatively isolated from much of the efforts of these social and community movements, they did raise important issues in relation to health services and had some significant success in changing services to reflect their concerns. Lay action from within the women's movement changed practices within the maternity services and lay concerns about the welfare of children in hospital were expressed through a campaign to allow parents to stay with their children in hospital – now regarded as normal good practice (Williamson 1992).

This section has attempted to demonstrate that lay action has played a significant part in contributing to the development of health and health services, but that this contribution has not always been explicitly recognized. Since the creation of the NHS in 1948 it seems that lay perspectives and lay action on health have been overshadowed by a belief held by professionals and the public alike that health is the exclusive domain of the NHS. The new policy framework for public involvement and its place in the modernization agenda for public services (see Chapter 2) requires a renewed understanding of lay perspectives on health.

Understanding lay perspectives

What is the lay perspective on health and illness? There is a large and respectable body of sociological literature which deals with the lay understanding of health. This may be influenced by professional perspectives, but it is very different to health professionals' understanding of health. Sociological studies of lay perspectives on health focus on people's experience of health and illness in the context of their overall life experience. They are therefore more diverse and complex than those of professionals whose focus is on their specific expertise.

For many people, health is integral to the way they live, something they appear to take for granted until they experience ill health. However, when time is taken to explore their perceptions of health, people demonstrate knowledge derived from a range of sources about what it means to be healthy and what kind of actions they should take to maintain good health. Such information is gained from their upbringing and family culture, peer groups and friendship networks, from the media as well as from health professionals. People also identify complex ways in which they manage their concerns about health and illness within their own personal understandings of the world and what is necessary to carry out their 'normal' daily routines.

Such decisions are influenced by their gender, their family responsibilities, age and cultural background. Blaxter (1990) identified differences in people's attitudes to their health at different times of their lives, with young men viewing health as physical fitness and middle aged people emphasizing the importance of mental and physical well being. Older people stress the importance of retaining physical functioning as well as seeing peace of mind and contentment regardless of levels of ill health. She found differences in social status in relation to people's ability to express their ideas about health in multidimensional ways.

Pill and Stott (1982) studied people's attitudes to ill health in a case study of working class women in Wales. They developed two broad categories:

- people who had a passive or 'fatalist' attitude towards their health status as something outside their direct control and who were content to accept the intervention of medical professionals when necessary; and

- people who viewed their health as something under their personal control and who were more likely to take actions to keep healthy as well as having a questioning attitude towards the interventions of health professionals.

Religious and other belief systems are often invoked to explain unexpected events including ill health and cure and they link to people's attitudes to their health status and to their attitudes to medical intervention.

Turner (1985) identifies distinct behaviour attached to when people decide to seek help and who they choose to seek help from. He describes the 'lay referral system', a process people may go through prior to seeking medical intervention. This included seeking advice from family and peers and others within their cultural systems.

Graham (1993) describes the reasons given for smoking among young mothers well aware of the negative health consequences of the activity. For them the short-term benefits of smoking as a stress reliever when coping with the care of young children in poor physical circumstances outweighed the longer-term effects. Studies of carers (Finch and Groves 1983) have repeatedly shown that they ignore their own symptoms of ill health in order to maintain their caring roles.

Studies of whole communities and their attitudes to health and well being are also part of the sociological tradition. Cornwall (1984) carried one significant study of community attitudes to health and illness in East London which illustrated the impact of historical perspectives and networks of support in influencing people's health behaviour.

Lay knowledge vs. medical knowledge

Williams and Poppay (2002) identify the epistemological and political challenges of lay perspectives in understanding their relationship with health professionals. They show that lay knowledge about health is a completely different kind of knowledge to that of medical knowledge.

Lay knowledge cannot be understood by using the positivistic tradition of research underpinning medicine, including public health medicine. The positivistic tradition is based on the ability to control conditions to isolate a variable to be understood and measured. It is essentially a reductive approach to knowledge and creates an 'objectification' of the patient as the object to be 'done to'. Traditionally the role of the 'patient' was one of acceptance of this role in exchange for the interventions of medical expertise (Stacey 1976). While this role acceptance is still common, particularly for short-term patient experience, it has been challenged by people with long-term contact with medical experts as alienating and denying the totality of their experience (Morris 1991; Oliver 1996). The impartiality of scientific knowledge has been increasingly challenged, concealing specific professional interests and not always serving the interests they purport to serve. In the new modernity (Beck 1992) there are many 'competing truths' which need to be continually negotiated and public health partnerships are no exception.

The key characteristic of lay perspectives is the variety and combination of factors they identify as influencing their decisions on health. The sociological studies highlighted above can suggest and illuminate some of the characteristics of lay perspectives, but can only suggest possible connections between social characteristics and individuals and are unable to give definitive predictions of how any one individual will understand their own health status. Lay perspectives must be researched using methods such as ethnography and narrative analysis, methods very different from those traditionally used within the positivistic tradition.

Medical perspectives on lay involvement

Why does the history of lay action on health show that it has remained outside mainstream thinking within the NHS? This section looks at medical perspectives, and identifies some of the obstacles to lay involvement in public health.

Medical epidemiology vs. lay epidemiology

Epidemiology is the main basis for public health knowledge and is defined in the Oxford English Dictionary as the science of understanding epidemics and diseases as they affect a given population. Lay perspectives on disease are acknowledged to be an important part of epidemiological research (Ben-Shlomo et al. 1996; Bartley et al. 1997) but there are acknowledged problems in accessing these views. Other issues such as how lay perspectives inform the agenda for research and, more importantly, their contribution to how the results of research are acted upon are crucial aspects of public health. Don Nutbeam (2002) commented that the UK had a world class reputation in describing public health concerns, but had demonstrated a very limited capacity to do much about them. Clearly involving lay perspectives in the search for effective measures of improving health is crucial.

Frankel et al. (1991) define lay epidemiology as: 'The process by which a person interprets health risk through routine observation and discussion of illness and death in personal networks and in the public arena as well as from formal and informal evidence arising from other sources such as television and magazines'. One might also add 'and through their contacts with health and other welfare professionals'.

Fundamentally, epidemiology is based on experimental research methods which seek to establish direct relations of causality between factors and in doing so explain the patterns of disease and ill health in any given population (see Chapter 15). The lay person's perspectives on health are complex and influenced by a host of other circumstances. They are difficult to evidence and research and so have remained marginalized and unrecognized within mainstream public health discourse. 'Lay epidemiology remains marginalised information scarcely recognised beyond sociology as legitimate knowledge. Despite most health professionals recognising that lay people have ideas about the causes of ill health, these ideas tend to be viewed as interesting, but irrational' (Moon *et al.* 2000).

The above quotes indicate the dominance of the biomedical model in controlling and limiting the discourse in public health. Lay views are not judged as significant within this discourse or, more significantly, their very diversity makes them difficult to identify using the traditions of positivism at the heart of epidemiology. Even when lay people are included in partnerships they will experience difficulties in getting their perspectives recognized and taken seriously. The tradition of the passive patient in receipt of expertise still influences the discourses of public health where the public are viewed as recipients of advice and expertise in relation to their health and lifestyles. Discourse within health care is littered with references to 'patient information', 'patient education' and 'patient compliance', implying that the only issue in relation to lay people using the NHS is to tackle their lack of understanding about health and health related issues as defined by biomedical discourse. The underlying assumption is that people are 'empty vessels to be filled' in relation to their health.

The dominance of the biomedical model

The underlying tensions of professionalism and the quest for exclusive expertise is a powerful factor in understanding the difficulties faced by lay people in public health partnerships. The biomedical model is concerned to reduce the encounter with the lay person, to isolate the problem to specific and achievable intervention within the sphere of specific medical expertise, so retaining the power and status in the encounter.

Even if the patient wants to work with a holistic view, wanting to understand the specific medical issue within the wider context of their lives, they find this blocked within the medical consultation. The result of these encounters, often taking place at a time of individual vulnerability, ensures that the public acquiesce to the dominant medical interpretation, they remain passive in relation to their own health and any views they have about their health remain within private and informal discourse.

GPs and primary care professionals, as the agencies of universal open access, are often at the 'sharp end' of this relationship, overloaded with people seeking expert advice for all kinds of health concerns, only some of which can be dealt with by medical intervention. Many have responded by prescribing medicines when they know that another type of support or service might be more appropriate. Or in referring on to other agencies they retain the separation between the medical intervention and other support which could influence health. The result of these encounters is to attain the goal of professionalism – for the public to see health as entirely defined by health professionals and to which they have little to contribute.

There is evidence to show that people will not feel able to express their real views in normal one off encounters with health professionals or in one off interviews, but need time and trust to open up (Hogg 1999). Attempts to stimulate discussion about health with lay people will often first focus on their concerns about current NHS services rather than ways in which they manage their own health (Taylor *et al.* 1998). Interviews with individuals about their health will tend to reproduce medical discourse or reflect medical definitions of their conditions even when this is not explicitly requested (Mykhalovskiy and McCoy 2002).

Another concern of the new policy agenda is to open up the public health arena to a wider range of professional groups outside the medical profession. If this is successful it may help youth workers, teachers, social workers and community development workers to bring a wider understanding of what constitutes public health action and to widen access to groupings of the population outside their role as patients. It could, however, lead instead to an increase in the army of public health specialists or experts who continue 'doing public health' to people who continue to be unrecognized as actors in the debate. However, research has shown that this kind of interprofessional and interagency working often leads to a greater awareness and willingness to include lay people and local communities as active and equal participants in the public health debate (Taylor *et al.* 1998).

User movements have clearly identified barriers which can result in lay people being marginalized by professionals in partnership working (Beresford and Croft 1993; Barnes 1997).

- *Defining the agenda* – lay people tend to respond to questions about health in terms defined by health professionals. They tend to be able to participate more easily in areas which are not already in a professional domain – hence the often heard comment from a professional involved in public consultation 'all they wanted to talk about was dog dirt'.

- *Education* – emphasis can be put on the need for the public to be educated in order to participate. While the public may need relevant information and support to participate, the 'finding out' process should be two way. This two way process can begin by attending to the use of professional jargon which can block all forms of partnership working.

- *Involvement as a therapeutic process* – seeing involvement as a way of letting people 'have their say' as an end in itself and a way of ticking monitoring sheets without any intention of taking lay views seriously.

- *Incorporation* – putting lay representatives onto committees and projects within the organization and absorbing them into the organizational culture and taking no interest in how these lay representatives can connect to the communities or interests they came from.

- *Exploiting* – expecting lay representatives to give their time and effort voluntarily without engaging with their need to be resourced in ways appropriate to their situations.

- *Dismissing and discounting* – lay people who are prepared to take part in consultations and long-term involvement being taken as unrepresentative and too articulate to represent the 'average' member of the public, without showing much interest in the experiences of lay people who have taken this route.

Williamson (1992) gives an excellent account of the way lay people seeking change within certain aspects of the NHS had to build up complex and coordinated campaigns to deal with these barriers, support people involved and build up strategic alliances with key people within the system who would act as advocates and create the right opportunities for the lay representatives to make their contribution most effectively. Increasingly some of these barriers have been recognized within the NHS in the new policy for public involvement and are now being recognized in good practice guidelines and in monitoring processes.

Promoting an effective lay contribution to public health

How can an effective lay contribution to public health be developed? First, it is helpful to consider the range of approaches to lay participation in public health, and the levels at which people are prepared to be involved.

Four approaches to public involvement

It is possible to identify four approaches to public involvement.

The consumerist approach
The first is a consumerist approach in which people are asked for their views on specific issues or services by those responsible for those services. This is focused on their specific relationship with the issue and service, and is often time limited with the boundaries decided by the service providers. It does not encourage any wider dialogue on health issues, but nevertheless may encourage an interest in greater participation if other opportunities exist to capture this (Winkler 1987; Lupton *et al.* 1998). Consumerist initiatives may take many forms from surveys and focus groups to patient panels and councils. They often attempt to address the issue of bias in their choice of participants.

The representatives approach
A second approach is the quasidemocratic approach of appointing public 'representatives' to sit on NHS trust boards and on different structures within health organizations. This supersedes the earlier inclusion of locally elected councillors on health authorities and in the past 20 years has been seen as a form of public accountability (Day and Klein 1987). The emphasis for these roles is to contribute to the development of their organization, by ensuring that public interests and perspectives are considered. The key issue for this kind of involvement is to ask how far these appointed 'representatives' are viewed as legitimate representatives by local communities and communities of interest and how well they can keep in touch with their communities.

These first two approaches lend themselves to an organizational agenda requiring specific evidence of public involvement. It allows the organization to define the terms of the encounter and be able to control the level of feedback

The interest group approach

A third approach is through the activities of organized interest groups who have an independent status, though this may be greatly influenced by the availability of funding. Such groups develop their own agendas which they then attempt to promote using whatever means available to them. They can be small self-help groups or part of a much larger network of groups within a national network or voluntary organization. Participants in these groups are likely to have developed skills over time in taking part in consultations and organized involvement events and may have developed their own research to underpin their perspectives.

As discussed in the earlier section, interest groups who challenge accepted professional opinions are often viewed by health professionals as unrepresentative and are seen as isolated and unconnected to wider 'public opinion'. However, another perspective may be that such groups represent the articulated tips of icebergs of public opinion which is hidden and undeveloped. Interest groups who may now seem well organized and articulate probably started as small groups of like minded people (often as informal discussion and self-help groups) which over time have developed into networks and larger organizations able to raise funding and lead campaigns for social change. They are interested in not only improving resources and services but often aim to change or transform society's attitudes to the issues they raise. They can be viewed as genuine tips of large icebergs of lay opinion. They are the public expression of much larger bodies of lay opinion which may still be difficult for individuals to fully articulate in their individual encounters with professionals. However, it remains a perfectly valid concern to check how far such groups are representative of more general public opinion. This can be done by surveys and other consumerist methods or it can be developed through the network approach identified below.

The network approach

A final approach to public involvement is to access the informal networks and activities within communities to find out the way people understand and live their lives and to find ways to help them articulate their perspectives and influence the development and delivery of services. Chapter 9 discusses the realities and spread of networks in greater detail and the ways in which they can be fostered and worked with. The need for public health to address inequalities as a priority implies that it needs to have good sources of information into all parts of local communities using as many information sources as possible.

Figure 8.1 provides a way of thinking about levels of public involvement. People come in and out of this kind of action as their personal circumstances allow. One individual has limited capacity to be active in all aspects of life so while they might be active in one issue they may be a non-participator in others, happy for others to speak on their behalf. However, the experience and skills built up in campaigning in one arena will broaden an individual's experience and knowledge of how 'things are done' and may lead to broader participation in other areas. Individual circumstances, wider opportunities, timing, attitudes and social support all influence an individual's

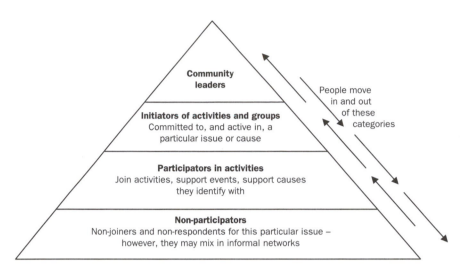

Figure 8.1 Levels of public involvement

decision to participate, as illustrated in the case study in Box 8.1. This level of activity within communities has been identified as 'social capital' and has recently been identified as important in promoting health and addressing inequalities (Gillies 1998c; Campbell *et al.* 1999). (Chapter 9 looks at social capital in more detail.)

Box 8.1 Case study example of lay involvement in public health

A young mothers' group on a housing estate has been meeting weekly at a local community centre for the past three years. The group was started by a local health visitor as a postnatal support group but has run independently for two years. There is a core group of eight women who maintain activities through an informal committee structure; about 25 other women attend the group with fluctuating levels of commitment. The group receive funding for their crèche worker from the local community association and are able to use the premises free of charge. The group raise funds for their activities by charging members, running a stall at the local community festival each year and doing occasional car boot sales. Over the past two years the group have organized children's activities and outings during the summer and Easter holidays and run a successful babysitting network. Their meetings alternate between organized sessions with speakers and informal coffee get togethers.

Individual members take part in other activities in the area and report back to the group. Several members attended an information session on the 'five a day' initiative (to encourage people to eat five portions of fruit and vegetables a day) at their children's school, run by the school nurse. When this was reported back to the group it stimulated a lot of discussion about the difficulties of buying affordable fresh food in their area. One of the mothers discussed this concern with the school nurse who put them in touch with a fruit and vegetable cooperative in a neighbouring town. After a group visit to this coop several members of the group became enthusiastic about starting a similar one on their estate. Five women from the group are now working with other people from the community association, two local farmers and the local allotment group to set up this initiative and have recently run a one off 'farmers' market' to publicize their project.

This work on healthy food has stimulated a more general interest in health. A small sub-group have begun to support each other to lose weight and take regular exercise, committing themselves to a 'weigh in' (known in the group as the 'naming and shaming session') each month; this has been a great success, with the sub-group gaining more members as weight goals were reached. At one of the meetings two of the slimming group commented that now they are exercising regularly they are feeling the effects of their smoking. This stimulated a heated debate about smoking and whether people should believe all the publicity about smoking and health.

The group decided to approach the local health centre to ask a GP to come and speak at their meeting. The GPs passed on the request to their health visitors, one of whom offered to go along to the group. But her colleagues were concerned that in the current climate of staff shortages they should not take on new work. Instead, they decided to send information to the group about the smoking cessation clinic which runs at the health centre every Tuesday evening and where new clients would be welcome.

The group received this response with comments like, 'I told you those doctors aren't interested in our estate', 'You wouldn't catch me going to the health centre when it isn't necessary', 'How can I get out on Tuesday evening with two small children to look after' and 'I'm not keen on going out after dark'. The subject of smoking was dropped and the group moved on to planning their summer outings. The original slimmer who raised the topic decided to use the babysitting network and to go to the clinic, but not to tell the others of her decision at this stage.

This case study illustrates

- the way in which health awareness was built up incrementally in this group of lay people;
- the group as a mechanism for informal discussion and information processing as well as a focus for organizing activities;
- the importance of building up skills based on what people feel they can do and are interested in within a 'safe' environment of trust and with people in the same situation;
- the acceptance of different levels of involvement for different issues; and
- the impact of contact with health professionals.

Conclusion – challenges and opportunities

This chapter has attempted to demonstrate that lay perspectives have always been integral to public health and historically have had greater recognition. As discussed in the sections on lay and medical perspectives on involvement, there are many and often conflicting opinions on what influences health improvement. The power of biomedical discourse in defining the terms of engagement for health and illness is a significant barrier for lay participation in health improvement. It both limits the boundaries of discourse in health and further seeks to control and limit any efforts made to link lay perspectives into the public debates about health and illness.

This chapter has offered a framework of four approaches to public involvement and has tried to identify and explain the connections between them. In using any one approach it is important to understand what the other approaches might offer. Anyone seeking to understand what lay perspectives have to offer public health may need to realize that lay perspectives are likely to be hidden and outside the public domain except where there has been concerted attempts to bring the lay perspective into the public arena through campaigning and the action of self-help, voluntary and community organizations. Inevitably these will be partial and sporadic – often the tips of much bigger icebergs of less articulated lay opinion and sometimes, though this chapter would argue less often, just unconnected pieces of driftwood, run by individuals without clear public support. Rather than make an instant judgement about whether these peaks of lay activity have any connection with what would be expressed by an individual in conversation with their health visitor or GP, it is important for more public health professionals to know how to check the links back into local communities. Public health needs to have clear strategies to link into networks and informal activities of local communities.

There are, of course, resource issues which need addressing. A constant concern for all lay activists is finding the resources, support and time to sustain their activities. They struggle to find people to become involved and willing to stay involved. Lay activity is sustained by an ever changing group of people who come in and out of involvement as their circumstances allow. Varied and diverse opportunities need to exist to maximize lay activity so that people can engage in particular areas of interest like the state of the pavements or the lack of fresh vegetables. Grassroot professionals who have day to day dealings with local people are an obvious resource for public health to access lay views if they are prepared to be open, non-judgemental and to listen. We have also outlined in this chapter that the inhibitions that local people may feel towards service providers, especially when they are particularly vulnerable or dependent, require consideration for professionals wanting to develop their access to lay views.

Developing an effective lay contribution poses challenges for people engaged in multidisciplinary public health. Health professionals must be able to understand, value and respect the way lay perspectives interact with professional interventions for individuals and communities in relation to health and illness. This must first involve medical professionals in accepting the political challenge to their traditional power to define and determine health knowledge and information. They must be prepared to accept and work in partnership with lay perspectives and those of other professionals to ensure that health interventions and health improvement can be made effective. It remains to be seen if the new arrangements for public involvement discussed at the beginning of this chapter will offer realistic opportunities for the range of lay perspectives needed for public health to be developed.

9

ALISON GILCHRIST
Community development and networking for health

Editors' introduction

Evidence suggests that people's social environment and the quality and diversity of their informal networks are important for their health. This chapter describes the role of networks within the voluntary and community sectors. It particularly looks at the role of networks in building 'social capital' and community participation in order to strengthen the community sector's contribution to partnership working. It provides helpful insights into social networks which will be of value to all public health workers who work with and for communities.

The author describes the nature of networks within communities and identifies the role they play in helping people share information, make sense of their experiences and articulate their collective needs. Understanding and nurturing personal and informal networks (weak ties) outside family and personal friendships (strong ties) is an essential prerequisite to community participation.

Networking is an integral part of many people's practice in paid and voluntary work, and is an essential feature of all aspects of partnership working. Community development practice and value base recognize the importance of networks within communities. Community development workers can connect 'weak tie' networks to foster greater cohesion and cooperation as well as countering the more negative aspects of elitism and exclusivity that can be characteristics of networks.

The author moves on to consider the way that social networks promote people's health by strengthening social relationships and combating social isolation, and how an understanding of networks can assist health promotion activity. She distinguishes between the activities that promote 'top-down' agendas and those that work with existing community generated concerns. Voluntary organizations, community groups and self-help activities are often underpinned by strong informal networks and these organizations will represent community and service user interests in partnerships. Opportunities for networking are stimulated by events and environments which encourage regular informal contact and interaction.

The author concludes by identifying the skills and activities necessary to promote and utilize networks. People with the responsibilities for fostering networks need to be able to work across organizational boundaries and have the skills and confidence to work in informal and unstructured ways, managing multiple accountabilities and issues of confidentiality.

Introduction

Public health has both personal and collective dimensions, reflecting individual as well as social circumstances and choices. The concept of 'community', although problematic in sociological and policy terms (Hoggett 1997; Nash 2002), similarly encapsulates the idea that people's behaviour and well being is influenced by interactions with others. Informal social networks contribute significantly to our quality of life, shaping our identities and sense of belonging, while enhancing many aspects of our health.

This chapter considers how networks provide important foundations for public health strategies, and argues that simply strengthening and diversifying social networks will improve health, as well as making health provision more effective. It explores the links between social capital, networks and community development, examining recent evidence connecting the quality of a person's relationships and social interaction with their levels of health. The chapter describes the role of networks within the voluntary and community sectors and, in particular, it looks at how networking is used to encourage community participation and to improve partnership working.

The concept of social capital

There has been a growing interest in the concept of 'social capital', a term first coined by Harifan (1916), and elaborated since then most notably by Jacobs (1961), Bourdieu (1993) and Putnam (2000). While there has been considerable discussion around the theoretical content of social capital and its application in practice (see for example Portes 1998; Fine 1999; Schuller *et al.* 2000), there is broad agreement that its core components consist of the 'shared understandings, levels of trust, associational memberships and informal networks of human relationships that facilitate social exchange, social order and underpin social institutions' (Richardson and Mumford 2002: 206). Some interpretations emphasize emotional aspects of these relationships, such as trust and mutuality, while others place more importance on processes of community participation and civic engagement. For the purposes of this chapter, social capital will be considered as a collective resource which is generated and maintained through networking interactions and voluntary associations, unmediated by formal contracts or financial exchange. The term displays considerable overlap with the concept of 'community' and it is no coincidence that a policy environment awash with 'community involvement initiatives' displays such a keen interest in the ideas of social capital (Halpern 2003 forthcoming).

Networks and community participation

Personal networks are vital to the sustainability and effectiveness of the community sector and community life generally. Informal connections create a web of links and relationships which support communication and cooperation between organizations and agencies and enable better coordination of community activity.

Networks are evolving configurations in which some participants cluster together (like families or members of a community group) forming dense linkages based on bonds of kinship and friendship. Other links operate across the whole network, forming 'bridges' between different sections of the community or between organizations. Granovetter (1973) makes a distinction between 'weak ties' and 'strong ties' among individuals who know each other very well. (Figure 9.1 shows this web of links diagrammatically.) Health professionals and social workers are more concerned with the latter, while community workers and activists often function as the 'weak tie' mechanisms which allow information, support and resources to be shared across boundaries. It is these that provide the basis for collective action and alliances, whether through formally constituted organizations or informal conversation and exchanges.

Our experience of 'community' is derived from these looser networks of neighbours, colleagues and fellow activists or associates (Wellman 1979), rather than more traditional (but often non-existent or overly intrusive) family connections. Social networks are used to identify and articulate collective needs and aspirations. People talk with one another, reflecting on their experience to share grievances, dreams and fears. They learn about different ways of seeing the world, new explanations for problems and, consequently, gain ideas for changing the status quo. This might involve taking risks in challenging vested interests or conventional ways of working. Networks help to spread the risk and enable people to anticipate potential obstacles or consequences by drawing on a wider range of perspectives. Networking builds trust and a sense of mutuality. It allows people to appreciate differences while also shaping people's sense of collective identity, building common cause and mobilizing resources for joint action (Marwell and Oliver 1993; Klandermans 1997).

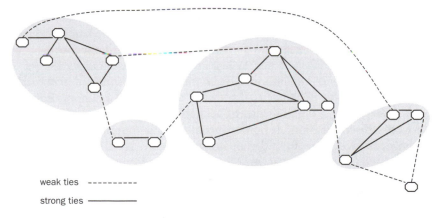

Figure 9.1 Diagrammatic representation of a network

People are largely recruited to community activities and volunteering through word of mouth or knowing someone who is already involved. They may develop their social networks through such activities. Indeed, this is often given as a reason for volunteering or joining clubs especially when people's circumstances change or they move to a new area. The 'grapevine' is a wonderful source of information about what is going on in people's lives, and it allows 'private' issues to emerge into the public arena. Relationships among people active in the voluntary sector have been revealed as important channels for influencing policy, for easing the sharing of facilities, for coordinating work and even for finding members of management committees (Taylor and Hoggett 1994). Effective community leaders are observed to have strong social networks, ensuring that they receive the support and feedback they need, and are held accountable by the people they claim to represent (Purdue et al. 2000).

However, networks can also perpetuate elite positions and exclude others from decision making (Skelcher et al. 1996). There is some evidence that participation in community activities has unhealthy consequences, for example, through stress, 'burn out' and feelings of helplessness when things go wrong or communities come up against intransigent authorities (Cattell and Herring 2002). Community leaders sometimes find themselves resented by other residents or undermined by rivals (Richardson and Mumford 2002). Strong social capital can be divisive, maintaining the dominant status of an established community against incomers. Conflicts and tensions within communities are well documented, though not so commonly recognized within policy pronouncements and practice guidelines. These antagonisms frequently arise as a result of different or competing lifestyles, and more powerful groups can unfairly occupy communal space and facilities. These forms of institutional discrimination are often unwitting, reflecting local norms and prevailing cultures, rather than deliberate intentions to exclude. Such inequalities can be tackled by proactive networking to develop positive and more tolerant relationships.

The 'community' dimension to health

There is an accumulating body of evidence suggesting that people's social environment (the quality and diversity of their informal networks) is an important determinant of actual and perceived health (Pilisuk and Parks 1986; Campbell et al. 1999). In recent years this approach has focused on economic inequalities (Wilkinson 1996; Kawachi et al. 1997; Acheson 1998) and social capital (Gillies 1998c; Cooper et al. 1999). As David Evans and Murray Stewart examine in their respective chapters on inequalities (Chapter 10), and regeneration and neighbourhood renewal strategies (Chapter 11), the government acknowledges that social exclusion, arising from poverty, discrimination and other life hazards is correlated with poor health. Wilkinson's research powerfully demonstrates that this is in part linked to relative income levels within a given (national) population, and he suggests that it might be due to the associated stress and discontent experienced by poorer sections of society who witness the relative wealth of their counterparts, but feel they can do little to close the gap (Wilkinson 1996, 2000).

Three recent government reports similarly make links between poverty and health inequalities, but suggest that this might arise from the varying quality of health provision across the country (Townsend *et al.* 1992) or to differential access to services between different areas or communities (Acheson 1998; Department of Health 1999a). Patterns of health are affected by factors such as physical impairment, mental distress, age and even the class status of previous generations. Smaje (1996) and Nazroo (1997) explore possible explanations of ethnic inequalities in health, including residence, culture, socio-economic status and genetic propensities. Issues around institutional racism also need to be considered (Macpherson 1998). Government policy has emphasized the importance of improving the quality of life for disadvantaged communities by reducing the gap between deprived areas and the average for the country as a whole (Social Exclusion Unit 2000).

A number of dissenting or more sceptical views argue that the case for a causal link between social capital and health has not yet been proven, and the correlation between such measures may reflect social and economic factors (Hawe and Shiell 2000). Evidence of an apparent decline in social capital in industrialized countries (which tends to be blamed on cultural factors) could equally be attributed to the negative impact of social and economic policies that erode collective solidarity, undermine public services and increase relative poverty. Each of these tendencies is likely to increase stress and isolation as well as having a deleterious effect on people's health and their willingness to develop trusting and cooperative relationships with people beyond the immediate circle of family and friends (Lupton and Power 2002).

However, those studies that have looked at the quality of people's informal networks and their participation in community life have discovered a clear link between these and levels of reported health. In a review of studies looking at early experiences within the family, Stewart-Brown *et al.* (2002) found that good quality relationships within the childhood household reduced their susceptibility to disease in later life. Green and Grimsley (2002) demonstrated that 'neighbourly' people and those who feel safe in their homes score higher in health self-assessment questionnaires. While the evidence for a meso-level explanation for health inequalities is more compelling for individuals than for whole communities, nevertheless the Health Development Agency was sufficiently persuaded to fund a programme of qualitative research examining the links between social capital and health – and this generated or encouraged the research cited above (Swann and Morgan 2002).

Promoting health 'in the community'

Well before these new developments in theory, public health professionals have recognized the value of a community-based approach and have looked to community development to provide them with tools and techniques for health education and health promotion projects (Labonte 1998).

Different approaches to health promotion are summarized in Figure 9.2. These approaches often take the form of services reaching out to or located in communities as a means of breaking down the formal boundaries between institutions and 'users'. Such schemes tend to work to an agenda set by health professionals or government priorities, but they may be designed and delivered according to the needs and wishes

Decision making	Mode of intervention	Example
Top–down	Service delivery	User involvement on mainstream partnerships
	Outreach services	Community-based clinic, home visiting
	Health education	Talks and material given to community groups
	Community development	Action research, setting up community led activities
Bottom–up	Collective action	Campaigns and user empowerment methods

Figure 9.2 Different approaches to health promotion

of the targeted populations. Two examples illustrate this approach: a campaign to raise awareness of heart disease among Asian people, and outreach work to schools and youth clubs by teenage mothers. Both of these are intended to increase people's knowledge of the risks involved in certain behaviours, with an expectation that habits will change as a result. Such health initiatives tend to be dominated by a medical discourse, using a deficit model which assumes that health problems occur because of some failing on the part of individuals or communities. Work programmes and spending priorities are disproportionately dominated by the views of the medical professions, bolstered by their own close networks and organizational culture.

In contrast, a community development approach would prioritize issues identified by communities themselves and seek holistic improvements in the quality of people's lives that indirectly would result in better health. Examples from this model might include the establishment of a community transport scheme, supporting an allotment association, campaigns for environmental improvement such as reducing the levels of dog dirt in the local park and helping a tenants group to persuade an intransigent landlord to carry out vital repairs to their homes. Achieving these would be important to the individuals, but the experience of working together, learning new skills and overcoming a sense of powerlessness might be just as significant for the long-term health of the community and its members.

Social networks sustain collective activity and informal mutual aid. By definition, they are rich in social capital and enhance people's health by strengthening the social relations between people. A community development approach to health is concerned not only with strengthening the 'strong ties' (between family, friends and neighbours), but also with nurturing the 'weak ties', ensuring that community members have access to facilities, information and influence beyond the normal boundaries. This is especially important for communities that experience high levels of deprivation and include many people who are socially excluded due to poverty or oppression. Working with individuals to boost their self-esteem, to improve confidence in social settings and to coax them out of, sometimes self-imposed, isolation is especially important for people with mental health problems or who enjoy only intermittent good health.

Community development and networking for health

In this context, community development is based on practices and policies that strengthen and extend people's networks, promote better health for individuals and benefit society as a whole (Campbell and Jovchelovitch 2000). Community development is usually understood to mean a professional intervention that helps people to help themselves by encouraging them to set up or be involved in collective activities which address shared problems or achieve some common goal.

As well as a range of useful methods of working with communities, community development incorporates key commitments and values as to *how* practitioners work with people and agreed principles about processes and outcomes. Perhaps the most significant among these is the need to address inequalities so as to ensure that more people are able to influence decisions that affect their lives. It is crucial that networking is used, not to perpetuate power and privilege among an elite group, but to open up channels of influence and allow for a more equitable distribution of resources. Empowerment is not merely a rhetorical term (which has become degraded through over use), but stands as a central goal of community development practice, tackling the disadvantage and discrimination that prevent people from achieving their potential. This applies to the fields of education, regeneration, employment and cultural activities as much as to health, and has important implications for professionals working for community benefit within and across all these policy areas. There is increasing emphasis for health improvements to be gained

Definition	Core values	Commitments
➤ Community development is about building active and sustainable communities based on social justice and mutual respect. ➤ It is about changing power structures to remove the barriers that prevent people from participating in the issues that affect their lives.	➤ Social justice ➤ Participation ➤ Equality ➤ Learning ➤ Cooperation	➤ Challenging discrimination and oppression. ➤ Encouraging networking. ➤ Ensuring access and choice-for-all groups. ➤ Influencing policy from community perspectives. ➤ Prioritizing concerns of people experiencing poverty and exclusion. ➤ Promoting long-term sustainable change. ➤ Reversing inequality and power imbalances. ➤ Protecting the environment.

Figure 9.3 Community development, core values and commitments
Source: Standing Conference for Community Development (SCCD) (2001)

through interdisciplinary, multiagency partnerships that have strong levels of community involvement, hence the importance of promoting networks which work across organizational boundaries.

Communities can be seen as complex and dynamic systems, in a state of constant flux and with boundaries only 'fuzzily' defined by the connections between informal networks. It is neither possible nor desirable to superimpose more formal structures on this web of unchoreographed interaction and spontaneous self-organization. Network models of organization are well suited to such turbulent environments, since tightly managed programmes accountable through more formal hierarchies tend to stifle the essence of an effective community, namely its vibrancy and flexibility (Gilchrist 2001). Health promotion strategies should support and complement community led initiatives, thereby invigorating community networks. This takes time and depends on long-term investment in generic community practitioners who can support a multiplicity of groups and activities, rather than just focusing on short-term or externally designed interventions.

Networking and partnerships

This broad approach has been incorporated into a raft of strategies and indicators, many of which are being implemented through interprofessional partnerships with a commitment to community participation. Multidisciplinary approaches to health improvement are relatively unfamiliar to most health workers but the experience of the health action zones (HAZs) indicates that much can be achieved by working across organizational and professional boundaries, despite initial difficulties and misunderstandings.

Building relationships

Multiagency working is found to be considerably easier if trusting relationships exist between the people involved (Goss and Kent 1995; Means *et al.* 1997). By facilitating more effective partnership working, networking contributes to directly measurable outcomes because it reduces duplication and unhelpful antagonisms. Informal conversation enables partners and participants to anticipate where opinions are likely to diverge, and to pre-empt tensions by suggesting possible forms of negotiation or compromise. Dissenting views are accommodated by developing new forms of service delivery or finding ways around apparent obstacles to joint working. Research indicates that networking can be effective in developing user or community orientated partnerships in service delivery (Beresford and Trevillion 1995; Taylor 1997).

Learning about other people's cultures and histories is an important aspect of networking, enabling people to empathize with perspectives which are different from their own and to operate appropriately in different settings. Being aware of suspicions and assumptions that may exist across the community–institution boundary usually ensures that conflicts can be anticipated, clarified and resolved quickly. As well as more formal arrangements, cooperation between organizations relies on a regular and reciprocal exchange of information, favours and occasionally resources. This cannot be arrived at overnight or through paper memoranda. It involves a more organic process of developing linkages between individuals, understanding different organizational cultures and addressing disagreements as and when they arise.

Building bridges across community barriers

Recent government policy has demanded a much stronger role for community representatives and for people who work in the voluntary and community sectors whether on a voluntary basis or as paid professionals. Such arrangements are fraught with difficulty, requiring major shifts in attitude and practice from all concerned if these partnerships are to operate on a truly equal and participatory basis (Hastings *et al.* 1996).

Health practitioners need to understand and work with informal networks, encouraging them to 'build bridges' across community boundaries and to use informal networking to select and support representatives who can express community views (Mondros and Wilson 1994). Networks enable community members to succeed in these roles, to build links with people operating in other sectors and to develop the confidence and status to challenge some of the power inequalities which exist between communities and statutory institutions, or within communities themselves.

Partnership working demands clarity of purpose alongside a willingness to respond to divergent interests, not least within local communities. Some of the recurring problems in cross-sectoral partnerships arise because of differences in the ways that communities operate, and the mismatch between their more fluid structures and processes, and the rigid protocols of formal institutions.

Power relationships

Numerous studies have shown that being connected to powerful individuals or agencies is itself a form of power (Laumann and Pappi 1976; Knoke 1990) and power relations are an important, although often neglected, aspect of social capital (Baum 2000). Consultation exercises can be enriched but also distorted by influential networks organizing to express particular views. Community representatives on partnership bodies benefit from being supported by formal democratic networks as well as through their informal connections in the community. Networks inevitably reflect personal circumstances and preferences as well as inequalities in our society. These biases need to be countered through positive action measures or, at the very least, acknowledged in formal deliberations and through proper accountability mechanisms.

Participation

In Chapter 8, Pat Taylor examines the contribution of lay people in greater detail and explores the value of community participation in the health service. It is worth remembering that individuals taking on the role of lay representative usually arrive in this position through participation in the voluntary and community sector, and that their expertise and legitimacy is derived from this. People can be encouraged to participate in community or civil activities if they feel their contributions will be valued and that there is a balance between what they give and what they get from their involvement. Participation can be seen as having three complementary interpretations in the current policy framework. It is about:

- taking part in communal activities as a citizen, a volunteer or community member;

- organizing collectively to deliver services through some kind of voluntary or self-help organization; or

- contributing as a lay person or service user to consultation exercises or to the decision making of partnership bodies as a representative of a particular community.

The community and voluntary sectors

General community activity is important in its own right but it is also the basis for community involvement in partnerships or consultation exercises (Taylor 1995). Just as people are persuaded to take part in communal activities and to serve on committees through their informal networks rather than through formal invitation, so networks are used to select representatives on more formal decision-making mechanisms. Community development is about empowerment, and network membership is an advantage for people wishing to influence policy or local democracy.

Community and voluntary organizations

Community-based activities take many forms. They may be organized by the local branches of national voluntary organizations to provide support, information and advocacy around specific illnesses or impairments. Well known examples include the National Schizophrenia Fellowship (now renamed Rethink) and the Terrence Higgins Trust, supporting people living with HIV/AIDS. These organizations offer care, advice and sometimes lobbying activities for people outside the auspices of the formal medical system. There are also many examples of groups which have formed around specific causes, such as to raise funds for equipment at their local hospice or to pay for pioneering treatment for a member of their own community. We have seen instances of groups organizing to send children abroad for transplants or for innovative (and as yet unproven) 'treatment' for various disorders.

Other bodies adopt a more overtly political stance, challenging medical orthodoxy or campaigning against the influence of the medical model of disability. Organizations of Disabled people have been particularly vociferous in this respect, arguing that they should receive help to meet their specific requirement as a right, rather than through charity or at the discretion of health professionals (Oliver and Barnes 1998). Their success in building alliances, uniting people with different impairments, has led to a greater understanding of the social model of disability, and awareness of the discrimination that Disabled people experience in all aspects of their lives. Networks are crucial to the effectiveness of modern 'user' led social movements, fostering solidarity and mobilizing for political change (Tarrow 1994).

Most voluntary organizations were established to highlight a perceived gap in provision or to address an injustice. The independence of the sector is therefore crucial to the ability of such bodies to represent the needs of their members and, where necessary, champion their rights. In the UK, the mixed economy of health depends on this pluralist model but it is based on a paradox. While many charities now receive government grants to provide important services in the community, they must try to remain relatively autonomous in order to preserve their campaigning role.

Indirect health outcomes

As well as the larger, well established voluntary organizations (which are often managed and run by paid professionals), there exist myriad groups and local organizations that make a contribution to health within neighbourhoods and communities of interest. Some of these provide self-help activities with an explicit focus on a particular illness (such as addiction); many are patient or 'survivor' support groups to be found through the Internet. There are also thousands of organizations that actively promote healthy living, for example, through keep fit classes and food coops. Many groups have a more tangential impact on health through activities which indirectly maintain both physical and mental health. These include sports and cultural associations, encouraging people to come together to run, dance, play games, sing and so on. There are obvious physical benefits, but also psychological benefits through the enhanced interaction and improved social networks that are developed as a result (Argyle 1996b).

Although some health centres are beginning to resurrect the 'Peckham experiment' (Pearce and Crocker 1943) by providing or prescribing activities for their patients, this preventative function of community participation is still undervalued by the formal health sector. One reason for this resistance is the paucity of scientific evidence from action research or project evaluation. It has not been easy to demonstrate links between the intangible processes of community networking and health outcomes. As a consequence there is plenty of anecdotal support for a positive link, but only limited and somewhat ambivalent hard evidence (Blaxter and Poland 2002). There is certainly more scope for communities to be involved in investigating the impact of social capital on health from their own experiences and perspectives, perhaps using methods of participatory appraisal and action research approaches as outlined in the LEAP framework described by Stuart Hashagen in Chapter 17.

Community networks and health

Empirical research indicates that relationships and regular interaction with others protects individuals against disease and mental distress. People with robust and diverse networks lead healthier and happier lives than those who are more isolated or whose networks are comparatively homogenous (Argyle 1989, 1996a; Yen and Syme 1999). They have stronger immune systems, suffer less from heart disease, recover more quickly from emotional traumas such as bereavement, and seem to be more resistant to the debilitating effects of illness, possibly because of some kind of emotional buffer which gives them a more positive outlook on life generally (Pilisuk and Parks 1986; Blane *et al.* 1996; Kawachi 1997). While the physiological mechanisms for this resilience are unclear, it is probable that social networks provide a variety of forms of support and affirmation, including practical advice around health matters. They may also maintain individuals in a more active lifestyle. Overall the evidence is not conclusive and relies to an extent on individual self-assessment of health, which tends to reflect a generalized sense of well being. It has been suggested that surveys purporting to demonstrate correlation between health and social capital are presenting tautological findings (Blaxter and Poland 2002).

However, the effect of peer pressure and social activities (especially for young people) in supporting unhealthy habits should not be underestimated, for example, in relation to unsafe sex, smoking or other forms of drug use, including alcohol abuse (Morrow 2002). Adolescent social networks have been implicated in the transmission of psychogenic epidemics, such as hysterical rashes or respiratory problems. Nevertheless, a positive association seems to exist between a person's social networks and their health. Informal conversations within trusting and egalitarian relationships supply non-stigmatized advice concerning medical or emotional matters, acting as a user friendly referral system (Hornby 1993). It is known that people will seek information from non-professional sources about difficult or risky issues before they will approach the appropriate agencies (Gabarino 1983). This understanding lays the basis for peer education methods and self-help projects, such as the tentative interest in men's health groups. Having knowledgeable people within one's social network is useful, assuming of course that any enquiries will be treated in confidence and not form the basis for gossip or disapproval. Similarly, role models and supporters can bolster self-esteem, enabling people to cope better during periods of distress and disaster. Neighbourhood networks provide practical assistance with a variety of tasks (Henning and Lieberg 1996; Williams and Windebank 2000) and family members can usually be relied on during a crisis and for long-term care (Bulmer 1987).

Notions of independence, personal pride and reciprocity are significant aspects of people's willingness to accept help, and it is these aspects of networking which deserve greater attention from health professionals. Relationships flourish when there is a balance of giving and receiving (Duck 1992). The 'gifted' time and skills of community members must be affirmed and encouraged by recognizing that volunteers, activists and carers are not merely unpaid staff, but individuals with needs, talents and sometimes considerable expertise.

Networking in practice

Networking is an ancient, perhaps instinctive feature of human societies, but the term has been over used in recent years, acquiring pejorative connotations as being manipulative and self-serving. I use the word more neutrally here to mean the practice of initiating, maintaining and using connections and relationships between individuals and between organizations.

Networking across boundaries should be recognized as difficult and sometimes risky work often requiring considerable ingenuity to find a connection or to step into unfamiliar cultural or organizational territory. Networking supports participation generally and can be used to reach and involve marginalized sections of the population. In particular, networking that is informed by an active commitment to inclusion, equality and anti-oppressive practices helps to build bridges and tackle barriers to participation. Working to extend and mend the weak ties across community and agency boundaries will promote greater integration and ultimately improve service delivery. This is important for achieving the government's neighbourhood renewal goals as well as its agenda around citizenship, civic renewal and community cohesion.

Informal networks are part of the infrastructure and capacity of communities and can be developed (or eroded) through skilful interventions and activities. In many areas, networks might appear to evolve and function 'naturally' without any obvious forms of support or intervention. Often these localities enjoy population stability and benefit from a history of collective organizing (Taylor 1995; Cattell and Herring 2002). They contain individuals who are skilled organizers or intuitive networkers, who seem to know everyone and have the knack of putting the right people in touch with one another. They do not necessarily occupy visible 'leadership' roles, but rather operate behind the scenes, soothing ruffled feathers, resolving conflicts, signposting others to the resources they need and generally acting as both 'connectors' and 'catalysts' to generate and maintain collective action (Gilchrist 1998). Such people are often unpaid and unproclaimed and yet their hidden networking is what weaves and mends the fabric of community life, especially in areas experiencing high levels of deprivation and population mobility where there may be a high proportion of individuals experiencing isolation, low self-esteem and mental health difficulties due to social exclusion. These communities are more likely to benefit from professional help from community-based practitioners who can support their networking and help people to organize collective action.

Skills of networking

Networking should be considered as a skilled and strategic aspect of community practice. It features strongly in the jobs or voluntary activity of many people working in communities (Gilchrist 2003). Networking to develop 'community' is not primarily about individuals using (and sometimes abusing) their connections with others. A recent research study looked at the skills and personal qualities that characterized effective networkers (Gilchrist 2001). It also examined the ethics of networking for community development and the strategies that community workers used in their practice to encourage networking among the people they worked with as well as to foster good working relationships between organizations. These have been dubbed 'the 11 Ms of networking' (Gilchrist 1998) – see Figure 9.4.

The study found that good networkers are gregarious, compassionate, curious about cultures other than their own, generous with their time and attention, diplomatic and sensitive to the emotional and political dynamics of situations. Networkers are well organized, preparing themselves for different settings and following up conversations reliably so that trust and mutual respect develop. Networkers are able to assimilate information from a variety of sources and to communicate in a range of styles and modes. They are versatile and flexible in their approach, able to seize

Mapping	Finding out who else might have an interest in a particular issue; gathering information about them, including existing connections.
Making contacts	Introducing oneself and organization; making referrals.
Maintaining connections	Organizing meetings; sending out information bulletins; keeping up-to-date records of names and contact details for key individuals.
Managing the web	Servicing networks; making sure that power and inclusion issues are addressed.
Monitoring changes	Introducing and inducting new 'players'; adjusting to shifts on the policy agenda or concerns arising in the community.
Mending	Identifying ruptures in the networks and addressing gaps that emerge through people leaving.
Merging	Helping separate groupings to recognize their common or overlapping interests; setting up joint organizational arrangements.
Mediating	Dealing with conflicts and misunderstandings; challenging prejudices and apprehensions.
Motivating	Persuading and encouraging people to link up with others; encouraging people to take on responsibilities and new roles.
Mobilizing	Using the network to form alliances and get involved in collective action.
Moving on	Making sure that network members have the confidence, information and support they need to sustain their own connections with one another.

Figure 9.4 Actions that facilitate and maintain networks

opportunities and use their imagination to conjure up exciting and innovative combinations, or simply to suggest interesting links between people from quite diverse backgrounds. Networkers demonstrate a confident awareness of self, and are able to convey their own identity and personal value system without being overassertive or arrogant. They appear non-judgemental in their attitudes, open to criticism but also willing to challenge unfair or inefficient practices. They value their autonomy, welcome opportunities to use their own initiative and consequently are less tolerant of organizational constraints, such as those imposed by bureaucratic procedures.

In many respects, networkers demonstrate the qualities of transformational leaders and social entrepreneurs in their ability to engender trust through their work in maintaining authentic relationships whether through formal arrangements or informal interaction (Bennis 1988).

Networking strategies

Networking strategies include taking particular care during the early phase of any potential relationship, thinking about self-presentation, using non-verbal cues to identify potential points of similarity and difference, and listening attentively to what the other person is saying. The initial contact often takes courage and networkers are assiduous in seeking out informal opportunities for conversation where the views divulged are more likely to express someone's real rather than official opinion.

Making space for humour and serendipity on these occasions is useful for opening up dialogue and allows unexpected connections to be made. Networkers consciously monitor the holes and breaches in the web, moving to plug gaps and mend severed ties.

Within community development, networkers also need to think about the principles of equality and empowerment, ensuring that the contacts they make address power differentials and that their networks reflect the diversity of the population around them, rather than their own interests and preferences. Personal passion and affinity will inevitably characterize one's networking practice, but these can be countered through a proactive and brave stance in building the more difficult or unfamiliar links.

Factors which influence community networking

The interactions of everyday life are vital to the growth of community networks. Many of these take place in quasi-public spaces, such as outside schools, around the local shops and in pubs or parks. Measures, such as alley-gating, which change the layout of neighbourhoods (and therefore the routes people take to local amenities) increase levels of social networking. This has been shown to enhance self-esteem among residents and is associated with decreases in depression, anxiety and other mental health problems.

The quality of a built environment can have a huge impact on the nature of casual interactions, for example, whether places feel safe, accessible and welcoming to everyone who wishes to use them. They are often areas where people from different backgrounds mingle, but may also feel territorial as if available only to certain sections of the population. Wherever possible this should be challenged, perhaps through cultural activities such as street festivals or murals.

Networking is facilitated by events that bring people together in semi-structured activity encouraging people who might not otherwise talk to one another to discover common interests.

Working at the margins of organizations and across the edges of networks that are aligned but not overlapping is important and can help communities to deal constructively with their own divisions by becoming more tolerant and cohesive, thus contributing to people's health and sense of well being (Stafford *et al*. 2002). This can be a difficult role in which workers face dilemmas around multiple accountability and confidentiality. Flexibility and honesty are needed to manage complex and diverse networks of relationships, but investment in such work pays significant dividends for public health.

Conclusions

Networking is an important tool for the modern welfare agenda. It is vital to the effective operation of multiagency partnerships, especially those involving people from very different disciplines and sectors. Extensive networks allow the identification and recruitment of useful allies and potential partners.

Informal interaction associated with meetings, training and other joint events will encourage the development of mutual understanding and respect, making it easier to explore and resolve conflicts, to reach consensus or compromise where necessary, and to clarify aims and objectives as these inevitably change over time. Networking encourages community participation in formal consultation and programme delivery, as well as in activities that nurture informal networks and release social capital.

Although it is proving hard to trace a causal relationship between social networks and health, community development experience indicates that people who feel connected, rather than isolated or excluded, tend to engage more in communal activities and to report that they feel more healthy as a consequence. The evidence briefly reviewed above suggests that these subjective feelings can be translated into objective statistics in morbidity and mortality levels, but more quantitative and qualitative research is needed to substantiate the 'community' dimension of health.

Acknowledgements

I would like to thank Amanda Inverarity, Janet Muir, Fiona Crawford, Paul Henderson and Thara Raj for their encouragement and helpful comments on an earlier version of this chapter.

PART 3

Major contemporary themes in public health

Editors' overview

What are the key challenging issues in public health at the beginning of the 21st century?

Public health resource and action has always had to address some all pervasive public health problems, such as the poor sanitation and lack of clean water tackled by the Victorians, and 'clean air' pollution control measures in the mid-20th century. Now, in the UK, public health faces new challenges. In this part of the book, we focus on four issues, selected because they are fundamental to today's task of improving public health: addressing inequalities in health; improving health and health inequality at a neighbourhood level; improving health in the cities of the world; and looking at the wider picture of global influences on health and health inequalities.

These four issues have a central place in recent change in public health policy, participation and practice. They will continue to do so, and compel us to redefine public health for the 21st century and to explain why change has to happen.

In Chapter 10 David Evans considers new directions in tackling inequalities in health. He provides evidence of the socio-economic inequalities in the health of the UK population and assesses the UK policy response from successive governments. He notes recent government recognition of the link between poverty, inequalities and social exclusion and its translation into policy initiatives. Evans discusses whether current government policy towards reducing inequalities is working. In the final section of this chapter he gives practical options for public health workers about methods they might use in their work to reduce health inequalities.

In Chapter 11 Murray Stewart examines the re-emergence of 'neighbourhoods' as a concern of public health professionals and policy makers and their role in addressing health inequalities and improving health and well being through 'neighbourhood renewal and regeneration'. Stewart outlines and assesses the success of national and local policy initiatives.

In Chapter 12 Colin Fudge takes an international perspective to discuss the implementation of sustainable futures in cities. He discusses the concept of 'sustainable development' and how urbanization and world population growth are threats to sustainable development and must be addressed in public health action. He provides case studies of his evaluative research in three Swedish cities. This gives useful pointers to public health workers and planners in growing urban city populations.

In Chapter 13 Stuart McClean debates the extent to which it is possible to rely upon nation state based institutions, such as a primary care led NHS, in the face of grassroots movements that flow from the forces of globalization. He examines the impact of globalization upon emerging public health risks, global health inequalities and international trade policy. He summarizes conflicting views concerning the future impact of globalization on public health, arguing that events at some geographical distance from home will impact upon public health agendas and actions.

10

DAVID EVANS

New directions in tackling inequalities in health

Editors' introduction

When looking at the health of populations in the UK, a key issue is that health is not evenly spread: some groups of people are healthier than other groups. In particular, poorer people are, on average, less healthy than better off people indicating an association between health and wealth. This uneven spread of health across populations is known as 'inequalities in health'. The existence of health inequalities challenges all public health workers to improve the health of less healthy groups of people so that it is as good as that of the healthiest; in other words to close the 'health gap' between rich and poor people.

Action to address health inequalities can take place at different levels of the population and the public health workforce. Policies can be implemented at different levels to tackle the root causes of ill health with, for example, actions to eliminate poverty, homelessness, lack of life chances and unemployment or by working directly to develop communities and individuals who have the worst health.

Reduction of health inequality should involve every public health worker, from those working for the government of the day in a health and public health capacity, the local authority, primary care trust members, social workers, community workers, nurses, environmental health officers, general practitioners, police and educators.

This chapter begins by looking at what we mean by 'inequalities' and whether they are always 'unfair'. It briefly examines the evidence for causes of health inequality between people in different socio-economic groups. Government policies over the past 25 years that aim to reduce health inequalities are assessed in terms of how successful they have been and what more could be done.

The author discusses five options for addressing health inequalities: lobbying, partnership working, community development, promoting healthy behaviours and improving access to health care. He concludes with practical pointers for the public health worker who wants to contribute to a reduction in health inequalities.

Introduction

Health inequalities have been observed and reported in the UK since the ground-breaking work of William Farr on vital statistics, first published in 1837 (Davey Smith *et al.* 2001a). More recently the term has also been used to describe inequalities in the health experience of black and minority ethnic groups in Britain, although there are methodological difficulties in disentangling the effects of ethnicity and socio-economic status (Davey Smith *et al.* 2000a). There are, for example, significantly different standardized mortality ratios for men aged 20–64 resident in England and Wales but coming from different countries of origin, with most but not all non-British born groups experiencing higher standardized mortality ratios than the total population. Inequalities in health also exist between geographical areas and between women and men.

'Inequalities in health' have been defined as 'the virtually universal phenomenon of variation in health indicators (infant and maternal mortality rates, mortality and incidence rates of many diseases, etc) associated with socio-economic status' (Last 1995). For almost every indicator, there is a clear positive correlation between health and wealth: on average, the wealthier people are, the better their health; the poorer, the worse their experience of health and disease, and the greater their risk of dying prematurely.

Inequality and inequity

A key aspect of inequalities in health, not always explicit in the literature, is that inequalities are variations that are perceived to be unfair. On average, younger people experience better health than older people, but these differences are not usually regarded as unfair or defined as inequalities in health.

In practice when commentators discuss inequalities in health, they often mean inequities in health: that is, those inequalities which are perceived to be unfair. Concepts of equity and inequity are thus value based, and refer to 'what should be' (Baggott 2000). As Baggott points out, they are therefore contestable, and there is much controversy about whether certain inequalities are actually inequitable and what should be done about them. Are we concerned simply with inequality of outcome as measured by our various health indicators? Or are we also seeking to ensure equity of access to services (which may or may not lead to equitable outcomes) or equity of opportunity for people to attain their full health potential (World Health Organisation 1981) which may require unequal input of resources towards poorer individuals and communities?

Causes of inequality in health

As well as debates on the extent to which inequalities are inequitable, there is a considerable literature seeking to explain the causes of inequality in health. This is a complex field, beset with conceptual and methodological difficulties in measuring inequality and in demonstrating causal pathways. Following a discussion in the Black Report (DHSS 1980), four major potential causes of the observed inequalities generally have been considered: artefact, social selection, behavioural/cultural and material (Macintyre 1997). Although these debates are unresolved (and possibly irresolvable, as the different explanations are not necessarily mutually exclusive), the vast majority of researchers and policy analysts accept that artefact and social selection account for relatively little of the observed differences in health experience between rich and poor. There is more continuing debate on the relative importance of material and psychosocial factors.

What is most notable about this literature, however, is how much of it is concerned with documenting and explaining inequalities of health and how little focuses on describing and evaluating interventions to reduce such inequalities (Mackenbach and Bakker 2002). This chapter is intended to help redress the balance by primarily focusing on what the evidence base tells us works in reducing inequalities in health, particularly from the perspective of public health practitioners working at a community level. Before doing so, however, it is necessary briefly to summarize what we know about socio-economic inequalities of health, and how UK health policy has responded to this knowledge.

The evidence for socio-economic inequalities in health

The last century has witnessed remarkable improvements in health both within Britain and in most other countries internationally. In developing countries, infant, child and maternal mortality have fallen dramatically. In the UK, Europe and the rest of the developed world mortality from the major killer diseases (chronic heart disease and cancer) has also been falling.

Despite these general improvements, however, socio-economic inequalities in health remain and are increasing between countries, regions, socio-economic groups and individuals. Inequalities in health are as obvious in Britain today as 100 years ago, despite the creation of the welfare state and the virtual abolition of absolute poverty. The health of the poorest has improved over time, but not as fast as for the rest of the population; thus the health gap between rich and poor has widened. This gap in health is of course only one aspect of the widening socio-economic gap between rich and poor which can also be seen in income, housing, education and other aspects of social life.

Health inequalities are much greater in some countries than in others; for example, inequalities in health are markedly smaller in absolute terms in Sweden (which for many years has pursued equality orientated social and Labour market polices) than in the UK, thus suggesting that social policy can impact on health inequalities.

The growing health gap in the UK

Health inequalities have been documented in the UK throughout the past 150 years. As well as the pioneering work of Farr, health inequalities were identified by Rowntree (1901), Booth (1902–03), Boyd Orr (1936), Titmuss (1943) and Tudor-Hart (1988) among many others (Davey Smith *et al.* 2001a). In 1977 the then Labour government commissioned Sir Douglas Black to lead a working group to review the evidence on inequalities in health and make policy recommendations (DHSS 1980). The conclusion of the Black Report was that:

> Most recent data show marked differences in mortality rates between the occupational classes, for both sexes and at all ages. At birth and in the first month of life, twice as many babies of 'unskilled manual' parents (class V) die as do babies of professional class parents (class I) and in the next eleven months nearly three times as many boys and more than three times as many girls . . . A class gradient can be observed for most causes of death, being particularly steep in the case of diseases of the respiratory system.
>
> (DHSS 1980)

The rejection of the Black Report by the incoming Conservative government stimulated additional research into inequalities in health, the vast majority of which confirmed the fundamental link between growing inequalities in wealth and health. Nearly 20 years later the new Labour government, elected in 1997, commissioned Sir Donald Acheson to chair an independent inquiry into inequalities in health (Acheson 1998). The Acheson Report not only confirmed the existence of the inequalities identified in the Black Report, but concluded that in the intervening period the differences in the rates had widened:

> For example, in the early 1970s, the mortality rate among men of working age was almost twice as high for those in class V (unskilled) as for those in class I (professional). By the early 1990s, it was almost three times higher. This increasing differential is because, although rates fell overall, they fell more among the high social classes than the low social classes. Between the early 1970s and the early 1990s, rates fell by about 40 per cent for classes I and II, about 30 per cent for classes IIIN, IIIM and IV, but by only 10 per cent for class V. So not only did the differential between the top and bottom increase, the increase happened across the whole spectrum of social classes.
>
> (Acheson 1998: 11)

Causal pathways

Some of the excess mortality and morbidity associated with poorer socio-economic position can be explained by recognized behavioural risk factors, in particular smoking, but also others including poor diet, high alcohol consumption and lack of physical exercise. Although such risk factors explain some of the inequality in health, particularly for cardiovascular disease where risk factors such as smoking, high serum cholesterol and high blood pressure play a part, they explain less than half of the socio-economic gradient in mortality (Mackenbach and Bakker 2002). Some commentators have sought to explain this finding through the psychological effects of income inequality (Wilkinson 1996) while others have stressed the cumulative impact of inequality over the life course (Davey Smith et al. 2001c).

The debates between these various schools of thought can be highly technical and difficult for non-specialists to assess. They are important because understanding the causal pathways leading to inequalities in health should help us plan interventions to reduce inequalities. But such understanding is advantageous rather than essential. The causal pathways are clearly complex and likely to be multifactoral. Recent research, for example, has demonstrated that there is significant variation in the association between socio-economic position and mortality for particular causes of ill health and death, with some risk factors having differing impacts at different stages of the life course (Davey Smith *et al.* 2001c). Nonetheless, there is clear evidence to support some policy interventions to reduce inequalities in health whether their specific causal pathways are fully understood or not.

The UK policy response

Conservative policy

Despite the publication of the Black Report and subsequent confirmatory research, for most of the 1980s and early 1990s the Conservative governments refused to accept the importance or even the existence of inequalities in health. From the mid-1990s the government grudgingly accepted what it termed 'variations in health' (Department of Health 1995a) and began to discuss what it might do about them. Work at this time included the commissioning of a systematic review of research on the effectiveness of health service interventions to reduce variations in health (Arblaster *et al.* 1995).

New Labour policy

However, it was not until the election of the new Labour government in 1997 that a comprehensive policy response to reduction of health inequalities was developed. Over its first term, the government launched a range of initiatives to tackle poverty, inequalities and social exclusion, including a specific focus on inequalities in health (Box 10.1). One of its first actions was to commission the Independent Inquiry into Inequalities in Health (Acheson 1998). The Acheson Report made a number of recommendations, but identified three key priorities:

- all policies likely to have an impact on health should be evaluated in terms of their impact on health inequalities;
- a high priority should be given to the health of families with children; and
- further steps should be taken to reduce income inequalities and improve the living standards of the poor.

The new government came to power with a commitment to tackle inequalities and a recognition that they needed to be tackled through 'joined up' thinking across both central government and local partnerships. Thus the prime minister established a Social Exclusion Unit reporting directly to his office with a remit to work across departmental boundaries. Local authorities and other agencies were required to establish local strategic partnerships and multiagency community strategies, with a range of national targets and performance indicators relating to inequalities. Following the

---

Box 10.1   Policies to tackle poverty, inequality and social exclusion

- Tackling low income through the national minimum wage, the Working Families Tax Credit, the Children's Tax Credit, income support for families and other changes to tax and benefit.

- Improving education by introducing policies to improve education standards, creating 500 Sure Start initiatives to improve early years' support to families and education action zones.

- Improving employment opportunities through New Deal programmes, employment zones, action teams for jobs and the Connexions strategy for 13–19-year-olds.

- Rebuilding local communities through Local Strategic Partnerships, community strategies, the National Strategy for Neighbourhood Renewal, New Deal for Communities and Sure Start.

- Reducing crime through crime and disorder partnerships and the Street Crime Initiative.

- Addressing the housing needs of deprived areas through new standards of decency for social housing.

- Strategy to reduce the number of people sleeping rough.

- Drug and alcohol misuse prevention programmes, in particular through drug action teams.

- Helping vulnerable young people avoid conception and teenage pregnancy through the Teenage Pregnancy Strategy.

- Tackling health inequalities through Health Action Zones, Healthy Living Centres, healthy community collaboratives and new national targets for reducing health inequalities.

Source: Department of Health (2001c)

---

priority given in both the Black Report and the Acheson Report, child and family poverty and child and family health are key policy priorities.

Within the health sector, the government published a public health strategy *Saving Lives: Our Healthier Nation* (Secretary of State for Health 1999) with an accompanying *Reducing Health Inequalities: An Action Report* (Department of Health 1999a) which laid out the range of government policies which addressed inequalities. *The NHS Plan* (Secretary of State for Health 2000) set out more concrete action and established two new national targets to reduce inequalities in life expectancy and infant mortality by 10 percent by 2010. Most recently, the government has been developing a plan for delivery which identifies six priorities for delivering action on health inequalities (see Box 10.2).

At the same time the government has implemented a major reorganization of the NHS in England with primary care trusts replacing health authorities as the major health sector player charged with tackling inequalities in health both through local strategic partnerships as well as action within the NHS.

Box 10.2   Six priorities for delivering action on health inequalities

---

- providing a sure foundation through a healthy pregnancy and early childhood;
- improving opportunity for children and young people;
- improving NHS primary care services;
- tackling the major killers: coronary heart disease and cancer;
- strengthening disadvantaged communities; and
- tackling the wider determinants of health inequalities through government policy.

Source: Department of Health (2001c)

(See also Chapters 1 and 2 for perspectives on government policy to tackle health inequalities.)

UK policy effectiveness

The evidence

What then is the evidence of the effectiveness of government policy in tackling inequalities in health? Given the complexity of the causal pathways and the long-term cumulative impact of health inequalities, it is unsurprising that definitive answers are not yet available. For many commentators, the key criterion is whether the government is successfully tackling poverty by redistributing income from rich to poor. Early evidence on this is equivocal. Shaw *et al.* (1999) argue that although most families gained from the first three Labour budgets, overall the poorest did not improve their relative position. Writing slightly later, the same research group (Davey Smith *et al.* 2002) found that the Gini coefficient for relative income inequality continued to rise in 1996–97 and 1998–99, that is, into the third year of the new government. By contrast, Benzeval *et al.* (2000) found that the government had been successful in redistributing from rich to poor, with the poorest income decile seeing almost a 10 percent increase in disposable income while the richest decile experienced a small decrease.

Davey Smith *et al.* (2002) also point to direct evidence that health inequalities are continuing to increase. They found that the poverty gradient in age and sex standardized mortality ratios for premature mortality (death before 75) increased over the period 1990–99, including between 1996–97 and 1998–99. As it may take many years for changes in policy to impact upon health, more data over a longer time period will be necessary before a definitive judgement can be made on the impact of government policy changes since 1997 on health inequalities.

Problems of policy

A number of commentators have analysed policy on tackling health inequalities and concluded that it is beset with limitations and contradictions. The Acheson

Report itself has been criticized for a lack of prioritization, a weak evidence base, being inadequately concrete and uncosted (Davey Smith *et al.* 2001b; Exworthy *et al.* 2002).

The government's focus on area-based initiatives has been criticized because the majority of poor people live outside the specified areas of deprivation. For example, two-thirds of children living in poverty are outside Sure Start areas. Even within targeted areas, the resources allocated to tackling inequality are relatively small compared to mainstream spend in public services. Thus the government has emphasized the need for neighbourhood renewal and other regeneration funds to be used to 'bend mainstream services'. However, there is little evidence of effective practice in doing this. Different local agencies continue to receive differing 'must do's' from central government; for example, the drive for improved academic attainment in the education sector does not encourage schools to engage in local partnerships to tackle the broader determinants of inequality. Other aspects of government policy, particularly the short timescales within which regeneration funding has to be spent, often militate against coherent interagency planning for long-term service change.

Within the NHS, the major central policy drivers focus on improving access (for example, reducing hospital waiting times) and quality in secondary and primary care rather than on tackling the wider determinants of health inequalities. Despite the government's rhetorical commitment to tackling health inequalities, a number of commentators have suggested that there has been a '*de facto* relegation of health inequalities' in central priorities, resource allocation and performance management decisions (Exworthy *et al.* 2002). As Exworthy and colleagues conclude, tackling health inequalities is a policy priority for the government, but local 'implementation is hampered by deficiencies in performance management, insufficient integration between policy sectors and contradictions between health inequalities and other policy imperatives'. It is too early to assess what the outcome of these contradictions will be on the health gap between rich and poor.

Potential policies for reducing inequalities in health

Upstream–downstream, universalist–selectivist policies

Interventions to reduce inequalities can be categorized as 'upstream' (tackling the fundamental causes of inequalities through national, social and economic policy) or 'downstream' (working directly with poor individuals and communities to tackle their immediate socio-economic and health problems). A second important distinction is between policies which are 'universalist' (ensuring everyone receives the same standard of service) and 'selectivist' (a means tested approach which targets benefits and services on those with greatest need). For some commentators the solution to health inequalities is clearly upstream and universalist:

> There is one central and fundamental policy that should be pursued: the reduction of income inequality and consequently the elimination of poverty. Ending poverty is the key to ending inequalities in health . . . Any child can tell you how this can be achieved: the poor have too little money so the solution to ending their

poverty is to give them more money. Poverty reduction really is something that can be achieved by 'throwing money at the problem'.

(Davey Smith *et al.* 1999)

Other commentators have suggested that while there is good evidence for such downstream interventions as smoking cessation, there is a paucity of good quality studies of 'upstream' interventions (Macintyre *et al.* 2001), even though they largely support such policies. Davey Smith *et al.* (2001c), however, have countered that such analysis inappropriately focuses on individual level determinants of health while ignoring more important macro level determinants: 'The *Cochrane Library* is unlikely ever to contain systematic reviews or trials of the effects of redistributive national fiscal policies, or of economic investment leading to reductions in unemployment, on health' (Davey Smith *et al.* 2001c).

A different type of evidence is needed to support macro-economic interventions to tackle poverty, an evidence base that Davey Smith and colleagues have sought to provide in numerous publications (Davey Smith *et al.* 1999, 2001b; Shaw *et al.* 1999).

Options for the public health practitioner

Such debates leave one with a conundrum: if the only fundamental way to tackle health inequalities is through national macro-economic policy, what can the public health practitioner working at the community level do? The choice is either to do nothing about inequalities which for most of us is ethically unacceptable – or to identify what can usefully be done at the local level. Fortunately, there is an increasing body of evidence to guide such decisions including reviews by Arblaster *et al.* (1995, 1996); Acheson (1998); Roberts' (2000) work on what works in reducing inequalities in child health; Mackenbach and Bakker's (2002) European survey; and the ever growing literature available online via the National Electronic Library for Health (www.NELH.nhs.uk). Essentially, there are five options for the individual practitioner: lobbying, partnership working, community development, promoting healthy behaviours and improving access to health care.

Lobbying

The practitioner can seek to influence how national policy addresses the upstream determinants of health inequalities by lobbying ministers, MPs, regulatory bodies and other national and local decision makers. Lobbying can be done on an individual basis (such as through letters to ministers and MPs) or through membership of national non-statutory organizations (for example, Child Poverty Action Group and the UK Public Health Association), professional organizations (such as the Community Practitioners and Health Visitors Association and the Faculty of Public Health), trade unions and/or political parties.

The media can be a very effective tool for public health lobbying (Chapman 2001). Lobbying national decision makers has the potential advantage of allowing the practitioner to address the upstream determinants of health and the decision makers who can shape policies to tackle these. At a local level the practitioner can act as an advocate for tackling inequalities within their own organization and across local partnerships.

It can be very difficult, however, to assess whether one is having an impact as a lobbyist or advocate. There has been little or no evaluative research on the impact or effectiveness of practitioners in lobbying for public health action to tackle health inequalities. However, an assessment of its value can be gleaned by examining the shifting national policy on health inequalities. Throughout the 1980s and early 1990s, the then government studiously ignored continued lobbying from the public health field on health inequalities. Most notably, the *Health of the Nation* White Paper (Secretary of State for Health 1992) did not address health inequalities despite this being the most common issue raised by those who responded to the preceding consultative Green Paper. However, a number of commentators are confident that the lobbying of the public health field was important in finally bringing the Conservative government to acknowledge and begin to address health 'variations', and for the new Labour government to have it as high upon its list of priorities as it did (Baggott 2000). Practical advice on how to lobby effectively for public health is given by Muir Gray (2001).

Partnership working

Government policy on tackling inequality emphasizes the need for intersectoral and multidisciplinary partnership between local agencies and communities through the formation of local strategic partnerships. There is an increasing body of evidence that such partnership is an important prerequisite for effective local action on health inequalities. Arblaster *et al.* (1996) identify a multidisciplinary approach as an important characteristic of successful interventions to improve the health of disadvantaged groups in areas including injury prevention, reducing smoking and chronic heart disease risk, pregnancy prevention and sexual health. Gillies (1998a, b) has reviewed a range of studies of alliances and partnerships for health promotion and concluded there is strong evidence for their effectiveness.

The public health practitioner can contribute to partnership working on inequalities both by representing their agency on relevant partnership groups (such as Local Strategic Partnership/community strategy groups, equalities action groups, neighbourhood partnerships, Healthy Living Centres) and by facilitating partnership action on specific health related issues (for example, promoting healthy eating, physical activity, tobacco control and so on).

Within such partnerships the practitioner can act as an advocate for local evidence-based, universalist and non-stigmatizing initiatives and services to tackle inequalities (such as universal preschool education, affordable high quality day care (Roberts 2000), vehicle speed reduction (Towner *et al.* 1993)) and targeted services where appropriate (for example, advice services to increase benefit uptake by disadvantaged groups (Arblaster *et al.* 1995)).

Practitioners may also have skills in needs assessment, ensuring interventions are multifaceted and culturally sensitive, skills development, training and other factors identified by Arblaster *et al.* (1996) as important for successful interventions.

Important as partnership working undoubtedly is, however, there is also a large opportunity cost in the time necessary to make partnerships work. There has been little robust evaluation of the relative benefits and costs of different models of partnership working or comparisons of their impact on inequalities. Published evaluations often focus on process issues (for example, see Evans and Killoran 2000) and give practitioners only partial guidance on how to prioritize their time between the range of potential initiatives to tackle health inequalities.

(Part 2 of this book looks in depth at participation in public health work, including discussion of partnership working.)

Community development

Community development has been defined as 'a process by which people are involved in collectively defining and taking action on issues that affect their lives' (Radford *et al.* 1997). For public health practitioners, it involves facilitating local communities to identify their own health needs and agenda, and to develop and implement their own solutions to improving health and reducing inequalities. (See Chapter 9 for discussion on community development approaches.)

Community development approaches have a long history in tackling inequalities and are often advocated (for example Benzeval *et al.* 1995). There is a substantial, diverse and mainly qualitative literature describing it (Stewart-Brown and Prothero 1988; Beattie 1991), which is methodologically very different from the experimental studies which form the basis for most of the reviews of interventions to tackle inequalities in health. Arblaster *et al.* (1996), for example, only included studies with an experimental design, and therefore unsurprisingly did not include any community development projects. The term 'community development' does not even feature in the indexes of two major recent collections on tackling inequalities in health (Leon and Walt 2000; Mackenbach and Bakker 2002). Health sector led community development projects have been reported to be critical catalysts for regeneration in a number of deprived communities (Hunt 1987; Smithies and Adams 1990; Roberts 1992; Whitehead 1995; Dalziel 2000; Roberts 2000).

Promoting healthy behaviours

There is an expanding literature on the effectiveness of health promotion programmes (such as for smoking cessation, injury prevention, social support, breast-feeding) specifically targeted on individuals in lower socio-economic groups who are at higher risk of poorer health and/or health damaging behaviours. The majority of the studies in Arblaster *et al.* (1995), Roberts (2000) and other reviews are experimental evaluations of these types of intervention. For example:

- Connett and Stamler (1984) have shown that interventions can be successfully carried out to reduce the incidence of smoking in deprived groups (in this case middle-aged black and white Americans of varying socio-economic backgrounds). A recent NHS report from the North-West region (in the UK) (Lowey *et al.* 2002) provides additional evidence that smoking cessation services can effectively reach and help smokers from deprived communities.

- Colver *et al.* (1982) showed that pre-arranged home visits to identify specific targets for change in families living in a deprived area of Newcastle encouraged them to make changes in their homes that would be expected to reduce the risk of childhood accidents.

- Oakley *et al.* (1990) demonstrated the effectiveness, appropriateness and safety of social support provided by midwives to women with high risk pregnancies.

- A recent review from the NHS Centre for Reviews and Dissemination (2000b) suggests that small group informal discussions appear to be the most effective way to encourage breastfeeding.

While many of these interventions have been shown to be effective, they are also largely focused downstream on individuals and their health problems associated with deprivation, rather than upstream on the determinants of health. Useful though this evidence base is, it does not offer practitioners guidance on how to balance their efforts between tackling inequalities through upstream determinants and downstream health problems.

Improving access to health care

Access to NHS health care is mainly free at the point of service (except for dental, ophthalmic, prescription and some equipment charges) and, in principle, universally accessible to everyone in the population regardless of socio-economic position or ethnicity. In primary care, recent studies have found that lower income groups were more likely than higher income groups to use GP services, and that this higher usage broadly reflected need (Patterson and Judge 2002). There is also a strong positive relationship between levels of deprivation and hospital outpatient and admission rates. There is, however, convincing evidence of socio-economic differences in the likelihood of receiving some specialist services and in survival. Several studies have found that men living in more affluent areas were more likely to receive coronary revascularization surgery than men from poorer areas, despite having less need as measured by mortality rates (Ben-Shlomo and Chaturvedi 1995; Payne and Saul 1997).

More equitable access to health care can be pursued either through universal initiatives, including developing explicit referral guidelines and standards, such as maximum two week waits for cancer referrals. The alternative is selectivist approaches targeted on more deprived groups, such as targeted home visiting for families in areas of deprivation. Paterson and Judge (2002) identify 36 interventions either aimed at lower income groups or which report separate results for them. Just over half (n = 19) report interventions aimed at lower income groups which were judged effective. These studies were mainly from the USA and included interventions for cancer screening, treating health risks such as hypertension or substance misuse, improving maternal health and child health outcomes. The interventions were diverse and included hospital-based education programmes, community outreach activities and home visiting.

Conclusion

The five options outlined above for practitioners to consider in tackling inequalities in health are not mutually exclusive and, indeed, many practitioners adopt several or all of these approaches in different contexts and/or at appropriate times. Unfortunately, there is no obvious evidence base on which to decide what level of effort it is sensible to put into each option or whether one should simply focus on universal health improvement and improved access, and not seek to specifically tackle inequalities at all. The evidence base for the last two options is the largest and easiest to interpret, simply because they are more amenable to the traditional randomized controlled trial method of evaluation.

There are a number of constructive responses to this uncertainty. First, the practitioner can seek to incorporate into their work Arblaster et al.'s (1996) characteristics of successful interventions to reduce inequalities in health:

- systematic and intensive approaches;
- improvements in access and prompts to encourage the use of services;
- multifaceted interventions;
- multidisciplinary approaches;
- ensuring interventions meet identified need of the target population; and
- involvement of peers in the delivery of interventions.

In addition, there are a small number of interventions which have a particularly strong evidence base for their effectiveness in tackling health inequalities including smoking cessation, breastfeeding support, early years day care, education and social support, and traffic speed reductions. Thus the practitioner can usefully begin by considering whether such interventions are in operation in their patch and, if not, work to put them in place.

The first steps in any initiative to tackle inequalities in health must be to identify the nature and extent of the inequality and then to search the literature to establish if any intervention has been shown to effectively reduce it. With the rapid expansion of Internet-based knowledge sources (in particular via the National Electronic Library for Health), evidence of effective interventions will increasingly be most accessible online. Other Internet-based sources of relevant knowledge on tackling inequalities include:

- the Department of Health (www.doh.gov.uk/inequalities);
- the Health Development Agency (www.hda-online.org);
- the network of Health Action Zones (www.haznet.org.uk);
- the Health Equity Network (www.ukhen.org.uk); and
- the *International Journal of Equity in Health* (www.equityhealthj.com).

On a professional level, the public health practitioner can ensure they have the underpinning competencies and knowledge to effectively tackle inequalities. Necessary competencies include health needs assessment, equity audit, literature searching, critical appraisal, health promotion, community development, partnership working and evaluation including economic evaluation. (See also Chapter 5 on capacity and capability in public health.)

Tackling inequalities cannot be done as a distinct and separate programme of work. It requires integration across the range of professional activities including continuing professional development, clinical governance, teaching, research and development, and work programme planning.

What is most fundamentally required is a new perspective, a new set of reflexive questions. To effectively tackle inequalities in health, the practitioner must continually test out their activity and programmes against the question 'What is the evidence that this will contribute to reducing inequalities in health?'

11

MURRAY STEWART
Neighbourhood renewal and regeneration

Editors' introduction

The future of deprived neighbourhoods and their problems of poor health, crime, drugs, unemployment, community breakdown, poor housing and quality of life have recently become more visible to government, regions and 'neighbourhoods' themselves. Government 'modernization' policies and public health interventions that occur at neighbourhood level, including empowerment of people living in such neighbourhoods, can be viewed as the cornerstone for regeneration and renewal at the beginning of the 21st century.

Action to regenerate and renew neighbourhoods (for example, New Deal for Communities initiatives) takes place at different levels of the public health work. Policies can be implemented to tackle the root causes of neighbourhood deprivation including partnerships such as local strategic partnerships.

Renewal and regeneration is the remit of many multidisciplinary public health workers. Professionals and policy makers working for central government and regional government are crucial to regeneration and renewal in neighbourhoods in terms of tackling the policy elements governing economic and psychosocial determinants of health and well being. Other people that are involved are local lay people, community leaders, local authority urban and transport planners, primary care trust health workers, social workers, community development workers, nurses, environmental health officers, general practitioners, police and educators.

In the first section of this chapter, the author traces the development of urban policy and neighbourhood renewal, highlighting the re-emergence of the neighbourhood and its rediscovery with the more holistic view of deprivation and disadvantage now evident in current urban policies. He then examines the link between neighbourhood policies and inequalities in health.

The last section explores the relationship between public health and the neighbourhood in depth, reflecting on the role of neighbourhood initiatives such as Health

Action Zones, New Deal for Communities and the importance of 'social capital' and 'partnership working' in bringing about change in neighbourhoods.

Urban policy and neighbourhood renewal: historical context

The history of cities has long been linked to concerns about public health. The record of town planning and housing is strewn with examples of the anti-urbanism which led so many to deplore the growth of cities and the conditions of life which they imposed on powerless populations. New Lanark, Saltaire, Bournville, Port Sunlight bear witness to the concerns of the 19th century community reformers whose benevolent, if paternalistic, initiatives sought to protect workers from the dangers of cramped and disease ridden city life. At the beginning of the 20th century Howard's garden cities aimed to expose residents to a healthy life style and to housing characterized by lower densities and public open space. In the 1950s the new towns movement was built around many of the principles of public health which half a century on we now seek to recreate.

It is against this anti-urbanism which runs so deep in the English psyche (Glass 1955) that we must understand the emergence of 'neighbourhood' as a foundation for regeneration and renewal at the beginning of the 21st century. We need to recognize the force both of those planning policies in supporting the ex-urban expansion and of a half century of ad hoc area-based initiatives which have represented urban policy (Stewart 2000). For many years after 1945 the physical and social reconstruction of cities was based on a belief that planning solutions – the new towns and similar overspill initiatives – would lead to improvement in the conditions of life in the inner city. The planned, and much greater unplanned, movement of population and jobs away from cities led, however, to recognition of a geographical concentration of 'deprivation' in both inner city and peripheral estates. This in turn led to the establishment of successive central government programmes targeting 'deprived' areas.

The initiatives of the late 1960s and early 1970s were characterized both by a philosophy which suggested that communities should help themselves and, later, by a drive towards the improved management and coordination of public services. An increased interest in public participation (often area-based) accompanied these shifts in thinking. Thus the educational priority areas, the community development projects, and the early urban programme, were accompanied or followed by moves towards wider participation in planning (Skeffington 1969) and by further area-based initiatives – general improvement area and housing action area legislation, comprehensive community programmes, the inner area studies, and area management trials.

Such initiatives were the antecedents of the rash of area-based initiatives – Health Action Zones included – of recent years. Educational priority areas were directed at similar issues as the current Education Action Zones – raising educational standards and supporting disadvantaged schools; the community development projects were directed towards community empowerment; the urban programme funded projects many of which would sit comfortably in current programmes. The community development projects threw up numerous useful projects on the ground but were above all characterized by their ability to raise the issue of whether/how far the structural, economic and social problems facing communities in local areas could be addressed by solutions based in those same areas. Evaluations of both the comprehensive community programme experiments in Gateshead and Bradford and the area management trials illustrated that area-based approaches attempt to deal with problems that are only partially spatially related, that political commitment to change is crucial and that traditional departmental structures are strongly resistant to change (Spencer 1982; Webster 1982).

In terms of formal policy area-based initiatives the comprehensive community programmes and area management experiments were overtaken by the inner city partnerships of the late 1970s within which vertical central–local partnership was pursued with ministers – chairing the partnerships – adopting a hands on approach to fostering joint working. The 1980s saw area-based urban policy sustained both in response to the 'riots' of 1980/81 and later 1985, and to the government's wish to introduce new instruments of regeneration – urban development corporations, task forces, city action teams, housing action trusts. The urban programme was refocused on 57 targeted areas. Emphasis was laid on policies to draw in private sector investment, with incentives (urban development grants, then city grants) for property and development led programmes.

In practice the 1980s represented a step backwards towards a reliance on single purpose agencies and the initiatives of that decade imposed fragmentation on urban policy. By 1991 relations between central and local government had improved and a new period of area-based working took off but this time characterized by the institutionalization of interurban competition. Two rounds of City Challenge, later superseded by the Challenge Fund element of Single Regeneration Budget funding supported a wide range of area-based initiatives, many (under the Single Regeneration Budget) in smaller towns and cities hitherto ineligible for and inexperienced in area-based working. By 2001, however, the circle had turned, with abolition of Single Regeneration Budget support for new schemes after six annual rounds, the transfer of regeneration responsibilities to the Department of Trade and Industry and the emergence of the Neighbourhood Renewal Unit and a national strategy for neighbourhood renewal.

There were successes and failures over this period, but the evidence is that disparities between richer and poorer areas increased (Robson *et al.* 1994) and that those neighbourhoods identified as the most disadvantaged (for example, by census data) remained disadvantaged over long periods (Power and Tunstall 1995). Successive initiatives seemed to have only temporary impacts. There were few signs of the emergence of an evidence-based urban policy (Harrison 2000; Lawless *et al.* 2000). Regeneration had stumbled from one initiative to another, driven by shifting political ideologies, institutional proliferation and fragmentation, and re-organization of the mechanisms for delivery. But successive programmes revealed the intransigence of urban problems and the continuing plight of communities of place and interest.

The development of the neighbourhood focus

The re-emergence of the neighbourhood

It was against this background of concern about the effectiveness of urban initiatives to counter disadvantage that the Labour government of 1997 sought to re-examine the assumptions upon which area-based intervention was based, and indeed to develop a more formal statement of urban policy as a whole. A White Paper – the first ever to address urban policy as a whole (DTLR 2002) – and the subsequent 2002 Urban Summit – encouraged urban stakeholders to talk up the prospects of cities, to recognize their potential as well as their weaknesses and to concentrate on the exploitation of urban assets. It recognized the strengths of urban life – variety, community, diversity of faiths and cultures – and conveyed a new perception of cities from government, promising indeed 'a new focus for urban issues at the heart of government'. The White Paper did not introduce a new urban policy or programme per se. Rather, it represented a framework for policies across a wide range, reflecting several strands of thinking about regeneration and renewal which had emerged over the previous five years.

The Rogers Report (Department of the Environment, Transport and the Regions 2000b) had examined the ways in which there could be a renaissance in cities and an enhancement of the quality of urban life. Strongly influenced by considerations of urban design but also by the government's need to find space in cities for increased numbers of households, Rogers created a new climate for thinking about the future of cities, albeit a future smacking of architectural determinism.

A local government modernization programme (Department of Transport, Local Government and the Regions 2000c; 2001b) set out the principles which would support the enhancement of local democracy and the protection of standards of conduct in public life. It would assure the more effective delivery of services and demand from local authorities a community leadership role within a broader based local governance. Embedded in this modernization programme, through best value and local public service agreements, for example, was a commitment to a more responsive and community orientated approach to service planning and delivery in disadvantaged neighbourhoods. Equally central was the drive for more integrated working across sectoral boundaries in order to link local government with both central government agencies and other non-departmental public bodies in health, policing, training and employment, and housing. Better joined up government within White-hall was a further prerogative of reform (Cabinet Office 2000a). Indeed, from the work of the Central Policy Review Staff in the 1970s (Blackstone and Plowden 1988; Challis *et al.* 1988) to the analysis of cross-cutting failure in the 1990s (Richards *et al.* 1999; Stewart *et al.* 1999), there has been a saga of evidence about the fragmented nature of governmental activity at all levels, and about the tendency for departments and professions to operate within vertical silos with central and local levels combining to protect their particular domains and the budgets and responsibilities that go with them. (See also Chapter 2 on public health and the government modernization agenda.)

The emergence of a new regionalism together with the establishment of regional development agencies saw economic regeneration linked more closely to the competitiveness debate. Responsibility for the Single Regeneration Budget was passed to regional development agencies. At the same time the government was concerned about the role and function of government in the regions and in local areas and a further Cabinet Office report (2000b) heralded the arrival of the Regional Coordination Unit with a remit both to rationalize the web of area-based initiatives and to support the integration of government work at regional level.

The spatial dimension of social reform was reflected in the work of the Social Exclusion Unit. The Social Exclusion Unit had produced a series of reports (for example, on rough sleeping, truancy and school exclusions, and teenage pregnancy), but its most influential work has been around the future of the deprived neighbourhood. In 1997 the prime minister gave the Social Exclusion Unit the remit to examine 'how to develop integrated and sustainable approaches to the problems of the worst housing estates including crime, drugs, unemployment, community breakdown and bad housing' (Social Exclusion Unit 2001b: 74).

Bringing Britain Together (Social Exclusion Unit 1998) provided a thorough and sophisticated analysis of the issues confronting deprived neighbourhoods reinforcing the observation that past policies had failed to arrest their relative decline. Over the next two years, 18 Policy Action Teams drew together a wide range of interests to develop further analyses and recommendations for action which were captured in a national framework for consultation (Social Exclusion Unit 2001a), which in turn, after consultation, was developed into the National Strategy Action Plan (Social Exclusion Unit 2001b).

As far as the resource argument was concerned, a cross-cutting Treasury led review *Government Interventions in Deprived Areas* (HM Treasury 2000a), undertaken as background to the 2000 Comprehensive Spending Review, set out the spending and service delivery implications of the national neighbourhood renewal framework, establishing crucial principles for resource planning and programme delivery. The review concluded that main programmes should bear the primary responsibility for tackling deprivation. This would mean stipulating both national service standards and 'convergence' targets for tackling deprivation. Funding and process mechanisms might need to be changed. To combat the proliferation of partnerships and provide a single focus for setting local priorities, Local Strategic Partnerships should be established. Nevertheless, targeted initiatives including holistic regeneration programmes still had a role to play, but as part of a wider framework rather than as the main tool.

The *National Strategy Action Plan* for neighbourhoods embodies these principles. It rejects the proposition that deprivation can be combated solely through area-based initiatives. Instead (or, at least, as well) deprivation is to be tackled through the bending of main departmental programmes to focus more specifically on the most deprived areas.

Neighbourhood renewal thus advances on two fronts. On the one hand, there are moves towards the realignment of main programmes. This involves new 'floor targets' set for substandard social housing, for the reduction of burglary rates, for educational achievement, for longer life expectancy, for reduced teenage conception rates and for increased employment rates. At the same time local strategic partnerships carry responsibility at the local level for neighbourhood renewal strategies, for meeting floor targets, for the rationalization of existing partnerships, and for new community strategies.

On the other hand, there remain a raft of specific initiatives. The Community Empowerment Fund supports community and voluntary sector involvement on local strategic partnerships in the 88 areas eligible for a new Neighbourhood Renewal Fund. Neighbourhood Renewal Community Chests are providing small grants to formal and informal community groups to support community activity and mutual self-help in the 88 Neighbourhood Renewal Fund areas. The Neighbourhood Renewal Fund itself provides extra resources for 88 of the most deprived local authority districts. The neighbourhood management programme will help deprived communities and local service providers work together at the neighbourhood level to improve and 'join up' local services, while New Deal for Communities partnerships have been established in 39 neighbourhoods across England. Over the ten year duration of the New Deal for Communities programme they will receive funding totalling £1.9 billion. Neighbourhood wardens provide a uniformed, semi-official presence in residential areas with the aim of improving quality of life. Wardens may promote community safety, assist with environmental or housing improvements and they can assist with neighbourhood management as outlined above.

Across the whole neighbourhood strategy there is an emphasis on improving skills, learning and information. The Neighbourhood Renewal Unit is committed to ensuring a 'step change' in the level of skills and knowledge of everyone involved in neighbourhood renewal. To achieve this, there is a distinct skills and knowledge strand which runs throughout the Unit's work. This skills and knowledge element of neighbourhood renewal – the learning curve – aims to promote better sharing of knowledge about 'what works'; and to ensure that everyone involved in neighbourhood renewal has the skills to make a real difference (Neighbourhood Renewal Unit 2002).

Neighbourhoods and health

The key characteristic promised by the government in its rediscovery of the neighbourhood and its development of a new renewal/regeneration policy has been the departure from a predominantly physical and economic development focus to a more widely defined and holistic view of deprivation and disadvantage. The split of responsibilities between government offices in the regions and regional development agencies has led many observers to comment that there has been a separation rather than an integration between economic and social regeneration. It is clear at least in the social domain, however, that the neighbourhood agenda has stimulated a more holistic view of regeneration which both reflects the new thinking about public health (described in this book) and, at the same time, reinforces and helps to consolidate that thinking. In 1998 the Health Education Authority commissioned work which articulated clearly the links between health and regeneration (Russell and Killoran 1999). Drawing on the local government focused New Commitment to Regeneration on the one hand and the early years of Health Action Zones on the other, but at the same time firmly rooted in the health inequalities analysis (Department of Health 1998c), this work provided a stimulus to thinking about linkage and overlap between health and other policy areas. Evaluation of the New Commitment to Regeneration (Russell 2001) pointed out lessons for joined up working – joint planning, pooled resources, integrated service delivery – and, reinforced by the findings of the Social Exclusion Unit's Policy Action Team 17, paved the way for the development of local strategic partnerships.

The Health Act 1998 had already offered some scope for flexible working between health organizations and local government, but there is now a more explicit focus for developing joint action at neighbourhood level as a consequence of the Local Strategic Partnership responsibilities in relation to community planning (and the preparation of a community strategy) on the one hand, and the need to develop a neighbourhood renewal strategy to guide the allocation of the Neighbourhood Renewal Fund on the other. These requirements have stimulated much cross-sectoral activity (Hamer and Easton 2002; Hamer and Smithies 2002), activity further informed by the guidance issued by the Department of Health and the Neighbourhood Renewal Unit to stimulate good practice in the support of healthy neighbourhoods (Department of Health/Neighbourhood Renewal Unit 2002).

The guidance offers no new insights into the relationship between health and the neighbourhood. Indeed its main aims appear to be to inform non-health interests in neighbourhood partnerships – New Deal for Communities in particular but additionally neighbourhood management partnerships and local strategic partnerships – of the foundations upon which initiatives to counter health inequalities can be based.

Neighbourhood policies and health inequalities

In terms of the five layers of influence often argued to determine health (Dahlgren and Whitehead 1992), the neighbourhood is a mediator in relation to social and community networks and living and working conditions, although it is also the setting within which individual behaviour and lifestyles are worked out. Poor housing, work-lessness, crime and fear of crime, and low educational attainment are major features of disadvantaged neighbourhoods and, with poverty, are major determinants of health status. Improvements in these aspects of quality of life are thus a prerequisite of improved health outcomes. Neighbourhood renewal offers the potential for public health to work in conjunction with employment, education, housing and community safety policies to offer a holistic approach to reducing the gaps between the most disadvantaged neighbourhoods and other less deprived areas. (See also Chapter 10 for discussion of new directions for tackling health inequalities.)

Neighbourhood initiatives to address health inequalities

It is impossible to do justice to the volume and variety of the new initiatives which these policies have spawned. Community safety partnerships support projects to reduce burglary, to support schemes for vulnerable groups, to introduce CCTV, to sustain higher levels of local policing, to combat vehicle crime, to introduce local neighbourhood wardens, to reveal and counter domestic violence and to stamp out racial harassment. In the field of employment there is major investment not simply to attempt to create more jobs and not least in the local social economy, but to ensure that as many of these jobs as possible go to local people. Intermediate Labour market schemes, mentoring, work experience, support for employers and the whole employment New Deal programme aim to reduce worklessness and support the revival of an active local economy.

Transport

Transport provides an increasingly important example, although not one emphasized in the national neighbourhood strategy. A Social Exclusion Unit report on transport and exclusion (Social Exclusion Unit 2002) reinforces the messages from earlier research (Department of the Environment, Transport and the Regions 2000a; Hine and Mitchell 2001; Lucas *et al.* 2001), pointing to the fact that for those who rely on public transport, getting to hospitals is particularly difficult and can lead to missed health appointments. Thirty-one percent of people without a car have difficulties travelling to their local hospital, compared to 17 percent of people with a car. Seven percent of people without a car say they have missed, turned down or chosen not to seek medical help over the past 12 months because of transport problems – double the rate in the general population. Thus the health and transport interface for those in disadvantaged neighbourhoods involves better advice on how to get to hospital through mainstream transport, greater publicity for the Hospital Travel Costs Scheme, and greater choice over the timing of hospital appointments to fit in with travel needs. Children from the lowest social class are five times more likely to die in road accidents than those from the highest social class.

Housing

Above all, however, the neighbourhood is characterized by its housing circumstances. Molyneux and Palmer (2000) pointed to the accumulation of housing issues with health implications – homelessness, poor housing, the quality of the environment – and to the links between housing costs, poverty and poor housing. The relationship between house condition – disrepair, damp and cold – has long been understood to have health impacts, while housing type and, in particular, living off the ground has been known to have consequences for mental and physical health. More recent longitudinal analysis (Marsh *et al.* 2000) reinforces these conclusions and in addition argues that the impact of poor housing on children may emerge as ill health only decades afterwards. At the same time as there is growing recognition of, and research into, the important relationships between housing and health, so also is there a more active debate about the precise nature of these relationships and about the causal linkages. One obvious consideration here is whether the causal relationships are unilateral or whether health affects housing as well as housing affecting health. If health status has traditionally been reflected in medical priority access to social housing, there is now more attention to the role of health condition in determining access to owner occupation and to the effect of health on long-term healthy living (Easterlow *et al.* 2000).

The health impact of the renewal process

A different dimension is examined by Allen (2000) who suggests that the renewal process itself may have health impacts and that the experience of renewal –

uncertainty, upheaval, displacement cost, noise – can cause stress which induces health damage and mental illness. The possibility that regeneration may exacerbate health inequalities by imposing detrimental effects on already impoverished communities should not be ignored (Curtis *et al.* 2002). Crucial to this is the relationship between tenant and landlord with the distribution of control and power being dominant factors. It is interesting to juxtapose this point about the potential stress of regeneration/renewal with the now common observation of regeneration fatigue among community active members of area regeneration partnerships (Purdue *et al.* 2000), and to suggest that the pace and complexity of current renewal activity places unreasonable demands on communities. Seldom is the need for 'community capacity building' couched in health terms. (Chapter 18 examines the process of health impact assessment in depth.)

Understanding inequalities in localities

What a neighbourhood approach demands is examination of the nature of the experience of residence within a particular locality and of the relationship with others in the home, with others in the building, with the immediate external environment and with neighbours and the neighbourhood. The residential experience may vary according to tenure, length of residence in the area, the condition of the building, neighbours and the connections from that residence to other activities – work, transport, shops and leisure. Experience of living will be dependent on sense of shelter, identity, status and security (Kearns *et al.* 2000).

Despite this and much more evidence about life and living within the neighbourhood, health inequalities cannot be addressed exclusively in the neighbourhood, and 'many are the outcome of causal factors that run back into and from the basic structure of society' (Acheson 1998). The parameters of such inequalities lie in poverty and income deprivation, in poorly maintained, cold and wet housing, in poor schooling and low educational attainment, in temporary and insecure employment, in vulnerability to crime and/or fear of it, in the absence of means of transport, and in the stress and mental ill health caused by one or more of the above. The work of the Social Exclusion Unit (1998) has illustrated graphically the relative deprivation experienced in the most deprived neighbourhoods and the *Indices of Deprivation* (Department of the Environment, Transport and the Regions 2000f) also highlights the worse position of certain neighbourhoods. Closing the gap between both disadvantaged localities and disadvantaged groups is a major objective of policy and there is extensive guidance about how best to approach the tasks of understanding inequalities in health, establishing a common language for expressing these inequalities and setting practical targets for meeting local needs (Bull and Hamer 2002).

Health inequalities often mirror other inequalities, but this is not always the case. In Bristol, for example, looking at the *Index of Local Conditions 2000*, the wards which rank third and fifth most deprived in the health domain (Kingsweston and Henbury) rank eleventh and thirteenth respectively on the overall index. Easton ranks second most deprived on housing and eighteenth in health. This illustrates, of course, the vagaries of ward-based information. It also illustrates, however, the need to look closely at city wide, ward-based and neighbourhood information where available, to understand local inequalities, to identify those characteristics which may be amenable to local action and those which form part of a much wider upstream health inequalities agenda demanding national policies and action.

Inequalities in communities of interest

It is also important to recognize, however, that while an emphasis on deprived neighbourhoods is the key feature of much government policy this excludes a significant number of people who do not live in those areas. The neighbourhood as a community of place must share attention with communities of interest which may be widely spread across cities and regions rather than concentrated in particular localities. The Department of Health guidance on health action zones (Department of Health 1999a) identified black and minority ethnic groups, Disabled people, homeless people, travellers, single parents and their children, housebound older people, housebound Disabled people, unemployed people, mentally ill people, former prisoners and vulnerable young people.

The urban White Paper makes clear that the full range of policies must address the challenge of inequality and that spatially concentrated neighbourhood working is just one approach. Nevertheless, a focus on area-based initiatives has been a feature of the late 1990s and early 2000s and the relationship between health and other aspects of neighbourhood renewal in practice can be illustrated through the experience of two different initiatives – health action zones and New Deal for Communities.

The impact of neighbourhood initiatives

Health Action Zones (HAZs)

Twenty-six HAZs covering a population of over 13 million people have operated in a range of urban, rural, ex-coalfields communities. In contrast with many smaller area-based initiatives (Sure Start, Education Action Zones and many Single Regeneration Budget schemes, for example), their scale is such that they cover much larger areas than 'neighbourhoods'. Nevertheless, much of their work has been targeted onto specific localities where deprivation is widespread.

Their influence on policy and practice has been significant. They have been able to undertake a range of innovative and often community-based initiatives on mental health, drug abuse, smoking and alcoholism, diet, health at work and so on. HAZs have had sufficient resource and energy to lead interagency working on such issues and have been influential in transmitting some lessons to the mainstream.

They have acted as a catalyst for the integration of other programmes. In East London, for example, health gain work on the Ocean Estate led to the local primary care group being heavily involved in the Stepney New Deal for Communities after the realization that many local residents travelled good distances to access health services. In Plymouth the Programme Board for Children began to function as the single planning body for services to this group, integrating planning across providers. The Sandwell GrowWell and AgeWell programmes impacted on the main programmes of both health and other departments. Elsewhere the South Yorkshire Coalfields HAZ supported joint working with a Single Regeneration Budget scheme on a survey of social capital.

HAZs have been subject to national and local evaluations and the broad findings of these have been that there has been some success in embedding within the PCGs and latterly the PCTs the principles of public involvement, so much so that the PCTs have continued to fund the function post-HAZ funding (Barnes *et al.* 2003 forthcoming).

New Deal for Communities

The New Deal for Communities initiative operates in 39 localities with populations of around 8000–10,000 people and involves a ten year programme which allocates around £50 million over the period to each New Deal for Communities initiative together with the support of all the relevant mainstream agencies. The areas experience disadvantage and inequalities as compared to the rest of their cities and the rest of the country, and all New Deal for Communities initiatives have some form of thematic health programme built into their delivery plans. New Deal for Communities partnerships were encouraged to undertake local surveys and to develop baseline indicators appropriate both to national targets and to local circumstances (standardized mortality ratios by disease category, teenage pregnancies, smoking, drug misuse, mental health and 'satisfaction with services').

The health work in New Deal neighbourhoods was informed by a review of the emerging evidence base on community health initiatives (Bauld *et al.* 2001a). The national evaluation of New Deal initiatives showed, however, through a review of the initial delivery plans (Health Promotion Policy Unit 2002), that while New Deal for Communities initiatives had collected much information, there remained significant gaps not only in the basic data but in their consistency and in terms of the indicators selected, interpretation, timescales and age groups. The review also argued that there were question marks over whether the outcomes set in the delivery plans were realistic, measurable and meaningful, whether planned activities were well specified, resourced and targeted, and whether the health plans of New Deal initiatives were embedded within the wider plans and structures of the New Deal for Communities partnerships. This confirms the conclusions from other studies which point to the fact that new neighbourhood partnerships – whether these be health partnerships or local strategic partnerships – need learning and development time to settle into new languages, new information sources and new planning mechanisms, before sensible, integrated plans and programmes can be developed (Department of Transport, Local Government and the Regions 2002; Hamer and Easton 2002; Hamer and Smithies 2002).

Public health and the neighbourhood

What is the future direction of public health in the neighbourhood? What are the key issues which health professionals and communities need to address in conjunction with others? From the history of renewal and regeneration over many years and in the light of the policy context at the start of the 21st century a number of key issues emerge.

The neighbourhood effect

Although renewal and regeneration are increasingly focused at the spatial level of the neighbourhood, there remains considerable uncertainty about the precise nature of the neighbourhood effect. Several of the determinants of health lie in the external environment and while problems of ill health (and of unemployment, crime and poverty) are to be found *in* the neighbourhood, they are not necessarily *of* the neighbourhood in the sense of being brought about by a 'neighbourhood effect'. There is much evidence, for example, that black and minority ethnic groups experience health inequalities, and also that in many cities they are concentrated into particular neighbourhoods. This does not mean, however, that the health problems particular to black and minority ethnic groups are caused by the 'neighbourhood'. Regeneration interventions may be appropriately focused at a neighbourhood level – on housing, on the environment or on traffic, for example – but may equally well be focused on solutions which must be generated externally in national policies – fiscal policies, benefits policies, industrial and economic policies. At the spatial scale of the neighbourhood there is likely to be a sharp illustration of the incidence of disadvantage, but it is at other scales – city, region and nation – that remedies are most likely to be found.

But while the neighbourhood may not be a determinant of health inequalities it remains an important focus for policy and practice and an arena for the expression of community of place, and it is in the links between neighbourhood communities and the wider networks of urban life that the most fruitful connections may emerge. Social networks have long been regarded as the foundation for strong community (see for example Dennis *et al.* 1957; Frankenberg 1957; Stacey 1960; Willmott and Young 1960), with strong ties to relatives, immediate friends and neighbours providing the basis for social interaction (Granovetter 1973). Extensive new evidence about the nature of local social networks has come from the Joseph Rowntree Foundation research on neighbourhood images (Andersen and Munck 1999; Cattell and Evans 1999; Silburn *et al.* 1999; Wood and Vamplew 1999). This complements other work on the strengths of, and pressures on, family life – the Bristol-based study by Gill, Tanner and Bland (2000), for example – and on the nature of social cohesion in disadvantaged neighbourhoods (Forrest and Kearns 1999; Page 2000). Much of the evidence focuses on the role of children as a pivotal element with networks mobilizing around issues of childcare and schooling. Women play a crucial role. It is important, however, to remember that some of the negative aspects of neighbourhood life stem from relations of trust and dependence built around drugs, crime, abuse and the function of illicit and often illegal power structures in maintaining oppressive systems of social relations (Hoggett 1997).

Social capital

Much has been made in health literature of the role of social capital in fostering better health, and community-based preventative work has been a major strand of health initiatives such as Health Action Zones as well as of other area-based initiatives such as Sure Start and the New Deal for Communities. There is, however, a parallel strand of literature which points to the failure of initiatives predicated on community cohesion and community capacity building (Hastings 1996; Hastings *et al.* 1996), and to the difficulties inherent in generating genuine community engagement in the management of neighbourhoods and the provision of services. Why, after all, should communities be invited to take on responsibilities which professionals have been so lax in offering over decades? A key issue for public health in the 21st century therefore is to work through precisely which interventions to improve health may be best pursued through community-based initiatives and which through other routes.

This in turn relates to the function of 'weak ties' and of the social capital which provides access for disadvantaged communities to the mainstream of public service provision. Taylor recognizes the 'strong ties' interpretation of social capital but helpfully also points to the fact that what is needed for capacity building is exploration of the space between state and civil society, between levels of political power and decision making and the networks of everyday life (Taylor 2000).

Main programmes

A significant route through which these networks can be built involves the reshaping of major mainline service provision to address the needs of local communities. Mainstreaming is seen as crucial to the sustainability of neighbourhood strategies in the long term. It is recognized that specific initiatives (such as Health Action Zones or New Deal for Communities) may provide one off improvements, but that lasting change is dependent on the engagement of the much larger main programmes. Research on area-based initiatives (Department of Transport, Local Government and the Regions 2002: 31) argued that:

> there was relatively little evidence of successful mainstreaming, in the sense of a mainstream agency adopting and reproducing examples of effective practice from initiative activity. When interviewees talked about mainstreaming, it was often to explore the reasons why it was so slow. The mainstreaming that does happen tends to be piecemeal and opportunistic.

The Audit Commission (2002) identified similar constraints, many revolving around the inflexibility of organizational cultures to accommodate new ways of thinking and acting towards effective neighbourhood renewal.

Where initiatives such as HAZs have been successful in influencing the mainstream, it derives from the fact that they have combined a radical agenda (about partnership working, reducing inequalities, modernizing services) and staff dedicated to progressing this agenda, with close links to the bodies responsible for planning and delivering mainstream services. Recent research on area-based initiatives (DTLR 2002) illustrated that in Plymouth, the South Yorkshire Coalfields, Sandwell and East London there appeared to be strong 'ownership' of HAZs within the mainstream. This might at times be seen as a problem where the HAZ has been seen as a proxy for the health community and as having to pick up issues outside its immediate remit not yet being addressed by the new primary care trust. The HAZ experience thus confirms the tension in investing in innovative projects and then integrating them into mainstream services (Sandford 2001; Audit Commission 2002).

The experience of the Bradford HAZ illustrates this point. The development of new primary care organizations with a strong orientation towards the public and the capacity to link up with others to achieve health goals was a key goal of this initiative. To achieve this the HAZ funded a community involvement team whose job was to work with the four developing primary care groups in Bradford to help build their public involvement capacity. Each PCG had its own community involvement worker but the individual workers also had strong links with each other through a centrally coordinated team in order to maximize cross-fertilization of ideas and to provide support.

Other attempts to influence mainstream change have combined structural and cultural change, for example, Coventry's programme of area coordination. Each area in Coventry is the responsibility of a full-time area coordinator whose job involves bringing together a cross-sector group of local providers and voluntary and community organizations to identify local priorities and try to meet these through improved coordination as well as through bidding for external funds. The work of the areas is supported by a strategic level group that represents the key players in the city. Most recently the area coordination scheme has focused on the development of common data sets of area-based service performance indicators to try and develop the evidence base for their work (Sullivan 2001; Sullivan et al. 2001).

Partnership working

Mainstream change is a function of the interdependence of area-based, neighbourhood experience with the strategic capacity to alter the behaviour of the larger agencies. Partnership is now an over used, often abused, term for what occurs when two or more organizations sit down together. 'Talking shops' are perceived by many stakeholders to be wasteful – for the private sector because they divert from core business and for the voluntary and community sectors because they demand scarce time and energy, which again diverts from getting on with the 'real job'. Over the years there have been numerous studies looking at partnership working (Mackintosh 1993; Roberts et al.1995; Hastings 1996; Hastings et al. 1996; Geddes 1997; Harding 1998; Lowndes and Skelcher 1998), and there is now an extensive literature on collaborative working across boundaries (Huxham 1996; Sullivan 2001). The impact of partnerships is a function of a number of features of joint working – membership, status, structures, leadership, agendas and organizational cultures. Health stakeholders are expected to participate in the new partnership structures and following Department of Health guidance the links with Local Strategic Partnerships have been reinforced (through the National Service Framework for Older People, the disability White Paper, arrangements for children's planning and so on). The lead role for Primary Care Trusts in Local Strategic Partnerships has been messaged a number of times, for example, in the reform document *Shifting the Balance of Power* (Department of Health 2001a).

Participation in local strategic partnerships is one matter, active engagement with a range of neighbourhood partnerships is another and health organizations, like others, need to think through their contribution to partnership working at regional, city and neighbourhood levels to ensure that role and function are understood. The evidence of the past is of complexity in the arrangements for joint working both vertically between centre and periphery, and horizontally between organizations at the same level.

If the health input to neighbourhood working is to be effective then a much clearer view about the protocols of working in partnership need to be developed. The neighbourhood can be a powerful arena for the development of cross-sectoral working between agencies and community, but it can also be a battlefield of competition and conflict. The key challenge for the new public health is to ensure that it is the former not the latter.

12

COLIN FUDGE
Implementing sustainable futures in cities

Editors' introduction

'Sustainable development', put simply, means development which meets the needs of the present without damaging the health or environment of future generations. This is a huge challenge for cities.

The world contains hundreds of nations and thousands of cities at different stages of industrial development. Some of the features of increasing development are an ageing population in advanced industrialized countries, and a growing population with substantial movement of people into urban city living in less developed countries. What unites all cities and the citizens who inhabit them, whatever the level of their development, is whether the future can be guaranteed or is 'sustainable'. Public health workers can make an enormous contribution to creating sustainable futures in cities.

The tension between increased urbanization and a sustainable future for people living in cities reminds us of the origins of modern town planning and its close association with public health. In order for cities to be sustainable, town and transport planners and local authority employees, including health protection and environmental protection managers, must pay great attention to spatial planning, social housing and transport systems, and architects must consider the design of buildings. Central and local government politicians must tackle the problems of an ageing population and pension provision; the threat of terrorism in strategic buildings; quality of life; and that the governance of cities is appropriate for sustainability to be delivered.

This chapter begins by outlining some of the issues arising from increased urbanization, or movement of population into city living, against the backdrop of world and regional population change. It moves on to consider the policy approaches to creating sustainable futures in European cities. The author outlines some of his own evaluative research into sustainable futures in cities using some Swedish cities as examples. In the last part of the chapter he concludes with a number of strategic issues and propositions for the future sustainability of cities in the 21st century.

Introduction

In this chapter sustainable development is identified as a much broader concept than environmental protection. This chapter argues that sustainable development has economic and social as well as cultural, health and environmental dimensions and embraces notions of equity between people in the present and between generations. This argument implies that further development should only take place within the carrying capacity of natural and social systems. In relation to work on the ecological footprint of cities, it could be suggested that a sustainable city is one that is attempting to reduce its ecological footprint (Douglas 1995, private communication: Rees 1992).

The first section of this chapter outlines some of the issues implicated in the current and future health of populations arising from urbanization and urban change and development against the backdrop of world and regional population change. This section also considers policy approaches adopted in Europe to take forward the sustainability agenda for cities. The second section describes some evaluative research that I carried out in Sweden, presenting findings from a case study in sustainable futures in cities. The final section of the chapter concludes with a number of strategic issues and propositions for the future sustainability of cities in the 21st century.

Urbanization, urban change, development and policy

The concept of sustainable development

Although the conceptual origins of sustainable development go back many years, for example, to the garden city movement in the UK and the Regional Planning Association of America, the more recent revival of the term comes from the 1980 World Conservation Strategy (International Union for the Conservation of Nature 1980), which suggested sustainable development as a means of integrating economic development with the essential conservation of the environment. The work of the World Commission on Environment and Development followed, leading to the publication of the Brundtland Report in 1987. In broad terms, the World Commission on Environment and Development rejected the (then dominant) argument that economic growth and maintenance of environmental quality were mutually exclusive. The report argued that development could and should be sustainable: '[meeting] the needs of the present, without compromising the ability of future generations to meet their own needs' (Brundtland 1987).

Since the Brundtland Report there have been a number of significant policy debates and a range of reports addressing various aspects of sustainable development, as well as a growing body of practical experience in attempting to operationalize sustainability. The major stimulus has been the United Nation's Conference on Environment and Development (UNCED) in Rio in 1992, and the series of UN conferences that followed, culminating in the Habitat II conference in Istanbul in 1996. However, despite the widespread adoption internationally of the non-legally binding Agenda 21 action plan from Rio, many observers conclude that sustainable development is a challenge that remains to be confronted, and here the urban and regional level, as the interface between local and national, in an increasingly globalized environment of international interests and pressures, is of particular significance.

Population change and urbanization

This part of the chapter draws on statistical information from the UN Population Division, Department of Economic and Social Affairs and commentaries from the UN and academics specializing in the understanding of these statistics (United Nations 1996, 1998). The Population Division of the UN biennially prepares the official UN population estimates and projections for countries, urban and rural areas, and major cities. The summary information provides an overview for the reader illustrated by a number of graphs and tables.

World population growth

The rapid growth of the world population is a recent phenomenon in the history of the world. World population was estimated at 791 million in 1750, with 64 percent in Asia, 21 percent in Europe, 13 percent in Africa and 2 percent in North and Latin America. By 1900, 150 years later, the world population had only slightly more than doubled, to 1650 million. The major growth had been in Europe, whose share of world population had increased to 25 percent, and in North America and Latin America, whose share had increased to 5 percent each. Meanwhile the share of Asia had decreased to 57 percent and that of Africa to 8 percent. The growth of the world population accelerated after 1900, with 2520 million in 1950, a 53 percent increase in 50 years.

The rapid growth of the world population started in 1950, with a sharp reduction in mortality in the less developed regions, resulting in an estimated population of 6055 million in the year 2000, nearly two and a half times the population in 1950. With the declines in fertility in most of the world, the global annual growth rate of population has been decreasing since its peak of 2.0 percent in 1965–70. In 1998, the world's population stood at 5.9 billion and was growing at 1.3 percent per year, or an annual net addition of 78 million people.

By 2050 the world is expected to have 8909 million people, an increase of slightly less than half from the 2000 population. By then the share of Asia will have stabilized at 59 percent, that of Africa will have more than doubled to 20 percent, and that of North and Latin America nearly doubled to 9 percent. Meanwhile, the share of Europe will decline to 7 percent, less than one third its peak level. While in 1900 the population of Europe was three times that of Africa, in 2050 the population of Africa will be nearly three times that of Europe. The world population will continue to grow after 2050. Long range population projections of the United Nations indicate population growth well into the 22nd century.

United Nations' population revision

Some of the highlights of the UN's 1998 revision of the world population estimates and projections are summarized below:

- World population currently stands at 5.9 billion people and is growing at 1.33 percent per year, or an annual net addition of 78 million people. World population in the mid-21st century is expected to be in the range of 7.3 to 10.7 billion people. The medium fertility projection, which is usually considered as 'most likely', indicates that world population will reach 8.9 billion in 2050.

- The global average fertility level now stands at 2.7 births per woman; in contrast to early 1950 when the average number was 5 births per woman. Fertility is now declining in all regions of the world. For example, during the last 25 years, the number of children per couple has fallen from 6.6 to 5.1 in Africa, from 5.1 to 2.6 in Asia and from 5.0 to 2.7 in Latin America and the Caribbean.

- The 1998 revision demonstrates a devastating mortality toll from HIV/AIDS. For instance, in the 29 hardest hit African countries, the average life expectancy at birth is currently 7 years less than it would have been in the absence of AIDS.

- The results from the 1998 revision shed new light on the global population ageing process. In 1998, 66 million people in the world were aged 80 or over, that is about 1 in every 100 people. This number is expected to increase almost six fold by 2050 to reach 370 million people. The number of centenarians is projected to increase 16 fold by 2050 to reach 2.2 million people.

World urban and rural populations

The percentage of population living in urban areas in 1996 and 2030 is given in Figure 12.2. Broadly this shows the urbanization trends in different regions of the world. The most noticeable changes are the very substantial increases in Africa and Asia.

Large cities

In terms of the world's largest agglomerations (with populations of 10 million or more inhabitants) the UN Urban Agglomeration Statistics 1996 depicted in Figure 12.3 provide us with the evidence of the changes that have taken place from 1970 and the predictions for 2015.

Figure 12.4 is a graph demonstrating the growth in the number of urban agglomerations with one million or more inhabitants from 1950 to 2015. It shows dramatically the difference between the more developed and less developed regions.

The brief review of world population revised estimates and the urbanization trends from UN statistics demonstrate that there is a rapid shift for all regions of the world to becoming more and more urbanized. The growing urban agglomerations increasingly will be the focus for national economic performance and local and global environmental performance. The urban policies of governments and the planning, management and governance at the city level become critical in the realization of

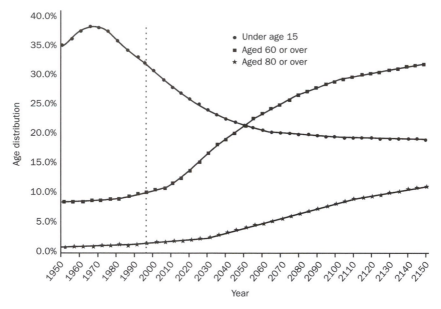

Figure 12.1 Percentage of world population 1950–2150 in three age categories and medium fertility scenario
Source: Population Division of the Department of Economic and Social Affairs at the United Nations Secretariat, World Population Projections to 2150 (United Nations, New York, 1998)

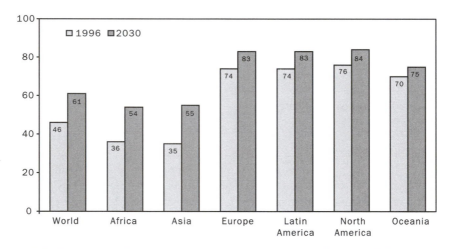

Figure 12.2 Percentage of population living in urban areas in 1996 and 2030
Source: Population Division of the Department of Economic and Social Affairs at the United Nations Secretariat, World Population Projections to 2150 (United Nations, New York, 1998)

sustainable urban futures and increasingly national competitiveness in global markets.

In Europe, which has been urbanized for a long time, there have been a number of significant policy developments that provide frameworks for urban policy so more sustainable futures can be developed in terms of energy use, transport, social

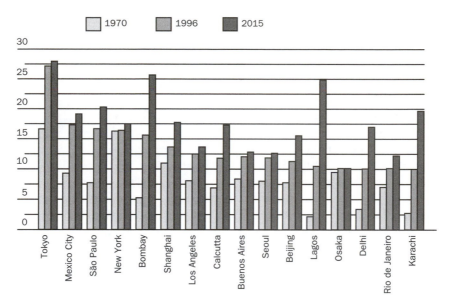

Figure 12.3 World's urban agglomerations with populations of 10 million or more inhabitants in selected years
Source: UN Urban Agglomeration Statistics, Population Division, United Nations (1996)

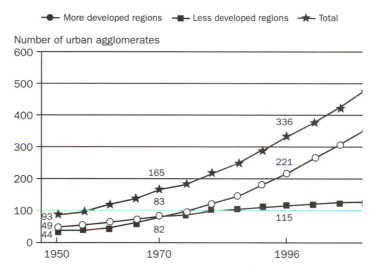

Figure 12.4 Number of urban agglomerations from 1950–2015 with one million or more inhabitants
Source: UN Urban Agglomeration Statistics, Population Division, United Nations (1996)

exclusion, economic regeneration, cultural heritage and governance. These policies take on board the sustainable development agenda; provide for the sharing of local practice in towns and cities across Europe; and are supported by an increasing research interest in the 'city of tomorrow'.

European urban focus

The European Union (currently with 15 member states) is one of the most urbanized continents in the world. The Union contains approximately 170 cities with more than 200,000 inhabitants, and 32 cities with more than one million inhabitants. London and Paris are the only two metropolises with populations approaching 10 million. Over 80 percent of the European population live in these towns and cities making them the cultural, economic and innovative centres of Europe. They function as the generators of local, regional and national economies, but together are the key localities in relation to European global competitiveness. They are also the centres of European social and cultural development and in recent times have undergone what is expressed as a 'renaissance' by some commentators. At the same time many of these localities are confronted with serious problems – high unemployment, social and spatial segregation, social exclusion; concerns over their future economy, crime and the general quality of life; negative impacts on health; and pressures on natural and historic assets. In addition they are handling wider global and societal changes due to the globalization of markets, shifts in demography and family structure and new technological innovations (see Chapter 13 for an in-depth discussion of globalization issues).

Along with cities worldwide, European cities are facing up to these challenges that are reshaping their futures. In work carried out for the European Commission and the World Health Organisation over the last ten years, a number of significant issues can be identified that are closely interrelated and that provide the agenda for policy development for both cities and member states, and for the European Union as a whole. These include increased competition among cities and regions both within the Union and between the Union and the rest of the world.

The accumulation of unemployment, poverty and social exclusion in larger cities are important issues for public health practitioners as urbanization is set to continue apace around the world. In-migration is an issue linked to these public health determinants. It is important that public health policy is directed towards sustainable urban development and reflects the influence of changes to public expenditure and social insurance on cities. Increasing concern over urban health; increasing inability to achieve access and mobility within and between cities; and concerns over the quality of local democracy appear to present many challenges for urban management, urban leadership and governance. Public health practitioners should be aware of such challenges in formulating their own actions and policy.

European urban policies for sustainable futures

Since 1991 the European Community, now the European Union, has sought consolidation of its actions for environmental protection and re-orientation of environment policy to promote the objectives of sustainable development in relation to towns and cities. These policy shifts have key implications for the urban environment. The principal developments are described and elaborated in *European Sustainable Cities* (Commission of the European Communities 1996). A selective policy history is provided in Table 12.1.

Table 12.1 Chronological policy history

1972	Stockholm Conference
1980	World Conservation Strategy
1987	Brundtland Report
1987	WHO Healthy Cities – Phase 1
1990	Green Paper on the Urban Environment (EU)
1991	Expert Group on the Urban Environment (EU)
1992	Rio Conference (Agenda 21)
1993	Sustainable Cities Project (EU)
1994	Aalborg Conference – Charter and Campaign
1996	European Sustainable Cities Report
	Lisbon Action Plan
	Habitat II Conference, Istanbul
1997	Urban Communications (EU)
	Kyoto Conference
1998	Vth Framework for Research
	'City of Tomorrow'
2000	Expert Group (new programme)
	Hanover Conference
2001	Habitat plus 5
2002	Rio plus 10

In the field of environmental policy, and by implication health, integration of the urban discussion has been extensively pursued. An integrated approach was first advocated in the Fourth Environmental Action Programme 1988–92; this led to the publication of the consultative *Green Paper on the Urban Environment* (Commission of the European Communities 1990) and in 1991 to the Council of Ministers establishing the Expert Group on the Urban Environment.

The rationale for detailed consideration of the urban environment is set out in the Green Paper, which was a response to pressures from three sources – the concern on the part of several European cities that a preoccupation with rural development within the European Commission was overshadowing the interests of urban areas; the commitment of the then environment commissioner; and a resolution from the European Parliament urging for more studies on the urban environment. The Green Paper is a significant milestone in thinking about the urban environment in Europe, principally because it advocated a holistic view of urban problems and a policy integration approach to their solution.

The Green Paper sparked a number of debates. Perhaps the most heated debate concerned different views on urban form and the relationship between notions of 'compact cities' and sustainable futures. While the urban form and density of cities are clearly important, discussions since have widened the debate to consider ways in which 'cities and their hinterlands', regions and urban society are to be governed and managed to achieve sustainable futures. The Expert Group on the Urban Environment, established in 1991, developed the European Sustainable Cities Project in 1993 which led to a wider policy discussion in the European Commission with an urban focus. This work has been published in *European Sustainable Cities* (Commission of the European Communities 1994b, 1996). The European Sustainable Towns and Cities Campaign, launched in Aalborg in 1994, now includes over 1700 local authorities as well as the major European local authority networks, the International Council for Local Environmental Initiatives and WHO.

European Sustainable Cities

In 1997 the European Commission published its communication *Towards an Urban Agenda in the European Union* (Commission of the European Communities 1997). This communication established a process of consultation culminating in the November 1998 conference in Vienna where the urban action plan, *Sustainable Urban Development in the European Union: A Framework for Action* (Commission of the European Communities 1998), was discussed. This framework was organized under four substantive policy aims. These were:

- strengthening economic prosperity and employment in towns and cities;
- promoting equality, social inclusion and regeneration in urban areas;
- protecting and improving the urban environment towards local and global sustainability; and
- contributing to good urban governance and local empowerment.

Further the Fifth Framework for Research in the European Union, which commenced in 1999 and continued for four years, contained a strong focus on urban issues and included a research area called the 'City of Tomorrow'. Fudge and Rowe (1997) in a report on the development of socio-economic environmental research for the European Commission suggested some of the priorities for urban research to be included in the Fifth Framework programme should be:

- how to upgrade (towards sustainability goals) current urban stock – which will also comprise the fabric of the 'City of Tomorrow';
- developing models for the future of access and mobility which are affordable and sustainable;
- how to reduce inequality and counteract unemployment and social exclusion;
- investigating methods of implementing healthy public policy including community safety;
- investigating how to reduce energy consumption in all aspects of production and consumption in cities;
- attuning urban economies to sustainability goals, at the appropriate scale and without exporting problems, thus the research agenda must include city and hinterland;
- underpinning research into the changing nature of urban and social values; and
- examining approaches to urban management and governance that are required for sustainable futures for cities.

Cities are increasingly at the centre of European policy thinking even though the legal and constitutional competence is less clear.

Multidisciplinary policy issues in sustainable futures

The problems with both conceptualizing sustainable development and applying the principles derive from the requirement to bridge the very different paradigms of the so called 'hard' disciplines associated with the environmental sciences, and those of management and social sciences. The extent to which different elements of the 'capital' of sustainability may be substitutable, for example whether an increase in human knowledge can compensate for resource losses, is also, by definition, unknown (see for example Pearce *et al.* 1990).

The concept of 'carrying capacity' seems to offer the possibility of setting objective limits upon the use of both natural and manmade resources. However, this concept too is interpreted differently by various users to reflect their own perceptions of value (see for example O'Neill 1996). Moreover, issues such as democratic probity have yet to be addressed at all (the majority may choose not to pay the price for sustainability policies and practice).

Tensions arise from the potential breadth and scope of sustainable develop-ment, both spatially (from global to local) and temporally (from 'as soon as possible' to the very long-term). Relevant policy areas include environment, transport, land use planning and practice, health, technology and business practice, as well as the frameworks for trade; the instruments which might be brought to bear thus range from legislation and market regulation to systems management and community action.

There are problems of definition, measurement, attribution of value and the use of indicators (see for example Local Government Management Board 1994b; Countryside Commission 1995. Work continues into green accounting (see for example Organisation for Economic Cooperation and Development 1996; Green Alliance 1997) and, particularly through the Organisation for Economic Cooperation and Development (OECD), alternatives to gross national product as measures of national well being.

However, it may be argued that the growth paradigm and the strength of business interests to a large extent still prevail. There is a dominant central commitment to international competitiveness which militates against business and capital engaging with more environmentally and socially beneficial forms of production and manage-ment (Welford 1995). Globalization, fostered by technological, informational and managerial change, proceeds apace; eco-efficiency may be superimposed but would require concerted international effort, of which there is little evidence (Fussler and James 1996). Localization, on the other hand, which underpins sustainability thinking in many countries emphasizes place, community and individual. The question which then arises is how urban and regional actors may most usefully resolve these dilemmas to make progress at the urban and regional level.

Swedish cities case study

Ecological modernization

Given these generic approaches emerging from both European and international experience, the chapter now examines in more detail the experience of implementation of policies for sustainable futures from Stockholm, Göteborg and Malmö in Sweden.

Sweden has long been an acknowledged leader in Europe in terms of its commitment to environmental protection linked with ecologically based technological innovation, and to social democratization and high levels of welfare provision. Following the 1992 UN Conference on Environment and Development in Rio, Agenda 21 was received warmly in Sweden as codifying an existing determination to pursue development that may be sustainable.

However, over the last decade the economy has come under increasing pressure from globalization and social change. Although the environmental agenda remains strong, a schism seems to be developing with key socio-economic drivers. The Swedish government has responded with a policy framework of ecological modernization, through which it hopes to regain the high ground economically, environmentally and socially. This is reported elsewhere in the evaluative study of the implementation of the national framework for sustainable development and how it is being interpreted in cities and towns in Sweden (Fudge and Rowe 2000, 2001).

Stockholm

The challenge for Stockholm (population 750,000) as capital lies in remaining a national leader in sustainable development in the face of rising consumer expectations in a globalizing society, ghettoization and developing 'edge crisis', and the ever increasing costs of implementing sustainability principles as the public ownership of land, housing and other resources diminishes.

Many of the difficulties it faces are reflected in the increasing inner-city traffic congestion and air quality deterioration which characterize all of Sweden's major conurbations. A thematic 'flagship' project has been developed through the partly EU funded programmes, Zero Emissions in Urban Societies and, more recently, Electric Vehicle City Distribution Systems. Standard traffic lights have been replaced with diode control systems, providing a significant energy saving. In the municipal fleet, 1500 petroleum and diesel vehicles are being replaced, or converted, to use methane from waste and sewage digestion, ethanol, rapeseed oil or electricity. Hybrid buses and heavy duty vehicles for waste management and food and goods distribution are also being introduced. Petroleum companies have cooperated in a new diverse fuelling infrastructure.

Evaluation of performance, the effectiveness of incentives and transferability are built into the programmes and many achievements have been noted. One of these is the ongoing cooperation that has been achieved between public and private sectors. The project focus, led by deputy mayors, has also meant that various players within municipal governance across sectors and levels have worked together. However, this mutual working has yet to be translated into significant institutional change. The approach remains heavily 'expert' and the community at large has been little involved. Road traffic continues to increase and the costliness of the programmes limits their expansion and transferability. More ambitious development of new transport nodes and routes, including light rail, is more problematic as public spending declines and public ownership of land and resources diminishes.

The project focus has also characterized neighbourhood regeneration projects in Stockholm. The adaptation of two 1960s suburbs to 'ecocycles principles' was the subject of an open ideas competition within the neighbourhoods themselves, among the professions and in senior school classes throughout Sweden, with the aims of inclusion and awareness raising. In what is intended to be an international prototype for inner-city regeneration an 'ecological neighbourhood', Hammarby Sjöstad (undated), is also being constructed on contaminated industrial land in south-central Stockholm. Aims include a halving of the usual environmental impacts of new-build housing. The neighbourhood will house 15,000 people in 8000 apartments within a mixed development of shops, offices, small businesses, schools and social and leisure facilities (Ministry of the Environment and Natural Resources 1992). Environmental and design objectives were agreed at the outset by a cross-sectoral partnership:

- to close resource loops at as local a level as possible;
- to minimize consumption of natural resources;
- to meet energy needs from renewable sources;
- to promote solutions that meet residents' and employers' needs; and
- to enhance social cooperation and ecological responsibility.

Technological solutions are already advanced. Thus, there will be district heating from heat recovery from local liquid biofuel fired boilers, supplemented by solar panels and heat pumps as necessary, and electricity supply in accordance with the Swedish Natural Environment Protection Agency's criteria for good environmental choice.

However, the commercial viability of the scheme is already under pressure. Its social inclusiveness, its feasibility in relation to the right to personal choice of its inhabitants, and its transferability are questionable. In this regard, an earlier experimental ecological neighbourhood, that of Ladugårdsängen in Örebro (Guinchard 1997), designed in 1989/90 for 3200 people and 500 businesses in public–private partnership, has to date largely survived commercial and ideological pressures. It continues to deliver successfully on waste and energy use minimization, and some transport parameters.

Göteborg

Göteborg (population 450,000) has an industrial past associated with the port and ferry industries and vehicle manufacturers (notably Volvo). Its reinvention of itself as a 'city of ideas' relies to a large extent on maintaining the close relationship between municipality, technological development and diversifying industry. Its early lead in Sweden in comprehensive planning (Bergrund 1994) aimed to reconcile what are seen as the contradictory drivers of ecocycles-based sustainability – competitiveness and citizen empowerment.

The city council's green procurement policy is a key tool in the (preregionaliza-tion) context of 60,000 employees, having a procurement budget of SKr7 billion (about 3.5 billion euro), and in the potential to influence a wide constituency in the private and community sectors (European Commission 1996). The procurement department, a municipal company wholly financed through commissions on con-tracts which works closely with the environment department, develops and adminis-ters lists of environmental life cycle efficiency criteria and approved companies within 250 fields. Companies must commit to ongoing improvement through annual reporting, which tends to impact positively on all their business practice. Although initial investment by both the city and private business was high, contract suppliers (often small companies, where growth is needed) have won significant market advantage.

Systematic auditing shows unambiguous reductions in the city's environmental impacts, through lower resource use in products and packaging, delivery planning and high volume supplies. However, the procurement model depends on political commitment and leadership, widely accepted methodology, and a comprehensive strategy of ongoing cross-sectoral research, development and information dissemi-nation, all of which are costly. In a changing political climate, and in the face of anti-competitiveness legislation from the EU and the dilution of local mutual responsibility (through regionalization as well as the globalization of markets), questions arise as to whether its devices and instruments will be strong enough to maintain it. In addition, the population's longer working hours allow less time for the political, environmental and community activity which has in the past assisted in holding together such policies. Priorities in a developing two-thirds (enfranchised) society are also changing as some districts remain as outsiders.

Malmö

Malmö (population 250,000) is at the forefront of the changes sweeping through Sweden. Its most pressing problem is unemployment, reaching more than 85 percent in one inner-city neighbourhood among immigrant communities.

It is the national pathfinder in integrating cultural and socio-economic change with traditional values, and innovative thinking is reflected in the development of the new University College (Malmö Högskola 1998). A key objective of the college is that it should make a significant contribution to the life of the city, and that its tuition and research should play a crucial part in the transition from a depleted industrial-based to a modern knowledge-based economy incorporating the highest environ-mental competencies. Development is publicly funded on publicly owned land on a complex disused shipyard/industrial site in the centre of Malmö, supported in part by parallel commercial development. Ecocycles thinking is being employed in both built form and curriculum development. The state programme for architecture and form underpins good functional and aesthetic design as well as sound, safe, manageable and ecologically durable technology at investment and operating costs appropriate to users' ability to pay. The college is expected to be self-sufficient in heating, with minimal electrical and cooling demands, and to incorporate systems to separate grey and foul water and waste close to source.

The curriculum is characterized by multidisciplinary and interdisciplinary activity. Departments and faculties are replaced by 'fields of training', all at basic, higher and research levels – for example, technology and economics, art and communication, health and community. Planning and implementation have been very rapid and thus strongly professional and 'top-down'.

The city's industrial, commercial and local communities generally have been little engaged. This is problematic both because the city is deeply divided socio-economically and politically, and because business remains strongly Conservative and tends to demand certain (sectoral) competencies in its potential employees. The extent to which the University College's ambitions can influence significantly the thinking and behaviour of the wider community remains in question.

Case study conclusion

The city case studies described above, implementing the national policy framework, provide compelling evidence of the progress Sweden has made towards sustainable development. In analytical work various needs were perceived in the municipality case studies (Fudge and Rowe 2001). These included:

- rebuilding power and trust in a new pluralist frame which can encompass the whole of the sustainable development agenda;

- strong and long-term leadership which may be able to survive the exigencies of party politics;

- clear methodologies, programmes and tools for vertical and horizontal integration in what remains a fragmented 'silo' culture; and

- a recognition of shifting public, private and community boundaries, so that expertise and experience at all levels in all sectors may be both governed and built upon.

Strategic issues for the future of sustainability

Following the opening discussion of the definitions and meanings of sustainable development, this chapter has examined world population estimates and urbanization trends. These demonstrate that the 21st century will be an 'urban century' and that the growth rate of cities in all regions, but particularly in Asia and Africa, presents major problems in terms of spatial planning, infrastructure, housing, transport and quality of life. It also leaves governments with major policy questions around the future of growing urban and declining rural populations; significant demographic questions concerning the growing population of the elderly and children in different regions of the world; and for the UN and governments, major concerns about global climate change and poverty.

These changes have been explored in relation to the European Union where a considerable urban policy history exists. Urban policy, spatial planning and sustainable development are being pursued at European, national and city levels of government, within supportive networks with considerable sharing of practice and the sense of being involved in a meta-urban, sustainable development project. The chapter then has examined ecological modernization in Sweden as a selected case study focusing on three cities – Stockholm, Göteborg and Malmö.

This concluding discussion aims to expand on the emerging policy and management orthodoxy to achieve more sustainable futures for urban areas and propose some steps for pursuing urban sustainability.

Emerging policy on urban management

Despite considerable work by towns and cities and by national governments, urban settlements continue to face economic and social problems, environmental degradation and ill health. New ways of managing the urban environment need to be found so that cities can both solve local problems and contribute to regional and global sustainability. At the same time an urban renaissance in parts of the world and policies for regeneration and renewal can be used to advance the sustainability agenda.

This chapter highlights the notion that sustainable development must be planned for and that market forces alone cannot achieve the necessary integration of environmental, social, health and economic concerns. A form of urban management and urban governance is emerging which provides a framework within which innovative approaches to the planning of sustainability can be explored. In this respect, a set of ecological, social, economic, organizational and democratic principles and tools for urban management can be identified which may be applied in a variety of urban settings and which could be used selectively as cities move from different starting points and different circumstances towards contributing to local and global sustainability. The case study examples from practice across Europe clearly demonstrate that an institutional as well as a policy focus is required. The capacity of different levels of government, and particularly local government, to deliver sustainability is seen as crucial.

This may require fundamental reviews of the internal structure and working of local authorities and their relationship with their communities, as well as an examination of the relationship between central and local governments. A further dimension is that thinking about cities is undergoing a reappraisal with a return to a view of the city as a complex system requiring a set of tools that can be applied in a range of settings. Although the system is complex, it is appropriate to seek practical solutions, especially solutions which solve more than one problem at a time, or several solutions that can be used in combination. Illustrative examples of this are numerous – a Sheffield, UK, example in housing captures the essence of the new approach (Fudge 1995; Price and Tsouros 1996).

The challenge of urban sustainable development involves both the problems experienced within cities, the problems caused by cities and the potential solutions that cities themselves may provide. Managers of cities, if they are to meet more sustainable futures, must seek to resolve the social, economic, cultural and health needs of urban residents while respecting local, regional and global natural systems, broadly solving problems locally where possible, rather than shifting them to other spatial locations or passing them on to future generations. This prescriptive advice must, however, be interpreted within the complexity of regional and global economic and environmental relationships. This interpretation may raise broader issues about the 'production of space' and the 'production of nature' (Harvey 1996) and the wider economic and social forces that influence these decisions.

The preceding overview of the changes argued to be necessary to achieve a more sustainable future for cities is proactive, coherent and potentially radical. However, for it to be implemented a number of deeper questions and issues are raised that must also be addressed. First, considerable local changes that support sustainable futures (environmental strategies, recycling, environment centres, Agenda 21 coordinators, Agenda 21 plans, increases in cycling provision and so on) have occurred, but there seems to be limits to furthering this early progress. The spread of ideas and ownership of issues are limited within the population of cities. Second, because the next developmental step cannot be accommodated alongside the existing economic functioning and economic relations within and between cities, it requires a more fundamental transformation of socio-ecological and political-economic processes and relations both within the locality and potentially at national and global levels.

Next steps

From policy development work and discussions with practitioners, general propositions include:

- Concerns of urban management and governance for sustainability are equally as important as the need for different substantive policies.
- Local authorities and their communities are crucial constituencies for sustainability, but regional and central government frameworks need to be supportive.
- Ecosystems thinking, particularly notions of resource flows, the recycling of land and buildings, the closing of resource loops, the principles of 'resource efficiency' and 'circularity' are the keys to adapting existing and designing new urban localities.
- Networks of actors engaging in this project are crucial to avoid duplication, share good practice and support problem solving (see network Winter Cities but also European Sustainable Cities and Towns Campaign network http://www.iclei.org/europe/la21/sustainable-cities.htm).
- Integration is needed between different sectors – economic, social, health, environmental and cultural; vertically between organizations and their communities; and horizontally within parts of organizations.
- Strategic planning and management, and infrastructure planning and provision at different spatial levels needs new approaches in terms of political leadership, technical competence, resource allocation and procurement.

- Conceptual and practical approaches need to be holistic at different spatial scales, not sectoral.

- Education and awareness need a strategic plan as well as 'bottom-up' initiatives and actions.

- Partnerships and collaboration between different sectors seem to provide more fruitful opportunities than relying on traditional categories of responsibilities.

- Demonstration projects are needed so that sustainable approaches can be experienced.

- Regular measurement of progress towards or away from sustainable futures related to baseline data is needed to understand progress and change.

- Democratic changes are implied through the involvement of communities (such as Agenda 21) and other factors.

- Action research is needed now to support and provide appropriate and timely feedback to practitioners.

- Longer-term developmental and evaluative programmes of research are needed to explore new ways of managing changing cities and evaluating existing policies and practices.

The focus on urbanization and the quality of life in cities in the 21st century raises issues of definition and scope for public health and public health interventions in society. It reminds us of the origins of modern town planning and its close association with public health and allows a closer relationship to be reconceptualized between health, town planning, global environmental change and the future of cities. In describing the urban context, the approaches to sustainable futures and the propositions for policy development and action, it is possible to see the implicit and explicit links to public health and indeed how mainline public health concerns may need to be reconceptualized to be able to take in the notion of sustainable development.

For the future the public health agenda, as well as concentrating on its core concerns, will probably have to engage with both the 'mitigation' and 'adaptation' responses to global climate change (Fudge and Antrobus 2002). In north-west European towns and cities, as in Japan and elsewhere, these 'new' concerns of the effects of global climate change will be coupled with the projected increase in the percentage of the population living until they are in their 80s or 90s, and the growing imbalance between those in work and providing services and a tax base, and those retired or in ill health. What then does the sustainable city look like and how will it be governed and managed? These questions give rise to further speculation on the nature of the public health agenda and current public health discourse.

Acknowledgements

I would like to acknowledge the assistance of my colleagues in the Faculty of the Built Environment at the University of the West of England, Bristol, particularly Dr Janet Rowe, and the work over the past ten years in the European Union from the Expert

Group on the Urban Environment, the European Sustainable Cities and Towns Campaign, and from colleagues in the research councils and in the universities in Sweden. The framework for this chapter was first given as a keynote paper for the Winter Cities Conference 2002, Aomori, Japan and I am grateful for the comments received there.

13

STUART McCLEAN
Globalization and health

Editors' introduction

Globalization or 'growing interdependence' between different peoples, regions and countries in the world is the term used to describe social and economic relationships that stretch worldwide and will continue to do so.

All 21st century public health practitioners, as defined in the Introduction to this book, should be aware of the conjecture attached to the positive and negative impact of globalization on future public health by today's writers and thinkers.

Positive impacts are the spread of communication and media across the globe creating a 'global village'. This increases opportunities for public health practitioners to join forces in confronting issues such as the spread of infectious disease, the threat of terrorism, trafficking in illegal drugs, environmental health issues, climate change and matters concerning food, including GM foods and animal diseases. Globalization also has negative implications for public health practitioners: as national boundaries and controls are weakened, the historical concerns of public health workers over the past 200 years, including problems from the movement of goods and people, re-emerge into a 21st century context.

The uneven spread of new technology across the globe leaves two-thirds of the world disenfranchised technologically, with no obvious means to redress the situation. The pattern of technological exclusion does not conform to nation states, but in time will exacerbate health inequality in ways not conducive to lateral or unilateral governmental action. Global public health action is thus inextricably linked by geography and ecology to economic growth through technology and this has numerous implications for 21st century public health workers.

This chapter begins by exploring the contested definitions of globalization. The author goes on to discuss the positive and negative impacts of globalization on public health, examining the role of key international institutions such as the World Bank, World Trade Organisation and World Health Organisation. The impact of global trade policy on public health in the UK and global health inequalities and global divisions are assessed. Finally, globalization and emerging public health risks are discussed. The author concludes with a summary of the challenges for public health in the 21st century.

Introduction

The aim of this chapter is to locate contemporary debates surrounding globalization and theories of global society within the domain of public health, and, in addition, to argue that these debates are central to the public health endeavour. A broad-based public health should take stock of significant social and political changes that define and shape people's health. The following sections therefore map a range of debates that the public health discussion of globalization has raised.

There has been a considerable increase in interest into the issue of globalization within public health, but this emerging field is a contested one, insofar as public health writers are undecided as to the impact of globalization on health. Nevertheless, I demonstrate how a key issue within public health is the need to understand the impact of macro processes of globalization on population health.

A theoretical approach to globalization is of key importance in helping us to understand the nature of contemporary social, economic and political changes, but at present globalization is generally undertheorized within the public health field. Therefore, by way of introduction, I shall briefly outline some of these issues as they are conceptualized within social science and consider how they illuminate wider debates within public health.

The globalization debate

The term globalization is a recent addition to academic circles and is only beginning to play a part in discussions within public health. Currently, it is argued that a key issue in 21st century public health is the challenge of globalization and how this affects individual and population level health (Zwi and Yach 2002: 1615). However, there has been a general shift in the awareness of globalization as a field of discussion, brought about partly by the public perception of events (such as war, conflict, famine and international level disputes) that occur at some distance from the recipient. As Hannerz states, 'Distances, and boundaries, are not what they used to be' (1996: 3). Globalization, then, undermines traditional perceptions and meanings of distance and national level boundaries.

Recent and high profile events that took place both in Seattle in November 1999 and New York in September 2001 have resulted in talk of globalization being no longer the sole preserve of lawyers, politicians, economists, sociologists and cultural theorists. These distant events, intensified and replayed through the role of the global media, have brought the 'new era' (United Nations Development Programme 1999) of globalization to public consciousness, although it is generally argued that globalization is not a phenomenon of the modern age, but predates this era (Held and McGrew 2000: 6). Insofar as the presence of a global society has been brought to the attention of individuals and communities through the global media lens, these recent high profile events have meant that globalization, as both a word and a social condition, has become ubiquitous in Western society.

Globalization – a contested term

Globalization is a greatly contested term in that it does not have a fixed meaning and therefore comes to mean different things to different people (Hannerz 1996; Held and McGrew 2000; Lee 2000b). Indeed, discussions that explore the nature of globalization also engender fierce disagreement among those within the field of public health. A good example can be seen in both the number and range of electronic responses to Feachem's (2001) article in the *British Medical Journal*.

During the 1950s and 1960s the term modernization was used (predominantly within the social sciences) to describe the changes that underdeveloped nations would pass through on their route to full industrialization (Rostow 1966; Held and McGrew 2000). Westernization as a term has also featured heavily, particularly as the early stage/era of globalization; industrial and capitalist were other terms synonymous with Western societies (Hannerz 1996: 8).

Globalization should not be interpreted as the imposition of Western modernity across the globe (Giddens 1990; Beck 2000a). Globalization does not just refer to the 'Americanization' or 'McDonaldization' of the global order (Ritzer 1993), a process that has also been referred to as the 'convergence of global culture' thesis (Beck 2000a: 42), in which what we are witness to is a greater uniformity of lifestyles and modes of behaviour. As a counter-trend to this 'McDonaldization', globalization can also refer to 'reverse colonization', where non-Western or 'developing' countries have some bearing on events that take place in the West (Giddens 1999). For example, this can be seen in the 'latinizing' of Los Angeles and the emergence of a highly innovatory high-tech sector in regions of India (Giddens 1999).

Others argue that globalization is itself problematic and ill-defined, and that either 'internationalization' or 'transnational' better describe these wider social, economic and political changes, particularly in relation to the erosion of state boundaries. Whereas internationalization refers to the continued primacy of the nation state in controlling territorial issues, transnational refers to the movement across bounded nation states that may not necessarily be global (Hannerz 1996), but trilateral (Giddens 1990).

Globalization is often seen to refer to 'interconnectedness' between individuals and communities across diverse and geopolitically separate nation states (McMichael and Beaglehole 2000; Stephens 2000). Moreover, globalization does not refer solely to processes which are remote from everyday personal lives (Giddens 1999). Individuals and communities can no longer consider themselves to be separate from wider global processes that have broader consequences for public health. As such, Giddens reiterates the interconnected nature of globalization when he refers to it as 'the intensification of worldwide social relations which link distant localities in such a way that local happenings are shaped by events occurring many miles away and vice versa' (1990: 64).

We shall see how this issue of distant events shaped by and shaping local happenings is thereby central to public health debates surrounding the global society.

Key features of globalization in relation to public health

Primarily, globalization has been brought about by, and is predominantly associated with manifestly economic processes (Waters 1995; Price *et al.* 1999; O'Keefe 2000; Baum 2001). Moreover, discussion surrounding the economic (as opposed to social, political or cultural) dimension of globalization has rather dominated the public health agenda. The argument here concerns the extent to which economic globalization has long been a feature of a world dominated by Western societies and ideology. Therefore, globalization in the economic context refers to a set of historical events which have their foundations in prior geopolitical events, such as the first period of European expansion from 1500 to 1800 (Feachem 2001: 506). As such, globalization is synonymous with the economic phenomenon of capitalism (Wallerstein 1979).

However, globalization does not refer merely to economic globalization: the economic integration of a global society has been over played (Turner 2001: 11). There are other spheres which we must take into account and are important in terms of public health. Globalization is engaged across a number of public and private spheres: the political, legal, military, socio-cultural and environmental as well as the economic (Held *et al.* 1999). These transformations within global society are central to contemporary social life and impact in both 'common sense' and unexpected ways on the health and well being of individuals and communities.

The Janus faces: positive and negative impacts on public health

Central to this debate is the effect of these wider economic and socio-cultural changes (understood as globalization) on the health of individuals and populations. Public health writers have weighed up the effects of key global processes and have considered the extent to which they are either beneficial or harmful to population health. Hannerz argues that ambiguity and contestation over the meaning of the term is at the heart of the debate concerning its effects: 'One almost expects any mention of globalization to be accompanied by either booing or cheering' (1996: 5). However, globalization is not intrinsically either beneficial or harmful to people's health, although it appears that proponents of both sides of this debate have become entrenched in their attitudes towards it (Lee 2001).

We can observe and illustrate the positive and negative consequences of global processes. Globalization is widely perceived as 'Janus-faced' (Bettcher and Wipfli 2001: 617), as there are perceived to be two sides to the process, one promising, the other threatening (Yach and Bettcher 1998). Positive consequences stem from the idea that globalization increases the sharing of information, ideas and forms of knowledge, and this has important benefits for public health. Bettcher and Wipfli (2001) argue that these opportunities are often missed from the analysis of global processes. For example, the collaboration between states over shared global public health issues such as tuberculosis or tobacco control can be an important experience: 'the ease and rapidity of communications have facilitated the diffusion of ideas and policy concerns relating to health care and public health . . . to areas of the world previously beyond the reach of the public health community' (Bettcher and Wipfli 2001: 617).

In addition, it is in the self-interest of high income countries to ensure that disenfranchised communities and nations do not become political vacuums of chaos in a globalizing world (Bettcher and Wipfli 2001: 617). In this respect political isolationism is seen as more of a threat to public health than openness to trade (Feachem 2001). The burgeoning of global travel, printed media and technologically enhanced media (such as the Internet) are viewed as positive aspects of global processes: 'Globalization of the world economy and the resulting increase in commerce, travel, and communication have benefited almost every country' (Howson et al. 1998: 586). Processes of technological innovation, for instance, have broader consequences for health. For example, the UK-based National Health Service has an Internet site called NHS Direct, and this is accessed by individuals and communities from all over the world as a resource for health.

For some writers within public health, globalization is something to be encouraged as it engenders 'openness' to ideas, people, trade and culture (Feachem 2001). This also seems to be the view of orthodox economists, in that globalization will lead to wealth accumulation. Such writers focus predominantly on the economic justification for globalization in terms of increased health equalling increased worker productivity: 'Healthy populations abroad represent growing markets for businesses of the industrial world. If developed countries invest in improving the health of other populations . . . their economic returns will be increased' (Howson et al. 1998: 589). The World Trade Organisation (WTO) and the World Bank (transnational and multinational level organizations) additionally support these views, and I explore these in more depth in the following section.

For others, however, globalization is creating rising social and health inequalities. Negative consequences are again viewed in terms of economic shifts; the market liberalization that global trade fosters: 'At the start of the 21st century one of the major threats to global health comes from the transnational financial interests who speculate against the world currencies' (Baum 2001: 613). Globalization is perceived as generating negative effects on national level health care systems, through the restrictive 'market promoting' policies of the WTO (Price et al. 1999), and that these policies have led to a disproportionate effect on the health of the vulnerable groups in the global society (Pollock and Price 2000: 13).

In addition, the public health concern has focused on equating globalization with direct health impacts, such as shifting disease patterns, climate change, poorer working conditions in the developing nation states and effects on food security. I will return to these issues in the final section examining contemporary public health risks.

The promoters of economic globalization and other key players

Global interconnectedness has been achieved largely on an economic scale, although we can also see that there has been significant erosion of boundaries in other spheres such as the cultural and political. Yet, economic globalization is not the serendipitous result of contemporary economic policy. This manifestation of globalization has long been a feature of Western states, and now the neoliberal economic agenda of the Organisation for Economic Cooperation and Development countries is given extra backing through the work and policy directives of the WTO, the World Bank and the International Monetary Fund. These organizations are widely regarded as the promoters of economic globalization (McMichael and Beaglehole 2000: 496).

However, we should recognize that the global health arena is a plural setting. For example, globally the health sector additionally consists of multinational companies, the independent sector, non-governmental organizations, WHO and the bilateral sector (Howson *et al.* 1998: 588). Yet the WTO, the World Bank, the International Monetary Fund and WHO take centre stage in discussions surrounding globalization and public health, so I will turn to these briefly.

The world trade organisation

A replacement for the General Agreement on Tariffs and Trade is the WTO, an international body based in Geneva which was created in 1995 to 'lower import taxes, remove barriers to free trade and resolve trade disputes' (Pollock and Price 2000: 12). The aim of the General Agreement on Tariffs and Trade was to reduce tariffs and thereby liberalize trade. It has also been perceived as an opportunity for the USA to create a trading system that best suited its interests during the post-war period (Waters 1995: 68).

A broader objective of the WTO has been to expand private markets by removing political/trade barriers to the global movement of goods, services and capital. A key component of these talks was that of public services. For example, a major aim of the WTO talks scheduled in Seattle in November 1999 was the restructuring of public services. Here, the focus was on prising open public funding streams that pay for public services. Therefore, the WTO is devising the international laws and regulatory frameworks that will allow it to open up public services to market forces: 'WTO plans are about dismantling public services in the interests of private sector corporations' (Pollock and Price 2000: 13).

Engagement with the promotion of economic globalization has been implemented through a number of strategies and trade laws, such as the promotion of free trade and the enforcement of structural adjustment policies (McMichael and Beaglehole 2000). Other strategies include the additional incentives that are offered to developing nations through a relaxation of wage controls and workplace standards (Daykin and Doyal 1999; McMichael and Beaglehole 2000). The specific role of the WTO is spelt out more clearly by O'Keefe (2000). O'Keefe argues that the WTO:

> sets the regulatory framework for the multi-lateral trading system including contractual obligations, which are legally binding on member states . . . It sets the rules applying to intellectual property rights, trade in goods and services, settles disputes and co-operates with other international agencies in developing global economic policy.

> (O'Keefe 2000: 174)

Some writers within public health interpret these trading obligations as a beneficial process. For example, Feachem argues that a key economic benefit of globalization is that countries that have gone through a process of trade liberalization will have an increase in GNP, and this has an equal effect on the health status of populations (Feacham 2001: 504). The notion of trade liberalization is crucial to the argument, and most commentators equate globalization with trade liberalization and the freeing of trade.

Trade liberalization refers to the relaxing of controls on the movement of capital, goods and services. The WTO website states it thus: 'one of the principles of the WTO system is for countries to lower their trade barriers and to allow trade to flow more freely. After all, countries benefit from the increased trade that results from lower trade barriers' (www.wto.org). However, the main questions that are posed in relation to trade liberalization are whether it promotes economic growth for poorer nations and whether it is equally practised (Labonte 2001: 620).

A good example of trade liberalization is the General Agreement on Trade in Services – one of the trade agreements devised by the WTO to encourage 'progressive liberalization' (Labonte 2002). Progressive liberalization essentially means that countries can only increase their commitments to free trade (Labonte 2002: 65). The WTO talks in Seattle were to focus on the revision of the General Agreement on Trade in Services: 'a system of international law intended to expand private-enterprise involvement in the increasingly important service sector' (Price et al. 1999: 1889).

Therefore, the General Agreement on Trade in Services opens up public service provision to foreign competition and ownership. This includes, for example, many service sectors such as health, education and housing (Price et al. 1999). The General Agreement on Trade in Services permits member countries to force the removal of barriers to foreign participation in the health services of other WTO members.

The world bank and the international monetary fund

Other organizations worth mentioning briefly are the World Bank and the International Monetary Fund. The World Bank is a source of financial assistance primarily for developing countries, and is seen as one of the largest multilateral funders of health care projects (O'Keefe 2000). The International Monetary Fund, based in Washington, also provides temporary economic assistance, but exists primarily to eliminate restrictions that hamper the promotion of free trade. The International Monetary Fund has been criticized particularly for its imposing of the structural adjustment programmes for developing countries that are in debt. The structural adjustment programmes exist in order to promote the private sector, and it is argued that this can lead to impaired population health (McMichael and Beaglehole 2000: 496). This is due to their part in driving for-profit insurance medical care, as opposed to encouraging developing nations to expand their public services (Navarro 1998). As a consequence, the combined result of debt repayment and structural adjustment programmes has resulted in developing nations dramatically cutting their social spending (Braveman and Tarimo 2002: 1627).

The World Health Organisation

The WHO additionally plays a crucial role in defining the field in terms of global institutions that have a stake in health. Generally, the WHO is viewed in positive terms in that its focus has been on reducing inequalities and identifying the inseparable nature of global-based inequalities in health. As O'Keefe explains: 'The World Health Organisation (WHO) has repeatedly insisted that policy at national and international levels should be linked and that we should be attempting to reduce inequalities between and within countries at the same time. A commitment to equity should guide health sector reform' (2000: 168).

Furthermore, the WHO has been influential in a number of forms of collaboration around health problems, such as tobacco consumption. As the WHO explains, tobacco consumption is a challenge to population health that 'cuts across national boundaries, cultures, societies and socio-economic strata' (www.who.int/en/). However, the WHO has not been exempt from criticism. Indeed, some have questioned its ability to address issues of global inequity when it has seen to become increasingly 'impotent' as a global player (Baum 2001: 615).

So far I have outlined the debates surrounding the role and influence of the international and transnational organizations, and have considered the extent to which economic/trade liberalization is exacerbating the gap between the rich and poor in the developing regions.

I now turn to examining the knock-on effect this will have on the vulnerable groups in the UK (the poor, the elderly, disabled and unemployed), due to privatization of public services, which is a product of key economic and political global trends.

Global trade policy and the UK health care context

National health systems are increasingly influenced by global factors that transcend state borders (Yach and Bettcher 1998). In addition, domestic policies have effects beyond the nation state: 'the domestic and international spheres of public health policy are becoming more intertwined and inseparable' (Yach and Bettcher 1998: 735).

A key issue here concerns the changing role of the state and the widening influence of the private sector. In this context, the UK is seen as an important domestic setting with which to discuss the changing relationship between global trade policies and public services (Price et al. 1999).

It is generally argued that the foundations of the NHS were based on a traditional nation state model of society. In addition, the NHS has been a public institution, but increasingly writers have argued that it is under threat due to the movement towards private enterprise. A key question is whether this form of global competition spells the end for the welfare state (Held and McGrew 2000: 19).

The UK is leading the way in restructuring and modernizing its public sector services, and this can be seen as a threat to the viability of the state. This restructuring is linked in the West to an increased use of experimentation with health care markets. Markets and quasi-markets for health care have been seen as a solution to rising health care expectations in the West, and as Braveman and Tarimo explain: 'Globally, there has been a downsizing of government and a marked trend towards privatization of many functions formally within the public health domain. To varying degrees, many countries have experienced a shift from centrally planned and regulated to market-dominated economies' (2002: 1627).

Pollock and Price (2000) explore some of the wider implications in addressing the reforming of public sector services, and these are also taken up in an article in the *Lancet* (Price *et al.* 1999). The example they give is that of the funding arrangements for public services. The NHS, they explain, has been funded on the basis of geographical area needs. Since 1991 and the creation of the internal market, funding is allocated as a payment per patient which follows them to the point of delivery. Pollock and Price argue that pro-liberalization organizations like the World Bank favour this 'capitation' payment as it allows the substitution of public for private sources of funding, such as private insurance and an incentive to withhold care (Price *et al.* 1999).

These authors argue that these wider structural changes in the delivery and funding of health care services hold key implications for public health. One of the most important of these is that of the effect on income and health inequalities in the UK, which are continuing to widen (Acheson 1998). It is argued that the WTO, through the General Agreement on Trade in Services, places restrictions on national sovereignty, although the wide ranging effects of these policies are yet to be explored in relation to inequalities in health.

Global inequalities in health: the local impact of global divisions

Some writers exploring the international health scene have argued that events like that of 11 September in New York symbolize the failure to address global inequities (Zwi and Yach 2002: 1618). Globalization is seen, on one hand, as exacerbating inequalities of resources. On the other hand, the World Bank and WTO have argued that economic globalization and trade liberalization (free trade) would bring benefits for all, and would act as a trigger for economic development within low income countries.

The impact of trade liberalization on health inequalities

The evidence largely points to the fact that trade liberalization has increased inequalities both between and within countries (see Navarro 1998; Walt 1998; Hurrell and Woods 1999; Lee 2000a; Rowson 2000). As Hurrell and Woods explain, 'Economic liberalization is exacerbating the gap between rich and poor within virtually all developing countries' (1999: 1). Moreover, these changes have effects wider than the developing nations. For example, Navarro argues that inequalities have increased substantially in both Western and non-Western societies. As he explains:

> These inequalities are growing at an unprecedented rate, not only among countries but also within most of the developed and developing countries . . . the globalization they extoll has meant an unprecedented growth in wealth and income, for others the process has meant an unprecedented deterioration in their standard of living, health, and well being.

> (Navarro 1998: 742)

Inequalities between and within countries

The United Nations Development Programme report 2001 produces some key data on inequalities between and within countries. On balance, global level inequality is very high. For example, in 1993 the poorest 10 percent of the world's population had only 1.6 percent of the income of the richest 10 percent. Conversely, the richest 10 percent of the US population had a combined income greater than that of the poorest 43 percent (United Nations Development Programme 2001: 19). However, as the report details, income deprivations are not limited to developing countries or regions. For example, within OECD countries more than 130 million are calculated as income poor and 34 million are unemployed (United Nations Development Programme 2001: 10), which raises some important questions regarding the relationship between global employment status and health (Daykin and Doyal 1999).

In addition, countries in eastern Europe and the CIS (former Soviet Union) have experienced some of the largest growths in income inequality and this has had a major impact on the recent resurgence of tuberculosis. Furthermore, since the political transition of the former Soviet Union and eastern European states, there has been a large and significant impact on life expectancy and personal security (United Nations Development Programme 2001: 13). For example, the report states, 'Globalization has created many opportunities for cross-border crime and the rise of multinational crime syndicates and networks' (United Nations Development Programme 2001: 13). This also has implications for the displacement of refugee populations across Europe.

More importantly, the report also notes that countries do not have to wait for economic prosperity to make progress in human development such as public health. This echoes some of the ideas of Wilkinson (1996) who argues that more egalitarian societies are healthier and more socially cohesive. Examples given such as South Korea and Costa Rica suggest that domestic social policies also contribute to and promote aspects of human development such as population health; this is not just the by-product of economic growth (United Nations Development Programme 2001: 13).

This also raises the issue of social capital, viewed by Putnam (1993) as stretching across four characteristics: existence of community networks, participation in networks (civil engagement), sense of local identity and solidarity, and norms of trust and reciprocity). The United Nations Development Programme report states that income inequality diminishes social capital (2001: 17). This also has major implications for public health: 'A deficiency of social capital (social networks and civic institutions) adversely affects the prospects of health by predisposing to widened rich–poor gaps, inner urban decay, increased drug trade, and weakened public-health systems' (McMichael and Beaglehole 2000: 497).

(Health inequalities in the UK are discussed in depth in Chapter 10.)

Technological inequalities

Another major factor raised by the United Nations Development Programme report (2001) is that of technological advance and its association with progress in human development. This is a moot point as inequalities of resources can draw attention to the technological capabilities of nation states. Sachs (2000), for example, argues that the world is split into regions that score highly on technological innovation and those that have limited technological expertise, although, interestingly, these regions that lack technological innovation do not necessarily conform to national borders (Sachs 2000). Sachs' argument is that technological inequality is synonymous with other risks, such as those connected with public health. However, unlike many economic-based arguments, Sachs explains that it is not the free market which can help provide technological innovations within these excluded regions, but partnerships and interaction between governments and scientific institutions (Sachs 2000).

The scope of contemporary public health is the reduction of social and health inequalities, and the striving for health sustaining environments (McMichael and Beaglehole 2000). In this way, we can see that exploring the effects of globalization on health inequalities is crucial. Additionally, it means that those professionals working within the broad gamut of public health may have to be more creative in exposing the multiple factors that contribute to continuing health inequalities.

Globalization and emerging public health risks

This section examines the wider impact of globalization on public health, particularly as it pertains to current key concerns within public health in the UK. It is argued by those in the public health field that people in the Western world are experiencing a major transition in the main causes of disease and must now address the challenges that these new public health risks bring to population health (McMichael and Beaglehole 2000: 495). (See also Chapter 7 for discussion on new threats to health and health protection issues in the UK.)

Non-communicable diseases

The 'epidemiological transition' brings new public health risks within the UK and the Western world in general (Gwatkin et al. 1999). For example, we see this with the rise of non-communicable diseases, such as coronary heart disease, cancers and forms of substance abuse such as alcoholism. A primary concern in terms of public health and in terms of the WHO agenda is that of tobacco related diseases (Lee 2000b). Although it could be argued that tobacco related markets are shrinking in Western Europe and North America, the impact of market/trade liberalization has meant that new markets have been fostered in Asia, Africa, South America, Eastern and Central Europe (Lee 2000b: 256). Other related public health issues such as substance abuse are also linked to emerging global trends, such as changing work patterns and lifestyles which are a result of the global economy (Lee 2000b: 257).

The greatest public health changes have been created through the global liberalization of trade (Walt 1998). As such, tobacco related morbidity and disease has been placed high on the WHO agenda. For example, WHO member states are involved in the negotiation of a law/treaty to assist in the regulation of tobacco companies – the Framework Convention on Tobacco Control (Bettcher and Wipfli 2001: 617).

Although the extent to which the WHO can set global policy on tobacco control has been perceived as heavily limited (*Lancet* 2002: 267), engagement with global and regional level public health policy has led to further debate and sharing of ideas. This highlights a point made earlier – that globalization encapsulates positive and negative expressions. For example, the negativity of the increase in tobacco related trade in Eastern and Central Europe contrasts with the increased cooperation among organizations on global public health issues. Globalization is both dynamic and contradictory (O'Keefe 2000: 172).

Communicable diseases

Non-communicable diseases aside, it is also true that globalization is changing the nature of infectious/communicable diseases (Lee 2000a: 14). Infectious diseases such as tuberculosis, malaria, the plague and cholera, are interpreted as 're-emerging'. For example, the WHO (1997) explains that the re-emergence of malaria is seen in areas where it had been thought it was eradicated, such as Azerbaijan, Iraq and Turkey.

Also, there are other newly emerging diseases like HIV, Ebola and nvCJD (WHO 1997). Indeed, the WHO claims that over the last 20 years 30 new infectious diseases have emerged (1997: 148). This is particularly the case among the low income countries, and regions which have experienced significant economic crises: 'Overall, communicable diseases were much more important for the poor than was suggested by global averages' (Gwatkin *et al.* 1999: 588).

It has also been argued that widening inequality within and between countries (identified by the United Nations Development Programme report 2001) is contributing to poorer people's vulnerability to infectious diseases, illustrated by the multi-drug resistant strains of tuberculosis and HIV (Farmer 1997; Howson *et al.* 1998; Lee 2000a). This is particularly interesting in the case of tuberculosis, where there has been a reversal of the trends in the West, with an increase of cases in particular with Multi-drug Resistant (MDR) TB (Farmer 1997). Furthermore, this has taken place in areas populated by the poor and most vulnerable groups in society: 'Significant outbreaks of MDR TB have been reported in homeless shelters, prisons and medical facilities from Washington D.C. to Boston to San Francisco' (Farmer 1997: 348). Tuberculosis increases in Russia and Eastern Europe during the 1990s have also been noted and this is seen as illustrative of the breakdown of the social order and social cohesion since the political fragmentation of the former Russian states.

Infectious diseases, therefore, have increased partly because of increased poverty and also because they are the product of widening inequalities. Infectious diseases are therefore treated as 'sociomedical phenomena' (Farmer 1997: 348). However, with the increase in global travel, tourism (to places like Africa, the Indian subcontinent and South America), population migration and displacement, other diseases like malaria and cholera are proving to be a public health threat once again (Lee 2000b: 256).

Food-borne disease

The increase and intensification of worldwide mobility in both people and trade also has key public health risks and implications for the transportation of food and the increased incidence of transborder food-borne disease (Lee 2000b: 258). This has led to certain authors claiming that we should source food from local farms – the 'proximity principle' (El Din 2000: 16). Other commentators such as Shiva (2000) argue that trade agreements like the Trade Related Intellectual Property Rights Agreement of the WTO have increased the patents on indigenous food varieties, which Shiva argues destroys the diversity of local food cultures and their rich biological heritage (Rowson and Koivusalo 2000; Shiva 2000).

Environmental change

Another key public health issue, in terms of risk, is that of global environmental change. It has long been argued that key global environmental changes, brought about by the intensity of modern consumer driven economics, hold risks for public health: 'These changes to the earth's basic life-supporting processes pose long-term risks to the health of populations' (McMichael and Beaglehole 2000: 497). McMichael and Beaglehole explore the potential risks of global climate change to health, for example, in the geographical range of vector-borne infectious diseases such as malaria. Strains of malaria have now been discovered in parts of south-east England, and this has been put down to global climate change (Brown 2001). Climate change can therefore bring about a greater spread in infectious diseases: 'many of the biological organisms and problems linked to the spread of infectious diseases are especially influenced by fluctuations in climate variables, notably temperature, precipitation and humidity' (WHO 1997: 124).

Health care organizations

I argued previously that the boundaries of the nation state are in the process of being eroded and challenged by the counter movement of globalization. One area in which there has been a key impact is that of health care organizations. We have witnessed one aspect of this in terms of the privatization of services and market orientated policies, such as the private finance initiative (Pollock and Price 2000: 12).

But there are other key issues regarding health care systems that pose potential risks as well as opportunities. Lee notes a particular movement in the UK, 'towards an increasingly transborder provision of healthcare through the physical migration of health professionals and the development of telemedicine and teleconsulting across national boundaries' (2000b: 259). For instance, the number of overseas trained nurses and midwives relocating to the UK has risen to record levels. The biggest overseas 'suppliers' of nursing staff are the Philippines, New Zealand, the West Indies, Zimbabwe and now Spain. It is argued that this is causing a 'brain drain' in these countries as the most skilled staff will often be recruited. In addition, instances of 'medical tourism' may increase as patients in the UK seek speedier or less expensive health care elsewhere (Walt 1998: 436).

Conclusion: the challenges for public health in a global era

In exploring the relationship between globalization and public health, two key issues can be identified. The first concerns that of the threats that global society and a global level trade system poses to public health. This issue throws up key questions surrounding inequalities, global climate change, global working conditions, regulations and so on. The second issue raises slightly different questions as it concerns the continued relevance of the nation state in relation to regional and global public health issues, particularly in the light of increased involvement of transnational and multi-national level organizations in the global health arena. I have expounded on the notion that globalization poses particular challenges (and opportunities) to public health workers. For example, writers such as Feachem (2001) remain largely positive about the long-term effects of globalization on population health, whereas others like Pollock and Price (2000) imply that globalization is an inherently unfair process and that markets are not the solution to rising health care needs. They suggest that the trade policies and ideology of the WTO and the World Bank are loaded in favour of private initiatives, and that these are having a detrimental impact on domestic health policy in the UK.

Further, their argument extends to the notion that this affects and restricts national sovereignty. However, discussions surrounding the decline of the welfare state and indeed the nation state may be premature (Turner 2001: 12); great importance continues to be attached to the notion of sovereignty and state legitimacy:

> While some feared that the intensification of globalisation would lead to greater diminution of state roles, others have argued that it is precisely because of globalisation that key state roles such as the promotion of equity, the development of a policy framework within which services can be provided, and the regulation of service and provider quality, need to be reinforced.
>
> (Zwi and Yach 2002)

Perhaps globalization is a trend we do not want to reverse, but merely to bring into play greater equity and adapt the rules and policies of the WTO, in short, to further democratize the transnational trade organizations. This proposal is supported by Labonte (2001: 621), who argues that the WTO should be reformed and not abolished. Others, such as Zwi and Yach (2002) argue that we should further support and extend the role of the WHO and the UN, as these are perceived as providing the widest fora for debate. This brings to light a question that should be raised in addressing the promotion of globalization – globalization for the benefit of whom? Therefore, we need to explore increasing the public health benefits of globalization for the disenfranchized and the poor, and not just the higher income nations and social groups.

Furthermore, globalization (as a movement that cuts across various spheres) should be linked to the notion of sustainability, and in particular sustainable development. This term had particular resonance within the 2002 Earth Summit debate in Johannesburg, and sustainability is certainly something desirable to those in the West. In this context, sustainable development can be seen as addressing the essential health needs of people in the present without threatening the health needs of those in the future. (See Chapter 12 for discussion on sustainability in urban environments.)

Nevertheless, for all the talk of globalization which has been addressed in this chapter, the key issue is how public health professionals in the UK will respond to these ever changing geopolitical events at the local level. Admittedly, local/regional issues are the most important and relevant to public health workers, although I have shown in this chapter how key events at some geographical distance from home will increasingly impact on the agenda of public health professionals in the UK.

PART 4

Evidence and evaluation in 21st century public health

Editors' overview

What actions should be taken in public health policy, participation and practice in the 21st century in order to improve health and well being? How can we demonstrate whether and why these actions are successful?

Some of the responses to these questions are tackled, by no means exhaustively, in Part 4 of this book. It explores new thinking about what should constitute the evidence base for contemporary multidisciplinary public health practice. It outlines four separate disciplinary approaches to evaluation from: epidemiology, economics, community health and well being, and health impact assessment, estimation and analysis. These disciplines were selected because of their traditional and emerging contributions to the questions that concern a multiprofessional workforce.

There is a growing requirement for robust, theory-based evaluation frameworks, appropriate for complex, context specific public health programmes. These requirements depart somewhat from the traditional, medically dominated evaluation questions in public health practice and have created a movement towards evidence informed public health or 'How and why do programmes work?' as opposed to evidenced-based public health or 'What interventions work?' These chapters will be useful to all public health practitioners who face the growing need to evaluate their work.

In Chapter 14 Tony Harrison explores the challenging question of developing an evidence-based multidisciplinary public health. He concludes with suggestions concerning the ways in which the professions and disciplines that constitute 21st century public health can work together and move forward.

In Chapter 15 Jon Pollock discusses the use of epidemiological evidence in public health. He reviews the role of classical epidemiology in public health before going on to examine the ways in which the discipline is responding to new challenges in public health. In particular he concentrates on methodological developments which attempt to disentangle the effect of different influences (such as environmental as opposed to genetic) on ill health and well being.

In Chapter 16 Jane Powell explains the key concepts, thinking and techniques of health economics for public health work. A new framework for economic evaluation of complex, context specific public health programmes is explained and assessed. Powell argues that the traditional 12 step economic evaluation framework applied in 'What interventions work?' type of evaluation questions is no longer appropriate for the majority of questions that concern today's public health practitioners.

In Chapter 17 Stuart Hashagen defines community health and well being work as a core area of 21st century public health, with a range of public health professionals acting in partnership, and communities themselves as one of the driving forces of change. He discusses the tensions between non-traditional evaluations in the community health and well being field and more traditional evaluation frameworks, arguing that the established 'hierarchy of evidence' that dominates evidence-based public health practice is inappropriate for community health and well being work. He presents useful new frameworks for evaluating community health and well being work.

In Chapter 18 Jack Dowie raises questions concerning the disciplinary basis and production and use of evidence for 21st century public health, exploring the use of health impact estimation, assessment and analysis techniques. The author offers a critique of all three 'health impact' techniques and in so doing raises issues about how the disciplines that contribute to public health are to be brought together 'as disciplines and not just people'. Dowie distinguishes the 'hierarchy of evidence' from the 'hierarchy for policymaker's decisions' and argues for the worth of the centre ground in both hierarchies.

14

TONY HARRISON
Evidence-based multidisciplinary public health

Editors' introduction

What does 'evidence-based public health' mean? At its simplest, it is about ensuring that any intervention (such as a patient's treatment or a public health programme) can be backed up with evidence to show that the intervention is likely to be effective and successful. This is in contrast, for example, to giving treatments or running programmes just because they follow a historical pattern, or are based solely on beliefs or opinion. This evidence-based approach is widely accepted and adopted in the health field.

Creating an evidence-based multidisciplinary public health is difficult because the disciplines and practices that contribute to public health have different approaches to gathering and analysing evidence; also, many policies and practices are aimed at long-term improvements in health and it is difficult in the short term to demonstrate whether or not they are effective.

The movement towards an evidence-based approach to practice and policy has been dominated by a quantitative and statistical approach to demonstrating the effectiveness (or otherwise) of specific interventions. This has been particularly successful in medicine and health care. But in public health this quantitative and statistical approach could result in marginalizing some important areas of practice. This is true especially of interventions that address social and economic conditions. Here the context within which they are implemented may be particularly important and it is more difficult to describe this using quantitative and statistical data.

This chapter distinguishes between evidence-based public health (which specifically tries to measure the effectiveness of interventions), evidence informed public health (where evidence of a wider type informs judgements) and the evidence base for public health (which includes all evidence, however it is used).

The author looks at the development of evidence-based public health in the UK. He suggests that problems of incorporating different types of evidence into public health could be reduced by recognizing the essential tension between quantitative and qualitative approaches, and between those that aim to demonstrate the effectiveness of interventions regardless of context and those that emphasize the importance of context. The importance of theory, or identifying the mechanisms linking interventions to outcomes, in evidence-based public health is briefly reviewed.

Introduction

This chapter looks at the problems of developing an evidence-based *multidisciplinary* public health. This is defined as an evidence-based approach which all disciplines that contribute to public health can share. It is not, therefore, about a more restricted evidence-based public health medicine, neither is it a review of the movement towards evidence-based policy and practice in all those separate professional areas that arguably contribute to public health. It is about the problems of creating an approach to public health, which, while being evidence-based, does not place a boundary around the concept of evidence that results in the effective exclusion of some disciplines from public health. Its particular focus is the problem of extending the evidence-based approach to complex community based interventions which aim to impact on health in the longer run through improvements in the social and economic determinants of health.

The chapter is primarily based on UK material. Specific evidence databases are referred to in this chapter, but as this is about the problems of an evidence-based multidisciplinary public health they are discussed only in terms of what they say about criteria for inclusion in evidence bases. They are not reviewed for their detailed content. Website addresses were correct at the time of writing.

While there is considerable material on developments in evidence-based public health in general (for example Heller and Page 2002; Rychetnik *et al.* 2002), that which specifically addresses the issue of multidisciplinarity is more sparse. There is, though, a growing literature on evidence-based policy and practice across different sectors (Nutley *et al.* 2002) and on the general debate about the use of evidence in public policy and in health (McQueen 2002; Solesbury 2002; Young *et al.* 2002). The most interesting formal development towards creating an evidence base for multidisciplinary public health in the UK is associated with the establishment of the Health Development Agency in England. This is heavily drawn on to illustrate the issues that need addressing in an evidence-based multidisciplinary public health.

The argument in this chapter is essentially twofold. First, unless multidisciplinary public health is evidence-based, then it is open to the charge that while its intentions are well meaning, its prescriptions require better demonstration of their effectiveness. Second, because the disciplines that contribute to multidisciplinary public health have such different research traditions and even conceptions of what is meant by evidence, the main prerequisite for multidisciplinary work is a common understanding of where each comes from and of the strength and limitations of each other's evidence. This, it is argued, is essential if partnerships (a key vehicle through which new public health is to be delivered) are to work in the manner hoped and expected of them. If the evidence on which policy and practice is based in different sectors remains part of their specialist preserve, then the understanding by different disciplines of what each has to offer by way of improving public health will elude policy makers and practitioners alike.

The structure of this chapter

This chapter is structured in the following way:

- First, because the term evidence-based public health is open to some ambiguity it is defined and contrasted with the broader ideas of evidence informed public health decisions, and the evidence base for public health.

- Second, because the chapter is specifically about multidisciplinary public health, the development of the wider evidence-based policy and practice movement in the UK is reviewed. This section looks at some of the major developments in the creation of an infrastructure to support evidence-based policy and practice. It also looks at how far this has gone in multidisciplinary public health. It concludes by setting out a simple model of evidence-based policy and practice.

- Third, the central part of the chapter considers the problems of producing evidence for a multidisciplinary public health and getting it accepted as useful and valid. It reviews the methodological problems involved, shows how these are reflected in the debates about the criteria for inclusion in evidence databases. It examines controversies around the concept of a hierarchy of evidence, which is widely accepted in evidence-based medicine but questioned elsewhere. This section proposes a framework for resolving disputes around the idea of a hierarchy and for clarifying the contributions that different disciplines can make to public health.

- Fourth, the next section briefly reviews some of the arguments about the role of theory in evidence-based policy and practice, and relates these to public health.

- Finally, the chapter concludes by arguing that if multidisciplinary public health is ever to become truly evidence-based, a number of difficult conditions need to be satisfied. But it also argues that evidence-based public health can only be a part of a wider public health.

Defining evidence-based multidisciplinary public health

Evidence-based policy and practice in general has come to take on a particular meaning. This is that interventions (acts designed to bring about an outcome that would not have happened in their absence) should be based on clear and rigorous evidence about their efficacy (in other words, on whether or not they work). Interventions may be at the level of the individual (for example, the use of a drug or therapy), a group (a school class being taught skills associated with literacy or numeracy) or of a community. Examples of the latter would be local policies designed to reduce crime or regenerate neighbourhoods, or to reduce the incidence of disease through behavioural changes induced by a health promotion campaign.

The evidence base for interventions may come from prospective trials conducted under rigorous conditions that leave little room for doubt that it was the intervention and not something else that brought about any improvement in outcomes. In medicine, greatest emphasis is placed on randomized controlled trials, and on systematic reviews that amalgamate the results of different randomized controlled trials. Where prospective trials are not possible then the evidence may be based on retrospective evaluations of interventions and observational studies. Often sophisticated statistical methods are employed in an attempt to measure the extent to which improved outcomes may be due to chance as opposed to being a direct result of the intervention.

Whatever methodologies are used, evidence-based policy and practice as characterized here rely on the ability to set up 'counterfactuals' (or clear predictions of what would have happened in the absence of the intervention). It depends, obviously, on the ability to measure outcomes (an issue of potential controversy, especially in public health where some would dispute that the traditional epidemiological outcome measures of mortality and morbidity should enjoy the dominance that they do). It also relies on the ability to isolate interventions (and in some conceptions of evidence-based policy to reduce these to single, simple actions) as part of this process of eliminating other possible causes of any change in outcomes.

Evidence-based policy and practice as outlined above also have another very important characteristic. That is the generalizability of the evidence (or the ability to replicate the effect of the intervention in different places at different times). In other words, one criterion for evidence-based policy and practice as seen by some is that the effect of an intervention should be independent of context. This is a major issue for an evidence-based multidisciplinary public health where many interventions at the community level (for example, those designed to promote community safety and reduce crime, or to provide social and economic regeneration in neighbourhoods) are so clearly highly context dependent.

A spectrum of use of evidence

The concept of evidence-based policy and practice implies a somewhat mechanistic process leading from the identification of a problem, to the selection of a preferred intervention, to implementation. Of course things are never this simple. Choice and judgement is involved at all stages. However, for the purposes of this chapter a distinction is made between the use of evidence in decision making at different points along a spectrum where the differences involve the level of judgement and an associated risk that the intervention may not work. In this chapter:

- Evidence-*based* policy and practice refer to a situation where least judgement and risk is involved in the decision to use a specific intervention. The decision is based on clear evidence as to what the effectiveness of the intervention is likely to be; the evidence is most likely to be of an experimental nature. This is most likely to be relevant to practice decisions, or to policy decisions which are specific to a defined group or locality.

- Evidence-*informed* policy and practice refer to a situation where evidence has been used as a basis for a more complex judgement. The evidence may be of a wider nature, including, for example, evidence of social and economic conditions, and of the links between these and health (the social and economic determinants of health). (See Chapter 10 for discussion about socio-economic determinants of health and health inequalities.)

- The evidence base for public health is the broadest term, including all the evidence that may be used in one way or another for public health decisions. It includes evidence of conditions (including, for example, health inequalities) as well as of the effectiveness of interventions. It carries no particular implications as to *how* it may be used – it could be as part of health impact assessments (for example Jaffe and Mindell 2002), or even to inform legislative change in a very broad way. (Health impact assessment is discussed in Chapter 18.)

The development of evidence-based public policy and public health

The development of evidence-based policy and practice has been an important feature of public sector policy in the United Kingdom over the last decade. The significance and breadth of this development is illustrated in important publications (see for example Davies *et al.* 2000), the establishment of collaborations for systematic reviews of studies of the effectiveness of interventions (for example, the Cochrane and Campbell collaborations), and a network for the development of evidence-based policy and practice by the Economic and Social Research Council. Few policy sectors have been left untouched by the evidence-based idea. It is best developed (both in terms of methodologies for providing and validating the evidence, and of the associated infrastructure for disseminating it to the policy community and practitioners) in medicine and health care. It has also influenced policy and practice in areas as diverse as crime prevention and community safety, education, social work, transport and many others (for example, Macdonald *et al.* 1992; Terry 1999; Coe *et al.* 2000; Davies *et al.* 2000: part 2; Sherman *et al.* 2002; Tilley and Laycock 2002), and generated debate about the extent to which existing housing policy is evidence based (for example Maclennan and More 1999).

The Cochrane and Campbell collaborations

The best known development in evidence-based policy and practice is the Cochrane Collaboration (http://www.cochrane.org/). This international collaboration concentrates on the preparation, maintenance and dissemination of systematic reviews of the effects of health care interventions. In many respects it sets a 'gold standard' for evidence-based policy and practice. The collaboration is international and its coverage correspondingly wide, it specifies rigorous criteria for reviewing and synthesizing studies as part of systematic reviews, and has developed an accessible infrastructure (including the use of web technology) for the dissemination of its work. It includes centres in countries in all continents.

It is structured around review groups which cover different areas of health care.

Currently there are over 30 of these – examples are the Heart Group, Oral Health Group and Schizophrenia Group. Methods groups deal with methodological aspects of systematic reviews (including, for example, health economics, health related quality of life and statistical methods) and fields/networks are organized around areas of interest which extend across different health problems. Examples are child health, health promotion and public health, and primary health care.

The more recent Campbell Collaboration (C2 Steering Group and Secretariat 2001) has developed from the Cochrane initiative and concentrates on systematic reviews of studies of the effectiveness of social and behavioural interventions, including education (http:www.campbellcollaboration.org). This was inaugurated in 2000 and consequently is at a relatively early stage of development, but its structure suggests its usefulness to public health. Sub-groups include those concerned with methods (including statistics, quasi-experiments and process and implementation), crime and justice, social welfare, and education.

An early paper produced by the Campbell Collaboration (C2 Steering Group and Secretariat 2001) is instructive in identifying both the ambitions of the evidence-based movement and some of the associated problems. C2's aim is 'to produce reviews that are useful to policymakers, practitioners and the public'. In doing this it seeks to challenge a situation in which 'scepticism if not outright cynicism' exists about the use of evidence in some policy sectors. It sees this scepticism as resulting from advocacy groups using evidence which they claim supports their positions, even though their positions are in conflict, and by a number of characteristics of social research that appear to diminish its value as evidence for public policy. These include the fact that policy and practice are implemented in a real world in which context and circumstance matter, whereas experiments often take place in an altogether different context under artificial and controlled conditions. Also, it is argued, the inevitable flaws in social research mean that there is invariably more than one explanation for the outcome of policy.

C2 seeks to guarantee the quality of its output by, among other things, ensuring the integrity of the methods it employs by the adoption of transparent and uniform standards of evidence and the use of rigorous procedures to avoid bias in the screening of studies and in producing reviews. Coverage is international and access to its findings is facilitated by the combination of new technologies with conventional methods and the development of end user networks.

UK Economic and Social Research Council evidence network

The further extension of the evidence-based movement is well illustrated by the establishment by the UK Economic and Social Research Council of an 'evidence network' in 1999. The remit and approach of this reflects some of the tensions in the social sciences about the concept of evidence-based policy and practice – particularly in relation to the question of whether any particular research methodology deserves a privileged position. Thus it states that research should 'play to its strengths as one kind of evidence among others'. But it also recognizes the advantages of 'greater rigour, replicability and independence' (http://www.evidencenetwork.org/history.asp) and the need for agreed standards for policy research. The interests of the node organizations that make up the network illustrate the scope of this. These include 'What Works for Children', a centre for neighbourhood research, a centre for evidence-based public health policy, a centre for evidence in ethnicity, health and diversity, systematic reviews in social policy and social care, and a research unit for research utilization (http://www.evidencenetwork.org.org/nodes.asp). The spread of this initiative illustrates its potential for multidisciplinary public health.

UK developments in public health

If we look more specifically at evidence-based public health in the UK, two developments are interesting. First, the House of Commons Health Select Committee's work and report on public health in 2001 (House of Commons Health Select Committee 2001a, b) included both evidence from expert witnesses and a comment in its report on evidence-based public health. This arose from the earlier White Paper, *Saving Lives: Our Healthier Nation* (Secretary of State for Health 1999) in which public health and the reduction in health inequalities were seen as central to health policy. Given the range of factors implicated in these, the intention here would seem to be that public health should be a multidisciplinary activity. The Committee's terms of reference included specific mention of initiatives that cut across departmental and disciplinary lines such as Health Action Zones, Employment Action Zones, Education Action Zones and Community Plans. (See Chapters 1 and 2 for detailed discussions of public health policy.)

In a written memorandum, Professor Sally Macintyre illustrated some of the problems of an evidence-based public health which covers such complex interventions (Macintyre 2001). She argued that in spite of the richness of research analysing health inequalities in Britain, there was a dearth of research into the effectiveness of interventions designed to reduce these, and that 'one reason for this is the perceived difficulty in applying experimental methods to the evaluation of social or public health interventions'. She went on to suggest that it should be possible to use such methods and find out something about their effectiveness if area-based interventions (initiatives based on defined geographical areas, such as inner-city areas or housing estates, with specific characteristics) were set up specifically to test these. This, she suggested, may involve identifying twice as many areas as money was available for, randomly allocating these to 'trial' and 'control' (no intervention) categories, and then rigorously evaluating outcomes in the two.

In other words, she was suggesting the possibility of a kind of randomized controlled trial to provide good evidence on whether this sort of area-based initiative works in reducing health inequalities. In its report the Committee cast doubt on the practicality of this idea, but acknowledged that there was a void in relation to evidence of the effectiveness of public health interventions which it hoped could be filled, at least in part, by the Health Development Agency (HDA).

The Health Development Agency's evidence-based public health database

The second development in evidence-based public health in the UK is the development of the HDA's database and its associated infrastructure since the House of

Commons report. This is in effect multidisciplinary, as part of the HDA's remit is to identify 'evidence of what works to improve people's health and reduce health inequalities'. It advises and supports policy makers and practitioners, helping them to get evidence into practice (www.hda-online.org.uk/). While this may sound clear cut it quickly becomes evident that the ambition of this project in addressing long standing health inequalities and the complex of causes that lie behind these, gives rise to fundamental problems of what is meant by evidence. Thus, the website introduction to the HDA's evidence base says:

> What 'counts' as good quality evidence for health promotion and health improvement is not a clear-cut issue, and there are a number of different arguments as to what constitutes appropriate or reliable forms of evidence. Initially HDA Evidence Base will not attempt to derive consensus as to what constitutes evidence, but will aim to present a wide range of information that could be used to inform public health. Information about 'what works' can be drawn from a range of sources including systematic reviews, research reports and journal articles, internet sites, expert opinion, Government guidance and unpublished research databases. Topics covered in these sources span a wide range of factors, interventions, policies and practices that impact on public health and reduce health inequalities.
>
> (http://194.83.94.80/hda/docs/evidence/eb2000/corehtml/intro.htm)

The HDA's evidence base (http://www.hdaonline.org.uk/evidence) contains two types of information: a database containing files of systematic and other reviews of effectiveness, and evidence-based briefing documents. The former is the core evidence base and the latter a series of briefings for professionals and policy makers which are designed to identify and review the evidence on specific topics, highlight conflicting evidence and gaps, and suggest future work (Swann *et al.* 2002). Given the emphasis on quality evidence in evidence-based public health, both these raise questions about the criteria for acceptance on the database. The difficulty of addressing this question in relation to multidisciplinary work is illustrated in a discussion on the HDA website on how the database and criteria for inclusion are currently developing.

The core database currently adopts an 'inclusive' approach that initially does not attempt to develop a consensus among professionals as to what constitutes 'best evidence'. This approach acknowledges the complex of factors, from social and economic to genetic and biological, that influence health outcomes. This means that approaches based on narrow questions and methodologies, designed to identify the effectiveness of very specific interventions, may be too restricted and only provide 'one piece of the jigsaw' of what works. Qualitative research, narrative accounts and expert groups may also provide relevant information about public health decisions. The range of sources of evidence which could potentially populate the HDA's evidence base thus includes:

- systematic reviews of effectiveness based on an explicit and systematic search methodology;

- reviews of effectiveness (without the systematic search methodology);
- expert group reports;
- meta-analyses (involving the collation of results from various sources and subjected to statistical analysis to measure the impact of an intervention); and
- maps of evidence (compendiums of all the above).

But this list does not address the issue of criteria that evidence has to meet to be included. Three criteria are currently identified. These are:

- transparency: showing how the evidence was collated, who was involved and how it was funded;
- a systematic approach (or systematicity): showing the process of evidence gathering and assessment; and
- relevance: it must be judged to be relevant to public health, and particularly to the strategy set out in *Saving Lives: Our Healthier Nation*.

The processes involved in producing evidence-based briefing documents further demonstrate the problems of selecting evidence for dissemination to practitioners and decision makers (Swann *et al.* 2002). This involves a number of key stages. These are:

- Prioritizing topics for briefings. This gives explicit recognition to the fact that evidence does not just emerge, but emanates from decisions about what is important and where resources should be spent. In this case it comes from the context for public health set by government and the HDA's own work plan.
- Setting up a research team of research and public health specialists to do the basic work, and a reference group of relevant stakeholders to guide the process and peer review draft briefings.
- Literature searching, which aims to identify reviews of sufficient quality to form part of the base of an evidence briefing.
- The selection and appraisal of data, which involves identifying relevant types of evidence, setting up 'threshold rules' for determining what should be included and critical appraisal for assisting judgements about how, or whether, material should be used.
- The synthesis of material and structuring it into an evidence briefing.
- An explicit schedule for the transfer of knowledge into practice and policy communities.

A model of evidence-based policy and practice

Figure 14.1 attempts to show in diagrammatic form different stages in the development and use of infrastructure to support evidence-based policy and practice. As it is specifically concerned with evidence of the effectiveness of interventions, and not

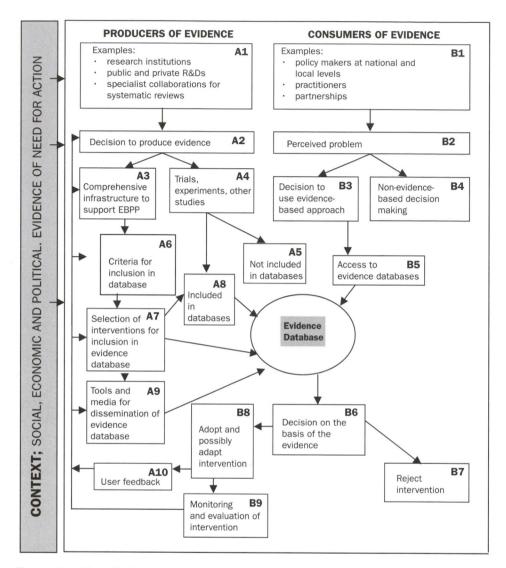

Figure 14.1 Simplified model of evidence-based policy and practice
(EBPP = evidence-based public health; R&Ds = researchers and developers)

evidence in the broader sense, it separates the external context which influences the development of evidence-based systems from the systems themselves and their use (vertical box to the left of the diagram). This includes not only political pressures, such as those currently evident in the UK, but evidence of need for policy or practice change.

Two aspects of evidence-based public health are shown inside the main box. One (boxes labelled A) outlines key stages in the decision to produce evidence in support of policy and practice, and the other (the Bs) stages in the decision to use it. The 'production' side of the diagram gives examples of the types of bodies that may produce evidence in support of evidence-based public health (A1), and distinguishes comprehensive systems (such as the Cochrane and Campbell collaborations, A3), from individual trials and studies (A4). At a later stage these may or may not become part of comprehensive databases (A5 or A8) depending on how these are set up and on the criteria for inclusion (A6, A7 and A9). These boxes show three key stages in setting up databases in support of evidence-based public health and in identifying their contents. A6 shows the criteria for including evidence from trial and studies – and this includes both search strategies and criteria based on methodologies (for example, whether to restrict the database to systematic reviews of randonized controlled trials, and these trials themselves). These criteria may be used at two levels. At the highest level, what kind of studies are accepted and, at a lower level, what kinds may be used in systematic reviews of studies. A7 shows that decisions have to be made about which interventions to include, and A9 about the type of media that will be used for dissemination to users. A10 shows how user feedback may influence the infrastructure and content of databases.

The user side of the diagram attempts to show key stages in the decision to use evidence-based public health. B1 gives examples of different kinds of users and B2 shows that decisions are made only in response to a perceived problem (influenced by the context of decision making). B3 and B4 distinguish between an evidence-based approach to decisions and other approaches, and B5 that if an evidence-based approach is adopted it requires access to some form of evidence database. B7 and B8 show different outcomes of the decision process, and B9 that a decision to use an evidence-based approach may feed back into an evidence database through monitoring and evaluation of the implementation of an intervention. Further user feedback may influence the form, structure and content of evidence-based systems; this is shown on the left-hand side of the diagram.

This simplified model helps make clear some of the central difficulties involved in the development of a multidisciplinary evidence-based public health. These are the issues of the criteria for the inclusion of evidence, the selection of interventions for which evidence of their effectiveness is provided, the mechanisms by which evidence is disseminated to users, and who the users are. These are considered in the next section.

Main problems of evidence-based systems for multidisciplinary public health

The first and central problem revolves around the debate about criteria for inclusion of evidence in databases and about the relative merits of data based on different methodologies.

A hierarchy of evidence

Evidence-based medicine and health care emphasize the concept of a hierarchy of evidence in which evidence from some methodologies is given higher status than that from others. The idea of a hierarchy of evidence has come to be widely accepted internationally in the health field.

Top of the hierarchy (type 1 evidence) is evidence from at least one good systematic review, including at least one randomized controlled trial. A systematic review, as the term implies, reviews and aggregates evidence from as many individual trials and experiments as are accepted by the criteria for inclusion in the review. The use of these criteria lies behind the adjective 'systematic', and distinguishes this type of review from other literature reviews where both the search criteria and the criteria for inclusion are less rigorously specified. One particular type of systematic review is a meta-analysis. This is a quantitative analysis, which aggregates the results of as many different studies as are found and accepted by the criteria, and then analyses these statistically. It thus increases the sample on which statistical statements of the strength of a relationship between an intervention and an outcome are made and in principle reduces the confidence intervals. It is thus designed to increase confidence in the efficacy of a specific intervention.

Mulrow (1995) explains the rationale behind systematic reviews and this provides the logic for their position at the top of the hierarchy. They reduce large quantities of information to useable dimensions and are an efficient scientific technique which may be both less time consuming and more reliable than instigating a new study. As a result of the diversity of circumstances in which individual studies are carried out they are generalizable across different contexts and have increased power when compared with individual studies as a result of the aggregation of data.

At the second level of the hierarchy comes type II evidence, the criteria for which is at least one good randomized controlled trial. Type III includes at least one well designed intervention study (that is a study that attempts to estimate the effect of an intervention compared with 'do nothing'), but without randomization. This would include, for example, retrospective studies that attempt to measure the impact of an intervention (such as improved domestic heating) on the health of a group subject to this intervention, compared with a control group with the same basic characteristics but which had not been subject to the intervention. Type IV evidence includes at least one well designed observational study. Bottom of the hierarchy comes expert opinion, including the opinions of service users and carers.

Applying the hierarchy to public health

The logic of this hierarchy is clear in relation to evidence-based medicine and health care. At the top of the hierarchy comes evidence that is objective and strives to eliminate bias. This has the greatest explanatory power in terms of its ability to measure the effectiveness of an intervention (and, conversely, the risk that it will not work) and thus gives decision makers the greatest confidence. At the bottom comes evidence that may be biased by the interests of those expressing opinions. This ordering within the hierarchy is not surprising given that one of the objectives of evidence-based practice is to not take the opinions of experts and others at face value, but to subject their practices to rigorous and independent testing.

However, the question is raised as to whether this hierarchy is appropriate for *all* aspects of evidence-based public health, particularly where we are talking not just about public health medicine but about a range of interventions that come from different professional practices and disciplines. The strength of the hierarchy lies in the ability to isolate discrete interventions, to identify measurable outcomes and assess the impact of interventions independent of context, and to measure the strength of a 'dose–response' relationship. As such it is based on a reductionist approach. But many interventions where there are grounds for believing there would be beneficial public health impacts do not fit this model. This would seem to apply particularly to the complex community-based initiatives associated with regeneration and neighbourhood renewal. There are three main reasons for this:

- First, the precise circumstances or context in which initiatives are being implemented is likely to have a significant effect on outcomes. Charismatic and energetic leadership, strong community bonds and the physical characteristics of an area, including its connectivity with other areas are likely to influence the success of such interventions.

- Second, the very principle of partnership is supposed to ensure that the details of projects are finely tuned to the local context, making generalization across different areas difficult.

- Third, initiatives commonly have long-term and complex aims. It may be optimistic to hope for measurable outcomes in relatively short periods of time.

The logic of these complex community-based interventions is based on well grounded research linking social and economic conditions (or the determinants of health) to health and the reduction in health inequalities (Acheson 1998; Wilkinson and Marmott 1998). This research is different in nature from evaluations of specific interventions. It is more complex, dealing with a multitude of factors that have a bearing on health. It is often based in the social sciences and on a range of methodologies. Its findings tend to be more provisional and context dependent, particularly where the work is case study based. This is particularly so with research into regeneration, housing and neighbourhood renewal where there are 'few high quality intervention studies which address the impact of housing and health (Thompson *et al.* 2002).

The tensions involved in attempting to absorb this disparate work into the evidence base for public health is well illustrated in a discussion paper on this topic for the King's Fund by Gowman and Coote (2000). This argues that 'in the first instance, it is essential that any new evidence base relates to the full range of public health objectives and activities', as set out in *Saving Lives: Our Healthier Nation.* These include specific disease-based targets for health improvement, as well as the broader goals to improve health and reduce health inequalities. The paper goes on to say:

> As visions of health have become increasingly broad, the range of activities encompassed by the public health umbrella has widened correspondingly. Initiatives and interventions across a range of sectors have a part to play in improving health, and a growing number are expected to link with the Government's public health strategy . . . Too narrow a definition of public health, or of what constitutes evidence, will work against joined-up thinking, and work against mainstreaming of health improvement . . . A medically oriented evidence base

will mean that evidence about health improvement remains the preserve of mainstream public health practitioners, excluding many others within local government or the voluntary and business sectors who have a significant part to play. A new framework for evidence needs to be based on a clear understanding of these different players and functions.

(Gowman and Coote 2000: 14)

Gowman and Coote's paper argues forcefully for an evidence base that is not restricted to medically orientated conceptions of a hierarchy of evidence. This, they say, would exclude much potentially valuable research and evidence from a new public health evidence base. They stress that a new framework has to recognize that 'in place of a hierarchy of evidence, it should be possible to accommodate different kinds of evidence, acknowledging their respective strengths in appropriate settings' (Gowman and Coote 2000).

Locating different research traditions in public health

One way out of what appears to be an impasse is to start by identifying the essential tensions between evidence that comes from different research traditions. Two such tensions are suggested:

- The first tension is between the quantitative and a qualitative tradition. The former seeks to establish measured relationships between variables, uses statistical analysis to estimate the likelihood that these relationships are due to chance, and uses a scientific and reductionist approach to isolate the influence of different variables. The latter's strengths lie more in its ability to convey meaning and the interpretation of complex situations including those involving attitudes and perceptions.
- The second tension is between approaches that seek to establish relationships that are independent of context and provide robust information about interventions which is replicable in different circumstances, and those which place much greater emphasis on the circumstances in which things happen.

These tensions are represented in Figure 14.2. In this the horizontal axis XY represents the spectrum from a wholly quantitative to qualitative approach, and the vertical axis AB, from one which attempts to generalize about cause and effect independently of context, to one which focuses on the effect of context on how things work.

It is possible to locate in this diagram different research methodologies. Thus, meta-analyses which attempt to establish measures of the effectiveness of interventions independent of context, would come towards the bottom left-hand corner of the south-east quadrant, and individual randomized controlled trials, further to the north. Observational studies, particularly those which are retrospective, come still further to the north. Case studies, with their emphasis on a variety of data, on the importance of context and on a process of triangulation to validate findings would come towards the top of the north-west quadrant.

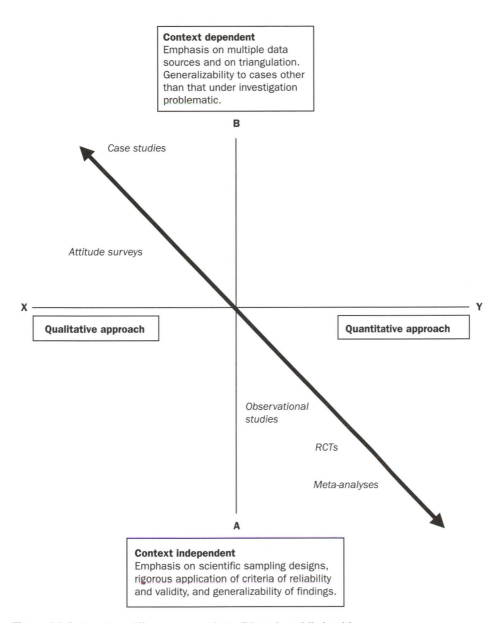

Figure 14.2 Locating different research traditions in public health

The heavy arrow in this diagram tentatively sets out the main line of tension in the current debate about evidence in public health. The validity of the concept of a hierarchy of evidence applies largely to the south-east quadrant. As one shifts to the north-west the idea of a hierarchy becomes more questionable for three reasons. First, there is greater reliance on different types of data based on different notions of evidence, for example, interviews, attitude surveys, demographic data, documentary historical data and narratives. This especially applies to case studies. Second, conclusions from research are based more on interpretation and judgement than on conventional scientific ideas of 'proof'. The whole notion of proof is a much more problematic concept in relation to this part of the diagram; evidence tends to be from the social sciences where there is much greater debate and controversy about methodology (Flyvbjerg 2001). Third, it is also notable that the critical appraisal skills (Critical Appraisal Skills Programme) that are increasingly now part of the training in evidence-based health are more easily applied to the lower right-hand part of the diagram than elsewhere.

In the diagram the south-west and north-east quadrants are shown as being empty. This is not to deny that there are qualitative research methodologies that come closer to quantitative, context independent studies in their approach. Indeed Silverman (1998) argues the case for greater emphasis on this type of qualitative work in health research and less on interviews.

The diagram is also suggestive of the ways in which evidence may be used to inform public health decisions – particularly along the north-south axis. At the lower end, where evidence is less context dependent, interventions for which evidence is available are likely to be discrete, controlled and at the individual level. It is also more likely to be outcome based – and consequently particularly useful for practitioners. At the top end, interventions are more likely to be complex, often at the community level and often concerned with processes rather than with final outcomes (for example, with public participation, capacity building and with developing social capital). Interventions in this area are more likely to deal with the environmental (in the wide sense) determinants of health, and evidence here is likely to be more provisional and so more likely to be used at the level of political interventions involving higher levels of uncertainty and greater judgement.

This diagram potentially offers a way forward in terms of identifying a common framework for the public health evidence base. The lower half of the diagram, with its emphasis on context independence and replicability is that to which the term 'evidence-based' public health in the conventional sense is best applied. The upper half of the diagram maps a different part of the evidence base for public health – particularly that concerned with evidence of the social, economic and environmental determinants of health. Interventions in this area are often long term in their intention, consequently it would be inappropriate to look for the sort of summative outcomes (such as changes in mortality and morbidity) in evaluation as are used towards the bottom of the diagram.

However, there is a potential link with the lower part through interventions that are designed to change behaviour (like journeys to work or school, exercise, diet and smoking) where there is plausible evidence that such behavioural change will in the longer term lead to health improvements. Here the behavioural change represents an intermediate outcome and one that is amenable to relatively short-term measurement. This suggests that the link between evidence-based public health and evidence of the determinants of health comes in the identification of short-term outcome indicators where there is an accepted theoretical link between these and a longer-term health gain. An example (below) from a complex multifaceted intervention like neighbourhood renewal may make this clear. (See Chapter 11 for more about neighbourhood renewal and regeneration.)

Example: neighbourhood renewal

Neighbourhood renewal strategies involve a range of objectives that depend heavily on the nature of the locality involved, on the outcome of processes of community participation and on processes of partnership working. The ultimate goal is improvement in the conditions in which people live their lives and may involve housing improvement, jobs and employment, skills enhancement, environmental improvement, community safety and crime reduction initiatives, and attempts to reduce feelings of social exclusion. The approach is holistic and involves cross-cutting/ joined up initiatives in which the contributions of different agencies and organizations to the fundamental goals of improvement are integrated through partnership working. This type of intervention does not readily lend itself to the reductionist, context independent, measurement-based approach of evidence-based policy and practice. However, it should be possible to identify process and intermediate outcomes from the improvement strategy which can be tested against evidence, where a link with health can be established.

A number of examples of intermediate and process outcomes, for which evidence of the link between neighbourhood improvement interventions and health may exist, can be given. Examples are housing improvements as measured by improvements in the internal environment (damp and temperature), young people brought into long-term employment through training and skills development, improvements in perceived safety from crime, and reductions in traffic noise. And the links between these and health is established by more fundamental research on the determinants of health (Acheson 1998).

It should be noted that there are two stages in connecting the evidence base from the top half of the diagram with evidence-based policy and practice in the lower half. One involves the identification of outcomes that can be measured and subject to the rigorous analytical treatment of evidence-based work, and the other involves the establishment of a sound theoretical link between these outcomes and longer-term health gains. This raises the issue of the role of theory in an evidence-based public health to which we now turn.

The role of theory in evidence-based public health

In an obvious sense all evidence-based policy and practice is theory driven. Even the most pragmatic trial that seeks to evaluate whether a specific intervention 'works' is based on a theory that links an action (the intervention) with an outcome (for example, reduced vulnerability to heart disease) through some intervening mechanism (a behavioural change, for example). In this sense it may seem surprising that a lively debate has arisen around the issue of theory in evaluations for evidence-based policy and practice (for example Pawson and Tilley 1997; Davies *et al.* 2000: 265–70).

The essence of this debate revolves around two linked issues. The first is the role of randomization in trials and its objective of isolating one factor (the intervention) from the circumstances or context in which it operates. A pragmatic view would be that what is important is the demonstration of effectiveness – not the underlying reason for it. Second, set against this, is a theoretically informed view that the real world is one of context and circumstances; these cannot be assumed away, and neither can it simply be assumed that the intervention will work everywhere. Therefore, what is important is to find out *why* an intervention works or does not work, what the mechanisms linking the intervention and the outcome are, and the ways in which context influences success or failure.

The importance of context and the dangers of pure empiricism are nicely characterized in Lytton Strachey's study of Florence Nightingale in his *Eminent Victorians* (1918). He says,

> she was simply an empiricist. She believed in what she saw and acted accordingly; beyond that she would not go . . . She had found that fresh air and light played an effective part in the prevention of the maladies with which she had to deal: and that was enough for her. What were the general principles underlying the fact – or even whether there were any she refused to consider . . . she had seen the good effects of fresh air, therefore there could be no doubt about them . . . the bedrooms of patients should be well ventilated. Such was her doctrine . . . But it was a purely empirical doctrine, and thus led to some unfortunate results.
>
> (Strachey 1918: 155–6)

Strachey goes on to relate how Nightingale tried to insist that the fresh air remedy, which proved to be successful in the Crimea, should be adopted in India. Those who understood Indian conditions knew this would be disastrous. In the end their wisdom prevailed, but the point of this is that the intelligent application of successful innovations requires understanding of *why* they work and the circumstances in which they both do and do not work. However, Florence Nightingale was not actually a pure empiricist. She was a miasmatist whose underlying theory was that illness came from bad air, rather than from 'germs'. Consequently this example demonstrates the dangers of elevating pure empiricism over theory. It may obscure an entirely false theory on which it is based.

Developments of the underlying theories associated with policy and practice evaluation can be found in Weiss (1995), Pawson and Tilley (1997), Connell and Kubisch (1998) under the title 'theories of change', and Pawson (2002a, b, c) under the heading 'realist evaluation'. These approaches are particularly appropriate to complex community-based interventions, and seek to uncover the actual mechanisms that link an intervention with what actually happens. Their relevance to this chapter lies in their application to complex community-based interventions, such as neighbourhood renewal strategies and Health Action Zones. In these the notion of replicability is problematic; conditions matter and the process of implementation is likely to influence outcomes. These theoretical developments provide a useful way forward in incorporating social scientific thinking into evidence-based policy and practice, while avoiding the dangers of pure empiricism so feared in the social sciences.

Conclusion

The challenge of developing an evidence-based multidisciplinary public health is considerable. It involves, among other things, complex theoretical and method-ological debates across disciplines, realignments of power and influence within the public health community, an open-mindedness combined with rigour about evidence among those training for public health practice, and the development of accessible mechanisms for the dissemination of evidence. The magnitude of this task should not be underestimated.

It could be argued that the complexity of the task raises questions about whether evidence-based multidisciplinary public health is actually necessary at all. Given that all the disciplines that arguably contribute in some way to the health of the public are, in themselves, being influenced by the evidence-based movement in its broadest sense, there may be an argument for leaving specialists in different fields to do their own thing and to capitalize on the division of Labour that this could bring. But the argument for evidence-based multidisciplinary public health is not an argument against specialisms and acknowledging the benefits this brings. It is an argument for recognizing the contributions of different disciplines to public health and for incorporating these into a framework that does not exclude. This should allow partnerships and other multidisciplinary teams to appraise and use evidence on the basis of its fitness for purpose rather than for its adherence to specific methodological traditions.

This is not to say that an evidence-based approach should dominate all aspects of public health. Public health is a complex activity, involving long-term goals and fundamental shifts in both policy and practice. This means that it is 'both an art and a science, but it shouldn't be an act of faith' (Gowman and Coote 2000). The role of evidence will in some cases be scientific, but in others it will be to inform complex decision making. Multidisciplinary evidence-based public health should help inform that decision making. It should make risks of failure clearer, encourage monitoring of outcomes so that corrective action can be taken when things turn out not to be as predicted and add to the constant improvement of the evidence base on which future informed decisions can be made.

15

JON POLLOCK
Epidemiology in 21st century public health

Editors' introduction

This chapter is probably the most technically demanding in the book. There are two reasons: first, epidemiology uses statistical methods and it is not possible to explain these within a relatively short chapter. Second, and as a consequence, the chapter has to assume some familiarity with statistics in outlining the contributions that new developments in epidemiology can make to contemporary public health.

Epidemiology has for a long time been a standard tool in public health. It is the discipline that has analysed the relationship between disease and ill health on the one hand, and causative factors like exposure to infected water, polluted air or contact with other individuals carrying infections on the other. It has resulted in major breakthroughs in public health, such as identifying the link between smoking and lung cancer. Epidemiology analyses patterns of disease in populations and attempts to identify causes by relating these patterns to known measurable risk factors. But as we become better informed and more sophisticated in our understanding of ill health, so we need more sophisticated and complex epidemiological methods to tell us something about the contribution that *different* factors (be they environmental, genetic, behavioural or life history) make to health and ill health.

This chapter reviews developments in epidemiology and looks at the contribution these do and can make to 21st century public health. First, the author reviews classical epidemiological approaches, their contribution to understanding the causes of ill health and the risks associated with exposure to different agents, and the effectiveness of therapies. Second, the chapter examines emerging demands that contemporary public health is placing on epidemiology as a tool. Third, it reviews the ways in which epidemiology is responding to these new demands by way of methodological developments. And fourth, the author looks at future developments: meta-analysis, Bayesian statistics, life course approaches and multilevel approaches.

The author concludes by saying that while epidemiology is only a tool for public health, public health workers have a responsibility to critically understand epidemiologists' advice.

Defining the scope

The use of epidemiological methods in public health has evolved in numerous ways since its original formulation as the science investigating patterns of disease within and between populations. In its classical form epidemiology developed as a method for exploiting the information content of natural variation in the prevalence of disease in order to generate testable hypotheses of aetiology and hence afford opportunities for prevention. The successful prosecution of an epidemiological investigation initially involved the systematic collection of numerical data on disease distribution and the identification of associative relationships with 'risk factors'. This was followed by postulating causative relationships between risk factors and disease in the form of hypotheses and proposing interventions which could break the relationships. Finally, the implementation of these interventions and the evaluation of their effects in reducing disease incidence would complete the task.

As such, classical epidemiological approaches involved the following skills and processes:

- classification, characterization, diagnosis and definition of disease states;
- insight and experience in identifying and defining potential risk factors;
- rigour and accuracy in recording disease risk factor distributions;
- quantitative skills in demonstrating relationships between disease states and risk factors;
- applying deductive processes in the formulation of testable hypotheses of aetiology;
- proposing measurable interventions and applying quantitative skills in their linkage with disease incidence; and
- formulation of mechanistic explanations and further hypotheses to account for patterns of diseases.

The classical epidemiological approach, therefore, primarily involves the application of precision in measurement and the identification of putative causal factors through the quantitative demonstration of associations that are unlikely to occur by chance or be accounted for by confounders. As such it involves clinical, scientific and statistical approaches that have been the dominating themes, to date, in the training of public health specialists. Both hypothetico-deductive (hypothesis testing using traditional frequentist statistics) and inductive (the selection of possible risk factors) mental processes are involved.

The identification, isolation and control of communicable diseases, while the traditional bread and butter work of the public health practitioner, is only part of the heritage of epidemiological work. (See Chapter 7 for more about health protection.) First, epidemiological risk factor analysis and, specifically, modelling risk, enables aetiological risk factor reduction programmes in public health to be proposed. This can range from the identification of a single key risk factor and the measurement of the risk attributable to it (for example, smoking as a risk factor for lung cancer), to the statistical creation, using multivariate statistical techniques, of scoring systems that enable a variety of modifiable risk factors to be addressed together as in, for example, cardiovascular event scoring systems (Shaper *et al.* 1987).

Second, the inclusion in epidemiology of the evaluation of therapeutic interventions other than those relating to the control and prevention of disease outbreaks has widely expanded its relevance into areas such as health service research, community-based programme evaluations, consumer satisfaction, social care and other areas. Traditionally, epidemiologists are involved in the quantification of effects attributable to clinical interventions of all kinds, ranging across the spectrum of surgical and medical practice. The classical clinical trial of a new drug or the comparison of radiotherapy and chemotherapy in the post-operative care of cancer patients are good examples. Skills required include an awareness and experience of the advantages and disadvantages of different designs in research methodology, and the knowledge of the increasingly complex medical statistical requirements of evaluative work. The distinction between the epidemiologist and the medical statistician has become increasingly blurred. These skills now need to be used in the more complex scenarios of the community setting, multifactor intervention in health and social care, and diverse outcomes that include concepts such as 'quality of life'.

Where then do classical epidemiology and public health epidemiology begin and end? Disease control in the community clearly remains a public health function. While the evaluation of new surgical techniques on its own might not constitute 'public health', the extension of epidemiological principles to the evaluation of virtually any health or social care related intervention (drugs, therapy, advice, education programme or community regeneration) in primary care or in the community can be considered as part of 'public health epidemiology' (see Table 15.1).

The purpose of this chapter is to draw attention to the changing requirements of data acquisition and analysis, and the broader methodology skill base required by epidemiologists working in the developing, wider arena of 21st century public health.

Identifying appropriate epidemiological approaches for contemporary public health

What then are the challenges for epidemiology in 21st century public health? As a tool there are three answers to this question.

- To guide and promote ways of using research and analytical methods for the investigation of broader sets of problems in the public health arena (McKee 2001).
- To evolve and disseminate new methodologies to cope with the particular demands of epidemiological investigation in the widening public health agenda.
- To inculcate good practice in the distribution of skills of evaluation and appraisal throughout the community of public health professionals in order to progress evidence-based health and, hopefully, social care (MacDonald 1998).

Table 15.1 Activity areas in classical and public health epidemiology

Classical epidemiology	21st century public health epidemiology
• Communicable disease outbreak control and surveillance	• Communicable disease outbreak control and surveillance
• Monitoring prevalence, incidence and trends in the social, demographic and geographic distribution of diseases and conditions	• Modelling disease risk and developmental outcome
	• Evaluating health and social care interventions and programmes within and across the community
• Identifying and quantifying disease risk factors	• Health service system evaluations
	• Health needs assessments
• Evaluating surgical and medical treatments	• Injury and accident prevention
	• Disseminating critical appraisal skills

Epidemiology depends on accurate, complete data; data limitations have a profound effect on the value and potential for epidemiological analysis in public health. Classical epidemiology has used disease recording systems to promote the surveillance (and hence control) of disease and the identification of risk factors (especially reversible risk factors) that introduce the possibility of making effective interventions. It should be pointed out, however, that much of the informational requirements of public health epidemiologists derives, with the exception of death certification, from information rooted in secondary and tertiary health care systems, rather than in the community or from social care sources.

While the NHS could provide the medium for structuring an integrated health and social care data collection system (and much important work has been successfully undertaken on registries and record linkage systems, and more recently the Electronic Patient Record) a strong case remains for the collection of standardized data on disease presentation and management in primary care to facilitate epidemiological studies in public health. With general practitioners' self-employed status this is restricted to voluntary schemes such as the Royal College of General Practitioners' 'spotter' practice scheme (www.rcgp-bru.demon.co.uk/) and the Royal College of General Practitioners' general practitioner national morbidity surveys (McCormick *et al.* 1995) that are used to monitor outbreaks and longer-term disease trends respectively. In addition, data are collected on prescribing practice by the Prescription Pricing Authority, on specific diseases from research networks such as the Medical Research Council's General Practice Research Framework, and the national notifiable disease system. The newly developed GP activity database (www.nhsia.nhs.uk/nhais/pages/products/vaprod/miquest/) may in time fulfil part of this primary public health monitoring role for providing data with an accuracy for epidemiological analysis. Of critical importance will be the success in developing a culture of research valuable data collection processes in the social care arena and the mechanisms for accurately linking health and social data together.

While classical epidemiological approaches to risk, disease surveillance and control, and clinical intervention evaluations remain important core components, the new public health demands assistance from methodologists in:

- specifying individual risk more accurately;
- understanding interactions between risk factors more deeply;
- investigating the proximal mechanisms for and wider ramifications of poor health on individuals, groups and societies; and, particularly,
- evaluating the impact of complex social/behavioural and/or community-based interventions in the wider public health.

As simple dose responsive aetiological explanations of disease (smoking and lung cancer, cholesterol and heart disease) become less common, as the more clear-cut relationships are understood, attention naturally turns to the more complex influences and interactions in which single agent models are insufficient to account for much of the individual variance in disease susceptibility. A prime example of this are the factors involved in the risk of stomach cancer. Here the proximal agent involved in most cases is a bacterium (Helicobacter pylori) but the individual risk of cancer is affected by both genetic variation between individuals (El-Omar et al. 2000) and dietary intake (Ekstrøm et al. 2000).

The larger the number of independent contributory factors, the larger the size of epidemiological investigation required to assess each factor's effect size and the more complicated the analysis. Hence epidemiology in the wider public health is likely not only to have to address a very much broader array of topics and settings but also to manage mixed health and social care settings and interventions with small effect sizes over long time periods involving complex interactions. The larger number of independent explanatory variables involved will increasingly use nominal or, at best, ordinal scales of measurement. Outcomes will more frequently include subjective factors such as quality of life, satisfaction, feelings, moods and attitudes – increasingly central measurements in public health as it widens towards more sociological and psychological horizons.

By way of example, consider a modern public health issue: the treatment of offenders to achieve a reduction in the physical abuse of others. A traditional approach would use mostly process evaluation methodologies to undertake an audit of management, mark instances of 'good practice' based on assumptions of efficacy or expert opinion (or both) and identify markers of offender behavioural change based on interviews with offenders themselves, corrective institution workers and other stakeholders. Long-term follow up would be unlikely (although the number of recidivists might be recorded). It is unlikely that information on the social and educational background of the offenders would be systematically collected and most of the evaluation would be undertaken at the level of the institution rather than the individual.

How could the further application of epidemiological methods be of benefit and what would be the consequences for costs and timings? First, detailed qualitative research would be required to identify examples of 'good practice' based on explicit criteria that, for firm theoretical reasons, were grounded in evidence and involved agreed outcome measures. Subsequent audit would categorize institutional activity as a function of such criteria so as to locate and identify those more likely to succeed. Longitudinal studies of a substantial number of individual offenders would be instigated, stratified across institutions, covering the range of practice variations and using prospective as well as retrospective data collection, starting as soon as possible on entry to the institution. Details would be obtained of offenders' social, economic and educational backgrounds, behavioural history and measures of psychological health. Sampling of offenders within and between institutions would involve multilevel approaches (see section below on multilevel approaches) and outcomes would be universally recorded by record linkage with police databases. Risk of discovered recidivism would be statistically related both to personal and institutional factors through multivariate analysis providing information on how different types of offenders respond to different forms of corrective care over the longer term.

Clearly the main disadvantage of this approach lies in the resources required for data collection over the longer term, for the large sample size required and for the need to plan for early baseline measures, expert statistical and analytical support. These considerations, however, need to be balanced against the adverse long-term fiscal and social costs of underfunded, poorly designed research which has to be repeated (Freiman *et al.* 1992).

How has epidemiology changed to support contemporary public health?

The epidemiological method can be traced, as an evolutionary course, back to investigations of the distribution patterns of disease such as cholera and the method of ecological epidemiology which depended heavily on accurate case definitions and reporting systems, the fabric of epidemiological study. Later studies involved monitoring cohorts prospectively, employing retrospective case control methodology as used in the seminal papers linking smoking with lung cancer, through to experimental trials of intervention to attribute causation in therapy.

These developments in method accompanied a conceptual shift in scientists' perceptions of the causes of ill health. The revolutionary changes in methods of hygiene, the disposal of sanitary waste and the prevention of contamination of drinking water that occurred from the middle of the 19th century were motivated initially by the avoidance of the putrefying and obnoxious smells of the 'miasma' that characterized diseased environments. As two eminent epidemiologists have pointed out in a seminal account of the history of epidemiology in public health (Susser and Susser 1996a), the transition from miasma to the bacteriological era led to the notion of disease specificity and the 'one agent (germ): one disease paradigm' that proved so successful in understanding infectious diseases, the development of methods of immunization through exposure and vaccination and, ultimately, antibiotic agents. It is noteworthy, however, that it was the *non-specificity* of the poisoning effected by the miasma that led to a multiplicity of major changes in public health as policies enabled improvements to be made in the collection and disposal of dangerous materials, the provision of clean drinking water, in housing and in personal hygiene, with many health benefits.

On the other hand it was the very *specificity* of the germ theory that encouraged disease susceptibility to be seen as more of an individual risk rather than as a measure to promote public health. The germ theory dominated medical thinking in public health from around the 1870s to the 1950s and, indeed, the practice of clinical epidemiology became very much the investigation of the health of the individual rather than the population – despite the clear benefits of mass vaccination and the evidence of declining mortality from infectious disease prior to the introduction of mass vaccination campaigns, presumably as a result of improved nutrition, social conditions and medical care (McKeown 1976).

The rise of mortality attributable to cancer and chronic diseases that has afflicted populations in developed countries since the Second World War led to epidemiologists using case control and cohort studies effectively to characterize individual risk without a deep understanding of the aetiological mechanisms involved. This 'black box' approach was accompanied by the notion of the 'web of causation' (MacMahon *et al.* 1960), the multi-causal nature of public health problems and the establishment of statistical measures of risk and odds to characterize disease susceptibility. Furthermore, substantial developments in quantitative methodologies have characterized the 'black box' era and substantiated the paradigm.

Eco-epidemiology and population level approaches

To this analysis has been recently added a new paradigm that returns epidemiology firmly in the direction of population health. The Sussers have termed this 'eco-epidemiology' (Susser and Susser 1996b) and have emphasized the need for modern epidemiology to embrace causal mechanisms and pathways at the societal level as well as at the molecular level, citing the HIV epidemic as an example. Here, while molecular level investigations are needed to understand the precise mechanisms and characteristics of infection and viral replication, details of the specific personal and sexual behaviour of individuals, and population mixing, is needed at other levels. The public health implications of HIV require understanding at all levels, demanding skills in biology, ecology, psychology, anthropology, population genetics and medical statistics, at the very least.

Consider sick person A in Group GA, part of population PA. Traditional epidemiological approaches might assess risk to A by measuring disease susceptibility in PA and approach prevention by identifying preventable risk factors in PA and applying them to A. The eco-epidemiological approach would prioritize the social and economic factors that predict risk, identify the personal factors that exacerbate risk within the social context and, with the knowledge of the biological mechanisms of disease contraction established, evaluate the efficacy of preventative measures targeted at the group and individuals within the group.

A number of epidemiologists have followed these eminent researchers' lead (Pearce 1996). The ecologic model for epidemiology has been supported by McMichael (1999), for example, who calls for replacing the preoccupation with individual level risk factors and cross-sectional measures of exposure with the development of 'dynamic, interactive, life-course models of disease risk acquisition' in a wider socio-ecological perspective.

One driving force for this redirection is dissatisfaction with the measured proportion of variation in disease explained by conventional, individual-based risk factors such as those measured on the British civil servants in the Whitehall study on heart disease (Marmot *et al.* 1984). A population-based public health epidemiology has probably been delayed not only by the understandable focus on individually targeted disease risk assessments but also by the fall from grace of ecological studies following the wide dissemination of 'ecological fallacy' arguments (see below). Concepts and measures of population health have been relegated in priority although the purpose of the Public Health Observatory system (www.pho.org.uk) might now be seen to include this brief.

Large randomized controlled trials and their meta-analysis form part of the evidence-based medicine move towards drawing generalizable, group level conclusions of efficacy of treatment. But while specific individual interventions can have large effects on individual health, it is also the case that small effect sizes in large populations can have substantial public health consequences. Modest population level reductions in blood pressure or blood cholesterol concentrations, or increases in exercise, can have substantive population level health effects and confer benefits on community health and reduce demands on health services (Morris 1975).

However, care is needed in integrating the results of individual level and population level studies. The 'ecological fallacy' emphasizes the differences in the determinants of disease between and within populations and cautions against interpreting the first as a mirror of the second (Rose 1985; Greenland and Robins 1994). Heavy smoking populations, for example, are likely to have lung cancer risk factors that differ from abstinent populations although the difference in risk of lung cancer between these populations will be largely attributed to smoking behaviour (Davey Smith and Ebrahim 2001). Population specific risk factors analysis has been recognized in less developed countries as an important epidemiological approach. Accordingly, optimal prevention measures are likely to vary between populations. The experience of individually targeted health promotion and health education programmes in failing to reduce chronic disease indices is an example (Ebrahim and Davey Smith 1997). Furthermore, ecological studies are being revisited as important sources of information on population level risk factors and on interactions between these and those operating solely at the individual level (Schwartz 1994; Mackenbach 1995). The other prime tool in population level epidemiological studies, the community trial, is discussed in more detail later in the chapter.

Genetic epidemiology

Other factors, to be discussed in more detail later, include the need for understanding more about the distribution of risk factors and combinations of risk factors within populations, the measurement of low or intermittent exposure rates over long periods of time, and the interactions between genetic, environmental and societal factors in the generation of disease (McKee 2001).

Genetic epidemiology, through the potential of the Human Genome Project, provides an additional new major opportunity for public health progress. Some of the hype surrounding the public health impact of this initiative seems excessive as even modest risk levels for disease attributable to specific genes or gene combinations generate great excitement in comparison to more conventional physical or behavioural characteristics (Davey Smith and Ebrahim 2001). Here the challenge lies in the analysis of interactions between genes and the environment and finding its significance in the context of the realities of public health such as the massive and increasing burden of ill health related to the rapid rise in obesity and diabetes.

As in the case of the 'ecological fallacy' an equivalent 'genetic fallacy' exists. This can demonstrate an individual risk *within populations* that varies substantially with individuals' genetic constitutions while these factors are not strongly correlated with variation *between populations* (Maes *et al.* 1997; Mokdad *et al.* 2000). It remains probable, therefore, that the ethical conundrum of providing a chemical solution to a lifestyle caused health problem, notwithstanding the exciting developments in the availability of genetic information, are probably unlikely to impact in a revolutionary way on public health in its wider context.

Other developments

Having considered the need for epidemiology to adopt a more ecological stance to service public health in the future, there are a number of other areas where technical and methodological development is occurring.

These other areas of development include the use of the Internet in data acquisition for a global approach to public health (LaPorte *et al.* 1994). It was envisaged in this initiative that international registries, surveys and disease monitoring programmes could be undertaken throughout the world using Internet-based technology. Disease distribution patterns, especially in more remote parts of the world can exploit the technical advances in spatial statistics based on geographical information systems (LaPorte *et al.* 1996; Robinson 2000). While email and web pages, user lists and the like undoubtedly foster communication patterns among epidemiologists, as they do for everyone, this approach is more immediately finding a particular niche in education and training. The SuperCourse in Epidemiology (www.pitt.edu/~super1/index.htm) is a new resource for those presenting public health orientated epidemiology courses around the world using well referenced materials including visual aids. Particularly suited to developing countries, the SuperCourse may prove to be a significant force for training the wider cadres of public health practitioners envisaged in coming decades.

Another area in which technical improvement is occurring is in the definition and classification of diseases and conditions of ill health, and the design and availability of health statistics. An example of excellence is the raw data on levels of pollutants in the air, as assessed by over 100 automated monitoring sites managed by the Department for the Environment and Rural Affairs, which is updated hourly and published freely on the Internet (www.airquality.co.uk). This provides a new level of accurate data on a few environmental exposures which are often so difficult to obtain.

In the area of health measurement major advances have been made with international agreements on definition such as the *International Statistical Classification of Diseases and Related Health Problems* whose tenth edition (*ICD10*) is now established within clinical epidemiology (www.who.int/whosis/icd10). But major faults remain in both voluntary and obligatory disease registration systems in the UK that confound their wider use for research purposes. These exist because of their development as structures of management (for example, hospital episode statistics) rather than specifically for disease monitoring or research. Limitations in primary care data sources have already been referred to. Much has been written about the strengths and weaknesses of these systems (Kerrison and MacFarlane 2000; Leadbetter 2000), but in general they cannot be used for dedicated 'case-wise' epidemiological studies in public health. The light might be appearing at the end of the tunnel, however, as the new electronic health record and electronic patient record which, in theory, will provide both the source data for aggregate statistics on health service provision and (suitably anonymized) case-wise, record linked epidemiological data for research.

Future developments in public health epidemiology: concepts and methods

For reasons already discussed it is probable that public health epidemiology will come to develop particular approaches and methods to satisfy demand for a better understanding of population-based measures of risk, integrating information from diverse sources, evaluation of complex interventions, and the challenges of life course exposure measurement and outcome assessments. In this section I shall visit four topics which, it is envisaged, will emerge as more prominent areas in future public health epidemiology. Two of these: meta-analysis and Bayesian methods, concern primarily statistical or mathematical progress more than, or at least as much as, conceptual and theoretical development. Life course approaches and community evaluations are areas demanding wider acceptance and understanding of the methods of design and analysis (and funding) required for their scientific development.

Meta-analysis

The statistical summation of different epidemiological studies on the same subject is becoming an essential tool in understanding the variation and complexities of research results. This is not only because of contradictory results of different studies of the same topic (Mayes et al. 1989) but because of variation or 'heterogeneity' of results due to chance effects or effects related to characteristics of the studies themselves. For example, separate meta-analyses of the effects of dietary beta-carotene intake on cardiovascular mortality conducted on cohorts and in trials indicate worrying discrepancies which are probably the result of inherent differences in study design (especially risk of selection bias in observational studies) as similar discrepancies have also been found in studies of cancer and in studies of other anti-oxidants (Davey Smith and Egger 1999; Egger et al. 2001).

In the wider public health, where observational studies are the norm and trials of intervention unusual, steps need to be taken to enable conclusions to be drawn from the widely ranging results of public health interventions. This area is controversial with opinions ranging from finding such meta-analytical systematic reviews of observational studies unacceptable (Shapiro 1994) to cautious conditional approval (Egger *et al.* 2001). The arguments governing this process include, first, the importance of avoiding selection and recall bias and confounding, particularly in observational studies, and second, concentration on investigating the sources of heterogeneity between observational studies rather than blindly presenting a single 'conclusive' meta-analytical result. The alternative, a cumbersome assessment of a set of narrative views, may be less useful. Ensuring that observational studies are undertaken with a rigorously scientific approach is likely to be helpful. One recommendation, that *individual* patient or client data (Altmann 2001) are utilized in a meta-analysis, while desirable, is unlikely to be achievable in the near future within the remit of the wider public health because of inherent non-conformity in the settings, researchers and interventions being employed.

Another developing role for meta-analysis in public health, where it has emerged from a careful process and where heterogeneity is limited, lies in identifying the realities of health behaviour impact as outcome, in contrast to interventionist studies of limited usefulness for broad health promotion or health education campaigns. For example, strong evidence that dietary changes effected in the animal or human laboratory setting have a marked effect on blood cholesterol concentration, may not be reflected in community-based populations with wide ranging prior risk profiles, baseline health behaviour activity and attitudes (Davey Smith and Ebrahim 1998). The 'context specific' differences in subject characteristics, compliance and overall diets may be of paramount importance, leading to disappointing results for the population as a whole (Brunner *et al.* 1997; Ebrahim and Davey Smith 1997). However, this finding is of great significance as broad spectrum health promotion campaigns might not be as effective as specific measures targeted at high risk individuals, suggesting that legislative or fiscal policies may be more effective (Davey Smith and Ebrahim 1998).

Bayesian approaches

One of the more challenging developments for epidemiologists to incorporate in their approach to the statistical treatment of public health data is Bayesian analysis (Bland and Altmann 1998). Traditional 'frequentist' statistics are used to ascribe probabilities to obtaining the sample data observed assuming that *no* association, difference or effect actually exists (the so-called Null hypothesis) in the underlying population made up of all possible samples. This is worthwhile doing because simply by chance unusual results can be obtained on a sample, just as we might – although it is unlikely – obtain 40 heads and 10 tails in a normal coin tossed 50 times.

If, for example, we are measuring the impact of an intervention such as nicotine replacement therapy our Null hypothesis would be that those receiving nicotine replacement therapy are equally likely to continue smoking as those not receiving it. If our *observed* data then seem to show that smoking rates are lower in the nicotine replacement therapy group we can use frequentist statistics to quantify the probability that such a result could occur by chance if, in fact, the underlying smoking rates in the population were equal. We then, to follow the frequentist paradigm, continue by judging whether this probability is acceptable or not. It is a convention, although in fact entirely arbitrary, to regard the probability (that the research sample data could have come from a population with equal smoking rates in the nicotine replacement therapy and no nicotine replacement therapy groups) as 'unreasonably low' if it is less than about 1 in 20 (or 0.05 or 5 percent). If the probability is below this criterion a decision is taken to reject the Null hypothesis as 'reasonably unlikely' and the result is taken to indicate a 'statistically significant difference'. It is an assumption of the frequentist method that, according to the Null hypothesis, the *expected* smoking rates in the nicotine replacement therapy group is fixed at the rate equivalent to those not receiving the therapy. In other words the data are being used to estimate the probability that a specific, and perhaps unreasonable hypothesis, is *unlikely to be correct*.

For decision making in health, however, we really want to follow a converse reasoning, that is, estimate the probability or risk that a (positive or negative) outcome *will occur* given the data we observe in the research study. In order to do this we may need to use all the information we have about the probable outcome rather than assume that a positive one is as likely as a negative one.

It is a central principle of the Bayesian approach in clinical medicine that the starting point for assessing therapeutic efficacy of some intervention is some probability that a specific outcome will be obtained (from all previous knowledge of the subject). Of course it may be that no such knowledge exists, but in many cases it does. This probability is called the 'prior probability' (or 'prior') and how the results of a new study might change this probability is the essence of Bayesian calculations. A major strength of the Bayesian approach is, as we shall see, that it naturally takes into consideration the incremental process of research evidence as more information, data and analysis emerge: these knowledges change the prior as research into a subject evolves and grows.

It is because the prior can vary according to information from previous studies that Bayesian statisticians regard the method as more realistic. To take the coin tossing example, most coins will have some (probably very small but nevertheless existent) bias (based on the uniformity of weight distribution and shape irregularities) and this should be taken into account. Furthermore, as many public health interventions or public policy changes are one off events, the probability of obtaining an advantageous outcome by chance is of limited meaningfulness using frequentist statistics that are based on the theory of multiple events or samples.

In public health, the need to incorporate information from *observational* studies, including specifically qualitative research, is of particular relevance in assessing the outcome of interventionist studies. In these cases the prior probability of an outcome is 'informed' by these sources of intelligence and the effects of the intervention judged against it in the 'posterior probability' (that is the probability of the event given the data observed and the assumed prior) using Bayesian techniques. For example, to assess the impact of a home-based rehabilitation programme for the elderly returning from hospital on independent functioning, pilot interviews and discussions could be used before the programme started to enable a set of possible priors to be estimated. It could be argued that such an approach provides a more reasonable baseline against which to assess intervention impact.

However, the difficulty lies in the validity of the estimate of the prior and this is one main thrust of the anti-Bayesian critics. Sensitivity analysis (incorporating a range of priors to cover a variety of contingencies) often accompany Bayesian estimates of probability. This makes results messier, conditional and continuous (rather than the apparently clear cut notion of statistical significance), albeit based on more realistic assumptions and theory (Spiegelhalter *et al.* 1999). Some modern statistical packages now include Bayesian programmes as use of the method had previously been compromised by the tedious nature of the calculations.

Another potentially important use of Bayes' theorem in public health lies in the methods of meta-analysis. Here it provides a conceptual and mathematical foundation for synthesizing research evidence and especially in moderating the quantitative influence of a large trial with unusual or unexpected results. As the results are presented in the form of probability distributions it naturally fits into the meta-analytical technique of 'random effects modelling', often used when research evidence on the same topic is internally discordant and heterogeneous.

Because Bayesian methods involve the interpretation of data in the light of existing evidence, it is particularly suited to policy makers (Lilford and Braunholtz 1996; Ashby and Smith 2000). It provides a method of analysis that allows the policy maker to formulate the questions they wish to ask: 'How does the new evidence of a recent study affect our current view that service X is most unlikely to have adverse effect Y?' or 'If we are dealing with the particular scenario S, what is the risk of Y being reduced by 25 percent?'. This is also equivalent to the doctor's assessment of the probability of a patient having a disease given the presence of certain symptoms. These computations are possible because the outcome is calculated as a *probability distribution* not as the 'p-value' for a fixed risk (Lilford and Braunholtz 2000).

For public health epidemiology where properly conducted community trials are required but prove to be resource sapping, expensive and lengthy, it is important to use the maximum amount of information available in designing and interpreting the study. In particular there is a need for decision making based on information which derives from some combination of routine data, observational studies and controlled trials (Ashby and Smith 2000). Inevitably this will necessitate the incorporation of lower hierarchy evidence into estimation of the design parameters such as overall sample size, acceptable statistical error rates, cluster size, cluster numbers, in addition to data interpretation. Here the value of the prior can be adjusted accordingly. Adjusting the prior enables valuable information to be gained about sub-groups on the basis of assumptions that can be informed from qualitative or observational evidence. As Freedman explains in a well written introduction (Freedman 1996), while Bayesian approaches might seem to be most useful in meta-analysis and assisting individual patient decision-making processes, its impact on public health may also lie in areas such as population screening (Eddy *et al.* 1990), assessing the cost effectiveness of trials (Detsky 1985) and sub-group analyses (Dixon and Simon 1992).

Life course approaches

Two methodological approaches typify developments of major interest in public health epidemiology. The first, which can be packaged under the generic term of 'life course epidemiology' encompasses long-term exposures, weak associations (Florey 1988), epidemiology of chronic conditions expressing themselves in older age and foetal programming. The common denominators here are, on the one hand, the determination of weak, longer-term adverse exposures affecting health and their inter-actions both with other environmental exposures and genetic factors and, on the other, early exposures during critical periods of development having major long-term effects.

The notion of single, acute exposures resulting in specific measurable outcomes after brief intervals may be paradise for the epidemiologist, but it is now an unrealistic model for elucidating the causes of major public health concerns such as the common chronic diseases of diabetes, asthma and other respiratory diseases, rheumatoid arthritis and the like. The reality, in complex, adaptive and responsive biological systems, is that temporal ordering, dose, exposure intervals, interactions between exposures, exposure duration, the presence of critical periods and interactions with genetic and social factors are all likely to alter the course of outcome expression. While the simultaneous modelling of all the influences is both conceptually and mathematically challenging, life course approaches to aetiological understanding can be initiated more simply.

By way of example, Ben-Schlomo and Kuh (2002) diagrammatically illustrate the biological and psychosocial exposures acting over a life time that may influence lung function/respiratory disease. These include, in chronological order, factors varying from genetic predisposition, to poor uterine growth to passive smoking and air pollution to occupational hazards, with socio-economic status, housing conditions and poor educational attainment also being contributory.

Such a life course model can incorporate 'critical periods', generally early develop-mental 'windows' which can irreversibly channel the structure and function of biological systems so that they are much more sensitive to risk factors in later life. Evidence that poor foetal growth, for example, can lead to non-insulin dependent diabetes, obesity, hypertension and cardiovascular disease as a result of 'biological programming' of metabolic physiology at early developmental stages of life form part of the so-called 'foetal origins of adult disease' hypothesis (Book and Whelan 1991; Barker 1998). This in turn owes part of its conception to seminal studies of the long-term effects on the infant and child of starvation at different stages of the mother's pregnancy (Stein *et al.* 1975). There remain, however, many careful clarifi-cations to be made in elucidating the mechanisms involved in foetal programming (Gillman 2002). The picture is made yet more complex by the existence of trans-generational effects on outcomes such as cardiovascular mortality, emphasizing that public health measures may require even longer acting programmes of research and prevention (Davey Smith *et al.* 2000b).

In contrast to the longer-term impact of acute events in critical periods are the weak exposures that accumulate over lengthy periods. The adverse effects of exposure to ionizing radiation are now known to be additive and not threshold specific, although their *impact* (for example, diagnosis of effects on function) may become evident rather suddenly. In the social context, epidemiological approaches can be used to characterize risk of, for example, depression following the accumula-tive impact over time of 'life events' such as mental breakdown, bereavement, unemployment and divorce (Brown and Harris 1978).

As populations age and knowledge of long-term risk factors and their interactions mature, public health professionals will increasingly require epidemiologists to steer them, using new methodologies, including sophisticated statistical techniques (such as meta-analysis and Bayesian approaches), in directions where meaningful policies can successfully be implemented. Life span perspectives will probably depend on the establishment, maintenance and full exploitation of large life course cohorts prospectively enrolled in previous generations (Golding *et al.* 2001). It is as apposite now as it always has been since the days of John Graunt's Bills of Mortality, to note that the foetal programming hypothesis which places new longer-term perspectives on public health and its causes, depends on accurate record keeping of birth weights, placental weights and maternal characteristics at a time when their ultimate usefulness could not have been foreseen. Investment in longitudinal data collection is likely to reap important public health benefits from the epidemiological analysis of cohorts in future years (Gillman 2002). The multiplicity of aetiological and contributory factors and the likely absence of large associations require such cohorts to be sizeable and, consequently, expensive to manage.

Multilevel approaches

The second methodological approach of increasing potential in public health lies in multilevel modelling and, specifically, the epidemiological analysis of community intervention trials. Many conventional medical statistics are based on the integrity of the individual as a unit of response to interventions to improve health. While this may be true in the individualistic treatment scenarios of the consultant's examination room, it is much less so in the field of public health. Here, individuals are physically arranged and characterized by clusters of spatial, social and genetic relationships. This non-random distribution also imparts non-independence of responsiveness to exposures and to public health measures. For example, individuals living in the same inner-city housing estate are more likely to be similarly affected by pollution from a nearby factory than those living in another, more distant, housing estate; or patients on the same GP list might be more likely to be given advice on smoking, exercise and weight control and, possibly, pursue a healthier lifestyle with health benefits, than those on another's list. Health measures in such common instances require evaluation to take into account the different levels of operation and this constitutes the principle of the process of multilevel approaches to the design and analysis of epidemiological studies.

The non-independence of individuals in many fields of public health measurement emphasizes the need for multilevel analysis. An eminent statistician recently drew attention to the general unawareness (including among experienced researchers) of the need to take the clustering of individuals in society into account in public health studies (Bland 2001). The problem concerns any situation where a health intervention, be it a preventative measure or a positive intervention – including health education, vaccination, provision of a clean water supply and so on – is applied at the level of a group or community but where outcomes are assessed individually. The effect of the correlation of outcomes within groups containing individuals similar in some way is to reduce the effective sample size of independent units and, hence, diminish the power of the study, thereby raising the risk of improperly detecting significant effects where there may be none.

What are the consequences of this apparent statistical nicety for epidemiology in 21st century public health? Unfortunately, the answer is that they are quite profound. This is because much public health work involves a few units of large size, such as the patients in two or three surgeries or a few large schools or housing estates. The practical implications of this have been simply and well presented by Ukoumunne and colleagues (Ukoumunne *et al.* 1999). They identified key considerations including the careful selection (and, generally, also the maximization) of numbers of clusters, cluster randomization and allowing for clustering effects at the time of analysis. It is in any case very common for the size of trials of intervention to be woefully under-estimated in public health interventions as well as in clinical medicine. This problem is exacerbated by the effects of clustering where, to maintain power, studies have to be increased in size by the 'design effect' (Donner and Klar 1994) – a quantity that takes into account the 'intra-class correlation coefficient', a measure of the non-independence of individuals within clusters. Properly including the design effect in power calculations can increase the required size of research studies two-fold or more. Probably of greater difficulty, however, will be the resource implications for increasing the number of clusters with some authors recommending an absolute minimum of six with strong indications for substantially increasing this number (Grossdkurth *et al.* 1995), especially where, as is the case for many modern public health interventions, the effect size is modest or small.

Multilevel regression analysis may also be required and, fortunately, software is now more widely available to assist in this endeavour. A more detailed discussion on the theory and practice of multilevel and cluster designed studies can be found in Von Korff *et al.* (1992) and Donner and Klar (2000).

Conclusion

Epidemiology is the main component in the public health practitioner's tool box and should remain as the primary form of methodological guidance for understanding the causes of poor health and to evaluate preventative and therapeutic measures. It can also be concerned with the elucidation of the mechanisms – from molecular to societal – of perturbation of health.

If a modern definition of public health such as 'the collective efforts organised by society to prevent premature death, illness, injury and disability and to promote the population's health' (Beaglehole and Bonita 1997) is adopted, then epidemiology must prepare for the task of developing methodologies to use in a much broader array of concerns such as poverty, war and global warming (*Lancet* 1997). There is little doubt that advantages would accrue were the development of a population orientated evidence-based public health to follow from the successes of the evolution of evidence-based medicine from clinical epidemiology (Heller and Page 2002). Indeed this is already happening specifically with the widening agenda of the Cochrane and Campbell collaborations into social care, educational methodologies and corrective behaviour, and an increasing focus on appropriate population-based measures of health (Aspinall 1999) such as those within the remit of the Public Health

Observatories (Ashton 2000). (See Chapter 13 on evidence-based public health for further discussion of these issues.)

The *methodological* changes that are foreseen to implement this re-orientation include the introduction of population services audit, dissemination of critical appraisal skills to managers and policy makers and improved population-based health data collection and dissemination (Davey Smith and Ebrahim 2001). Analytical innovation is also required, including further developing group and population orientated study designs and data analysis for health assessment and intervention evaluations.

Epidemiology is simply a tool to be used for public health as its practitioners demand. New focuses on evidence summations, ecological contexts, life course effects, health and social inequalities, and community health interventions must energize epidemiologists to develop the methodological and analytical skills to support these demands. Additionally, however, epidemiologists have the right to expect public health workers to listen to the advice they offer in appraising the evidence correctly and in designing research studies appropriately. This is of particular importance as the wider public health often requires more complex, more expensive and more resource hungry study designs than hitherto. These messages have passed from clinical medicine to traditional public health and now need to continue the journey towards the broader reaches of public health and social care.

16

JANE POWELL
Health economics and public health

Editors' introduction

Health economics is a way of thinking and a set of tools and techniques associated with this way of thinking. It is concerned with resources and how they are allocated and distributed in society.

This chapter outlines some of the tensions between economists and public health policy makers that arise from different ways of thinking about public health, resources in health, and economics. It gives public health practitioners a brief outline of 'how to do' an economic evaluation.

Most public health professionals will benefit from knowledge of the key concepts, thinking and techniques of health economics, as outlined in this chapter. The new framework for economic evaluation in social welfare is an especially helpful tool for evaluating public health programmes, because we need good public health programmes which incorporate a service user perspective and are effective, with beneficial outcomes outweighing costs for society as a whole.

In the first section of this chapter, the author focuses on economics as a discipline. She outlines key concepts from the perspective of public health professionals, and tools and techniques that are closely associated with the work of health economists. In the second section she argues that traditional evaluation techniques in health economics are increasingly out of step with the challenges presented by 21st century public health and its focus on 'equity'. The third section explores new directions for health economics input into public health, explaining why 'efficiency' continues to dominate economic thinking in economists' advice to public health evaluators.

The author concludes that the time is right to further develop the framework for economic evaluation in public health research and practice.

The role of economics in 21st century public health

Popular wisdom often suggests that a little knowledge is a dangerous thing in the wrong hands. In the case of public health professionals, a little knowledge of some of the key concepts, thinking and techniques of health economics, particularly their limitations, can be viewed as an important part of professional development in public health practice. This chapter will outline the economic approach to the allocation of public health resources and assess its relevance within 21st century public health for policy and practice.

Economic evaluation encompasses a well established set of techniques in the health care field of public health practice, but economic evaluation is scant in other areas of public health (Sefton *et al.* 2002). In recent years the demand for such evaluation has risen in response to the modernization agenda of government and the focus upon research aimed at reducing health inequalities. (See Chapter 2 for more on modernization, and Chapter 10 on inequalities.) In order to encourage greater use of economic evaluation, there is a need for economists to better understand the nature of public health as *action* or *intervention* and public health as a *resource*, in order to ensure that approaches they suggest public health evaluators adopt are useful and feasible.

The structure of this chapter

The first section of the chapter will focus on economics as a discipline, outlining the economics approach to thinking about problems of resource allocation. It will outline key concepts from the perspective of public health professionals, and tools and techniques that are closely associated with the work of health economists. The second section will argue that the evaluation techniques of health economics, focused as they are on the notion of efficiency, are increasingly out of step with the challenges presented by 21st century public health and its focus on equity. The third section will explore new directions for health economics input into the public health arena considering the reasons why health economists tend to find it difficult to re-orientate their thinking around the notion of equity. This third section will explain why the efficiency criterion continues to dominate economic thinking in economists' advice to public health evaluators, despite its lack of practicality for public health policy evaluation.

Key concepts, tools and techniques in health economics

Definition of economics

Economics is a discipline or a way of thinking (Cohen and Henderson 1988). A number of tools and techniques, such as economic appraisal, are associated with this discipline.

According to Paul Samuelson (1976) economics is:

> the study of how men and society end up choosing with and without the use of money, to employ [allocate] scarce productive resources, [which may have

alternative uses] for production and distribute them for consumption [efficiently and equitably], now and in the future, among various groups and people in society. It analyses the costs and benefits of improving patterns of resource allocation.

(Samuelson 1976: 5)

The health economics discipline

At the end of the 19th century, the basis for orthodox, economic theory was laid through the introduction of mathematical developments from the physical sciences into economics. These paradigms dominated the development of economics as a discipline and set the mainstream economic view that economic systems are rational, rule bound and mechanistic (Ormerod 1994). Mechanistic theories and models still pervade much economic theory to this day and have influenced profoundly the development of many economic techniques and tools such as programme budgeting, marginal analysis and all of the variants of economic appraisal techniques. These techniques are based upon a common approach that is systematic and conforms to certain strictures.

The sub-discipline of health economics developed around the late 1960s and early 1970s from the main discipline of economics. Health economics is at present based firmly in 'micro' (small) as opposed to 'macro' (large) economics and is concerned with the aggregate behaviour of individuals (people, and private and public sector businesses), as opposed to the aggregate macro- or whole economy. Economic or econometric analysis of the behaviour of people and organizations at an aggregate level has much in common with epidemiological population approaches to quantifying aggregate public health problems. In particular, they are similar in that assessments from average, aggregate data analysis of the population may not necessarily apply at an individual level. This has to be borne in mind when developing public health policy using the findings from economic evaluation as an aid to decision making.

Both the way of thinking and tools and techniques of health economics are borrowed mostly from the micro-economic branch of the mother discipline. Increasingly criticism has been directed towards shortcomings in mainstream micro-economic theory. In particular, rationality in behaviour of individual economic agents pervasive in micro-economic theory has been strongly questioned (North 1990; Earl 1995). Despite the ethical emphasis in economic approaches upon utilitarianism or the common good, economists have focused in the past upon outcomes for individuals, families and other agencies or third parties as separate groups. Prioritization of individual preference ignores outcomes relating to the complex interplay between each of these and the institutions with which they interact. In the process of abstraction from detail, and following a strict systematic framework that is endemic to an economic approach, some of the key elements of public health programme evaluation (for example, social capital, community values and infrastructure) are not reflected as adequately as is desirable in 21st century public health evaluation (Sefton *et al.* 2002).

Proponents of institutional economic approaches argue that economic evaluation should move away from a utilitarian framework and recognize the interactive relationship between individuals and their environment alters their behaviour (North 1990; Jan 1998; Sefton *et al.* 2002). This issue is returned to in the section on evaluating outcomes, but it is probably worth acknowledging that without some change, economic evaluation will continue to fall short as a potentially powerful evaluation technique to measure the worth of public health programmes (Shiell and Hawe 1996).

Key concepts in health economics for public health professionals

Orthodox economic theory is founded upon numerous principles and is full of jargon. Fortunately, for those in public health who have not had a thorough grounding in economic theory, explanation of a few key concepts will cover a substantial amount of what is needed to get by.

Efficiency and equity

We can relate the public health function directly to the definition of economics we discussed above. Resources are scarce or finite. Public health professionals cannot do everything for groups and populations that they would wish as demands are infinite and resources do not allow it. Therefore, they have to make choices about how to allocate scarce resources at their disposal.

Efficiency is a criterion for sharing out or allocating resources among all competing uses in public health. According to an economist's perspective, resources should be allocated in order to obtain the maximum 'health improvement' from the finite amount of resource. However, most public health professionals would be concerned to allocate resources equitably as well. Unfortunately, there is almost always a trade-off between efficiency and equity in allocating resources, so it is unlikely that in public health care, an efficient allocation of resources will also be an equitable allocation of resources (Dolan 1998). Nevertheless, this fact does not necessarily detract from the potential usefulness of economic techniques in any activity where scarce resources have to be employed and distributed efficiently, for example, priority setting of public health care activities, created by the combination of finite resources and infinite demand.

Quality adjusted life years (QALYs)

Despite their numerous difficulties, development of QALYs, as a tool for measuring outcome or the benefit of interventions, can be viewed in retrospect as one of the most well known, tangible contributions that health economists have made to the development of evaluation in health care.

A QALY is a number indicating the size of health gain from an intervention. It is created by combining quantitative information of length of survival with 'softer' information of patient perceptions of quality of life (Bush *et al.* 1972; Weinstein and Stason 1977) so that:

a QALY = estimate of length of life × estimate of quality of life (from service users' perspective).

QALYs can be estimated at an individual, group or population level and their main attraction has to be that they permit outcomes from different health care services, interventions and diverse specialisms in health to be measured in common terms. This circumvents the problem endemic in evaluation tasks of comparing 'apples and pears' in measuring outcomes or benefits.

But it also raises a host of other issues. Criticism of QALYs as an outcome tool relates to methodological problems in their construction and calibration. Probably the most important of these are the difficulties inherent in estimating survival after health care intervention which is hazardous enough at an individual level (readers are referred to the seminal study in economic evaluation by Alan Williams (1985) as an example of difficulties in medical practitioners estimating survival). Difficulties in estimating survival at group and population level encompass the issue of risk assessment that is also a complex estimation task.

However, the area that has received more critical attention from commentators is the quality adjusted part of the QALY measure. For example, how should different levels and dimensions of quality of life be measured? (Bowling 2001); how should different health states be valued? (Mooney 1992; Dolan 2001); how and from whom should values be elicited? (Carr-Hill 1989; Dolan 2001); and what do the resulting values mean? (Nord 1990; Dolan 2001), are all areas within this debate. Ethical concerns regarding alleged ageism and/or sexism endemic in QALY health gain measures have been made (Rawles 1989) and countered strongly (Mooney 1989). The full development of these arguments is outside the scope of this chapter, but interested readers are referred to Mooney (1989) for an excellent summary of the issues of constructing QALYs and applying them in health care evaluation.

Opportunity cost

In Samuelson's (1976) definition of economics there are added square brackets containing 'which may have alternative uses' in connection with resources. Resources are limited and if they are used in one way they are then not available to be used in another way. Very few activities are costless and costs can be incurred without money necessarily changing hands. For example, if a public health professional foregoes the opportunity to visit an elderly house accident victim in order to attend to an emergency road accident victim then there is a cost involved to the elderly patient, which is the benefit foregone in not having immediate emergency care. The value of the best opportunity foregone as a result of undertaking an activity or the sacrifice involved is the opportunity cost.

Usually money is used as a means of measuring opportunity cost. Definitions of cost in economics and accounting are different. The economist's notion of cost extends beyond the cost falling on the public health service. All sacrifices involved in pursuing a particular public health policy should be incorporated within any measure of opportunity cost, including those on other agencies in society, individuals and their families.

Economic evaluation

Systematic review of economic evaluation

A recent systematic review of published studies sought to uncover the number of economic evaluation studies in the field of social welfare (Sefton *et al.* 2002). It was based upon a search of electronic databases covering the major international journals for the period 1996–2000, using the search terms for each type of economic appraisal and social care, families and housing. Such terminology is not inclusive to public health action as it is used in this book because the terms environmental health and transport, among others, would need to be included. However, the results of this systematic review are nevertheless indicative of the current state of play of economic evaluation in the public health field.

This systematic review indicated an average of 30 studies per year published internationally within the field of social welfare. This figure compares with 450 studies published per year internationally between the years 1991–96 within the field of health care evaluation (Elixhauser *et al.* 1998) and this is a figure that is likely to have increased substantially since then.

Two-thirds of the 131 studies identified were conducted in the USA and two-thirds of the studies were of the cost–consequences type of evaluation. A further one quarter of studies were cost–effectiveness studies leaving a very small percentage of the cost–benefit variety and no cost–utility studies. This last piece of information is very revealing because cost–utility studies take the economic construct QALYs as their measure of outcome. The results of this systematic review seem to suggest that the social welfare evaluators of the present have found some difficulty incorporating the QALY into their evaluations, a state of affairs in contrast to the health care evaluators of the past.

Types of economic evaluation

Economic evaluation – sometimes known as option appraisal – is a generic term covering four main types of economic evaluation technique. These four types are:

- cost–consequences analysis;
- cost–effectiveness analysis;
- cost–utility analysis; and
- cost–benefit analysis.

Each is applicable to answering different types of public health questions. According to Cohen and Henderson (1988) three broad categories of economic evaluation can be categorized, namely cost–effectiveness analysis, cost–utility analysis and cost–benefit analysis. Drummond *et al.* (1997) add a further two categories of cost analysis and cost–consequences analysis.

All of these separate types belong to the same family of economic evaluation techniques, but they are applied in different circumstances to different questions.

Cost–effectiveness and cost–utility analysis are applied in circumstances where the available budget is fixed and the maximum benefits are sought, or the objective is fixed and the minimum cost method of achieving an objective is sought. Cost–consequences analysis is similar to cost–effectiveness analysis in terms of the questions addressed, but it is applied to evaluate interventions with more than one multidimensional outcome. Cost–consequences analysis does not attempt to combine measures of benefit into a single measure of effectiveness, so it cannot be used to rank interventions in terms of their effectiveness and efficiency. Nevertheless, it is a systematic technique that allows decision makers to weight and prioritize the outcomes of an evaluation.

Cost–consequences analysis
A general example of a question that would be answered by conducting cost–consequences analysis is: What is the least cost way of providing a public health programme that does a specified amount to solve or lessen a problem?

This cost–consequences question could be posed in a specific form as: What is the least cost way of reducing homelessness among all young people in the area covered by North Bristol Primary Care Trust?

In this question the objective of reducing homelessness among all young people is fixed, the budget to find a minimum cost method of providing a homeless service for young people is variable and there is more than one outcome. These include the behaviour and self-esteem of the young people, the net effect of intervention on the number of young homeless, the wider community, and the impact on relationships and government agencies among others.

Framework for economic evaluation of public health interventions

This section focuses on a new economic framework for evaluating public health interventions that has been developed by the Centre for Social Exclusion at London School of Economics and the Health Economics Unit at the Institute of Psychiatry. This approach is outlined in a very thoughtful and practical text-book, Sefton *et al.* (2002) and all readers are referred to this excellent source for more detailed exposition of this framework. Sefton *et al.* (2002) argue that many public health interventions are more complex and multilevel than interventions in health care, introducing problems for the application of 'traditional' economic evaluation techniques favoured by health economists. Readers are referred to the blue book by Drummond *et al.* (1997) and Drummond and McGuire (2001) for exposition of the traditional framework for economic evaluation in health care.

Figure 16.1 presents a schematic diagram of a developing framework for economic evaluation in public health care. This framework couches economic evaluation within an overall evaluation framework first articulated by the Medical Research Council (2000).

There are four stages in a thorough economic evaluation in public health and it is vital that the amount of resources that will be consumed during this process are not underestimated at the outset.

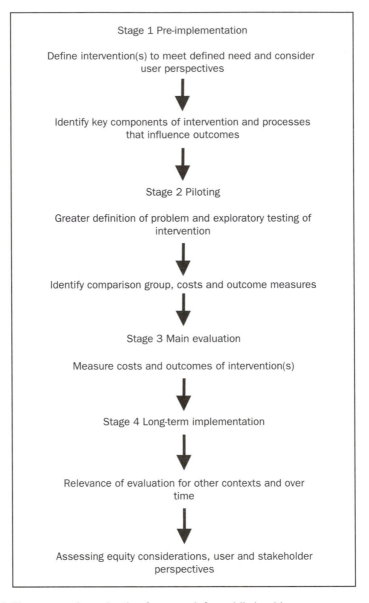

Figure 16.1 The economic evaluation framework for public health

Stage 1 Pre-implementation and thinking stage

Define intervention(s) to meet defined need and consider user perspectives   Economic evaluation in public health should be about designing effective programmes that meet the needs of a population group, community and wider society. Economic evaluation is not meant to be about validating decisions about expenditure that have already been taken, or take the form of a proposal to spend resources in a particular manner. It is not meant to be an exclusive or limiting approach; its tenor is non-limiting and non-exclusive. In conceiving the interventions or programmes that meet need, and feasible solutions to the problem that has been defined, no limit should be placed upon what is considered possible, and political motivations should be placed to one side.

The early, thinking stages of an economic evaluation are vital to the quality of the end product. Time should be allocated here for consultation with whoever might be affected by the issues encompassed in the appraisal, including all stakeholders and users of a programme. This is an area that economists of the past have been reluctant to embrace for fear of not remaining impartial in their analysis. It is vital that economic evaluators take a hands-on approach at both Stage 1 and Stage 2 of an evaluation in order to get a feel for the processes and outcomes that might be of importance at Stage 3 where they will become much more involved.

Identify key components of intervention and processes that influence outcomes, objectives and questions   In order to determine the outcome(s) of an evaluation it is important to first set the objective(s) of appraisal and to recognize that public health programmes are likely to have many outcomes at various levels. For example, the opening of breakfast clubs, community cafes, gardening projects and skill training centres will almost certainly benefit individuals who attend these projects. At one level their quality of life, employment status and self-esteem might be improved and each of these could be a designated objective of these programmes. In addition, communities might also benefit from the capacity building and community development and this might be another multilevel objective of these types of public health programmes.

Stage 2 Piloting

Greater definition of problem and exploratory testing of intervention   At the piloting stage of a public health economic evaluation it is important to re-clarify the original objectives of a programme as it is possible that the objectives of such programmes can change as they develop (or fail to develop) and improve (or worsen). For example, public health programmes that seek to reduce social exclusion might ask how this concept is viewed by various breakfast clubs, community cafes and gardening projects. It might be relevant to consider whether each of these projects differ in their attachment to the overall government objective of reducing social exclusion. Exploratory testing of a programme intervention would examine how the specific elements of breakfast clubs and so on operate, why each project is successful or unsuccessful and noting emergent 'best practice' in reducing social exclusion.

Identify comparison group, costs and outcome measures   Comparison group: Economists take the view that an evaluation study design should demonstrate the effectiveness of any programme or intervention, public health or otherwise, with respect to another programme or intervention. There are numerous methods for achieving a comparison group, for example, outcomes in one group that has received a programme compared with another group that has not, or the same group compared before and after a programme intervention.

Costs: There are four broad categories of cost that should be considered in a public health economic evaluation:

- Programme costs arise from the direct cost of providing a public health intervention.
- Direct costs include all of the individual elements of an intervention, such as staff, volunteer time, buildings, equipment, transport, support services and so on.
- Non-programme intangible costs (or savings) arise from the resultant programme effects, such as the savings that may result due to a reduction in the need for alternative programmes.
- Indirect costs, such as child, family and wider agency costs (or savings), for example, the salary of carers should also be included in economic evaluation.

Benefits: Economic evaluation should be comprehensive and have a societal perspective. It should therefore consider outcomes that may not be referred to in the objectives including the impact upon parties other than the main target group.

Outcome measures: Outcome evaluation will also recognize that programmes impact at different levels. It will be important to evaluate the impact of these programmes on the community and organization in which the programme is set as well as on individuals, in order to capture the full impact of a programme.

There are two types of outcomes to be evaluated:

- final outcomes arise from the populations impacted by a public health programme; and
- process outcomes arise from achievement of potential, actual joint working processes and partnership arrangements that arise from a public health programme.

Process outcomes relating to the manner in which an organization and its workers implement a programme are not part of traditional economic evaluation that focuses upon inputs and outputs. But it is difficult to ignore process outcomes within public health programme evaluation as it is essential to uncover the reasons why a public health programme succeeds or fails and add this knowledge to the analysis and findings (Sefton *et al.* 2002).

Stage 3 Main evaluation

Measure costs and outcomes   Traditionally economists have favoured measurement of final outcomes, for example, quality of life of people affected by an intervention. In public health intervention, however, there are very likely to be process variables that arise from the impact of the intervention on the community and the existence of organizations or networks that facilitate the intervention. Such impacts really need to be included in a comprehensive evaluation.

In addition, in a multiple outcome with different levels, it is important to recognize that a variety of 'hard' and 'soft' information might be incorporated into the measurement stage of an economic evaluation.

Strenuous efforts should be made within public health economic evaluations to ensure appropriate costing methodology is applied by considering resources used and their unit cost separately, following Beecham (2000). Readers are referred to Sefton *et al.* (2002) for an excellent summary of the relevant considerations in measuring costs and outcomes and some excellent suggestions of ways to capture 'hard' and 'soft' information to incorporate within an appraisal.

Stage 4 Implementation

Relevance of evaluation in other contexts and over time It is important to consider the context of an economic evaluation and to decide if there is anything about the particular context that might be generalized to other settings. Particular groups in a community may achieve better outcomes and others worse. The different levels of costs and outcomes and these impacts over time must be reflected in economic evaluation. Time differences in the occurrence of costs and outcomes can be reflected with discounting by the public sector discount rate. Sensitivity analysis can be applied to test the robustness of any data to assumptions that might underlie the production of cost and outcome information. This is important in economic evaluation because assumptions will most probably have to be made.

Assessing equity and user perspectives It might be the case that costs and outcomes and the interaction effects between organizations, individuals, communities and society may not be apparent at first or may quickly fall off. Evaluation should continue to take place once a public health intervention is in place to inform improvement and evaluation of interventions.

Again, it is important that economic evaluators embrace the users of services and become involved with the data generated, as it is then much more meaningful and provides richness to the process of interpreting the data generated.

An economist's natural instinct is to use quantitative data, but in public health interventions the usefulness of qualitative data should not be overlooked. It is usually a good source for trying to tease out what people actually mean by what they are saying and for gauging how and why public health programmes work as opposed to what works in evidenced-based public health. (See Chapter 14 for discussion of evidence-based public health.)

Strengths of economic evaluation

The great strength of economic evaluation as a technique is that it follows a systematic, rational and logical approach that leads beguilingly to an answer or, in public health, to a range of answers that can be applied with other types of analysis and information in decision-making processes. It is, when conducted as it should be, much more transparent than deployment of 'expert judgement' as a basis for making decisions about public health resource allocation. Decision-making processes in public health may still be very cloudy, but the evidence from economic evaluation should at least act to create some discussion about values, viewpoints and judgements before decisions are made.

The thinking, problem definition time of economic evaluation is also extremely worthwhile. If deficiencies in services and need have not been identified correctly or at all, then it becomes a rubber stamping exercise to support vested interest, which it is not meant to be.

New directions for health economics in public health action

The ethical stance of public health professionals

According to Mooney (1992) there are three principal ethical theories: virtue, duty and the common good. Virtue and duty are essentially individual ethical theories and the common good a societal ethical theory. Jonsen and Hellegers suggest that: 'traditionally medical ethics has dealt mostly within . . . the theories of virtue and of duty . . . the nature of contemporary medicine [new public health located in primary care] demands that they be complemented by the third essential theory – the common good' (Jonsen and Hellegers 1987: 4).

It can be argued that there is much more that can be identified as the doctrine of the common good in the contemporary ethics of 'new public health care' than the individual ethic that predominates in medical health care. This would imply that economics and public health care are likely to be more comfortable bedfellows than economics and health care and we will return to this issue later on in this chapter.

The ethical stance of economics

Utilitarianism forms the ethical basis of economics as a discipline. Utilitarian ideas, theories and techniques are concerned with 'the common good or the greatest happiness of the greatest number' and this philosophy is closely associated with the writings of Jeremy Bentham (1834). Vilfredo Pareto also brought concepts of social welfare into economics with his notion that improvement in the allocation of resources takes place if at least one person is made better off and nobody else worse off (Pareto 1935). The translation of utilitarian, social welfare concepts into economics revolves around the issue of distributive justice which is the ethical concept most relevant to choosing priorities. Application of the principle of utility is most relevant to the choosing of priorities per se, but its application in public health care poses many questions and creates many problems.

There are question marks over a number of issues, for example, whether it is possible to measure utility, health, ill health or social welfare. Another issue is whether the economic deprivation suffered by one group of individuals can be offset by the freedom from economic deprivation of another group of individuals. According to most economists, it is possible to measure these things and to make trade-offs between population groups. Economics is a 'positivist' discipline that takes an aggregate, societal view of resource allocation. From this perspective it concurs reasonably well with traditional population-based, health promotion approaches that form part of contemporary public health (Lupton 1995).

Efficiency and equity – difficult bedfellows

There are competing theories of social justice. Rawles (1972) is concerned with both liberty (equal for all) and social good, which he argues should be distributed to the advantage of those at the 'bottom of the pile'. He believes that given the choice any rational being would opt for a society run by his rules of social justice as opposed to a utilitarian-based society. The worst that could happen to you in a society run according to his maxims would be better than the worst that could happen to you under a utilitarian regime. Economic evaluation techniques highlight the importance of using scarce resources in the most efficient way possible to maximize overall health gain. Ideas of prioritization and rationing of health care are closely linked to concerns that health demand is infinite and yet resources are finite. The argument that a public, taxation funded NHS and primary care led public health system will never be able to meet all the demands of an expectant public, new expensive technologies, new drugs and an ageing population, stands despite a recent government report (Wanless 2002). (See Chapter 1 for a perspective on government policy for public health.)

Few people would argue against spending public health resources in the best way possible. The argument about what is the best way is a normative question that can be viewed from the perspective of maximizing health gain or addressing health inequalities. Current government policy gives a strong direction to the latter, particularly within a primary care led public health movement. But there are many more attendant difficulties attached to the notion of reducing health inequalities than there are to achieving efficiency or maximizing health gain. Reduction of health inequality requires that equity be defined for these purposes. Unfortunately, as Pereira (1993) notes, there are at least six main definitions of equity and it is this lack of focus in potential objective that may give rise to non-achievement of public health outcomes. (See Chapter 10 on approaches to tackling inequalities in health.)

However, the policy environment and thrust of the modernization agenda within which public health workers now operate (see Chapter 2) is a far cry from the 1980s and early 1990s when cost reduction was paramount and equitable shares of the distribution of health care were not considered viable objectives for professionals to pursue. Unfortunately, economic evaluation as a technique does not seem to have evolved in order to encompass renewed emphasis upon equity in public health policy and requirements to consider user perspectives in evaluating services. It can be argued, therefore, that economic evaluation techniques focusing as they do upon individual value do not adequately reflect social values (Dolan 1998) and are not an adequate guide to the distributional effects of a given course of action.

Economic evaluation is ethical from the standpoint of the utilitarian. In the utilitarian welfare function (Bergson 1938) that applies to health, 'happiness' is replaced by 'health gain' and the philosophy of spending resources to maximize health gain is applied. Using QALYs as the measure of maximizing health gain has been criticized on numerous fronts. Cost–utility analyses are reliant upon the QALY measure, other types of economic evaluation, for example, cost–consequences and cost–effectiveness analysis are much less so.

Equity as the objective of economic evaluation techniques

A review by Sassi *et al.* (2001) exploring how techniques of economic evaluation could be improved, commented that an attempt by Lindblom in Scandanavia to develop equity life years, a tool to weight QALYs to take regard of equity, was not a sufficiently robust method to warrant further investigation for application within economic evaluation. A recommendation was made to move away from cost–utility analyses towards cost–benefit analysis, using willingness to pay to help value the benefits in monetary terms. However, the authors considered this move to be also fraught with methodological issues. Economic evaluation in public health seems to have gravitated towards the application of cost–consequences analysis; it is probably within this technique that future developments will lie.

There are good things about using economic evaluation to aid decision making, but it has to be recognized that individual preferences manifest in the QALY measure do not adequately reflect societal preferences (Dolan 1998). In general, it can be argued that societal preferences are concerned with need, fair distributions and extra help for the most disadvantaged.

Sassi *et al.* (2001) found that while maximizing health gain is important to people, they are prepared to make trade-offs. These trade-offs are between the amount of health gain and the number of people treated; the total amount of future health and the degree of equity between groups; and the severity of illness and health gain. Nord (1999) have conducted some research in Norway to develop societal preferences in techniques such as the person trade-off. The future development of tools that reflect community values and preferences should be encouraged, as they would undoubtedly add to the scope of economic evaluation. Readers are referred to a paper by Nord on 'cost–value analysis' in health care to explore these ideas further (Nord 1999).

In their review, Sassi *et al.* (2001) recommend that all economic evaluation studies should include information in tabulated form concerning the differential benefit to different sub-groups of the population. This should indicate clinical, socio-economic and age characteristics, and other data that is deemed of distributional or 'fair shares' importance. They reason that in this way decision makers will have analysis concerning efficiency, and information and data concerning equity in front of them when they make policy decisions.

Nevertheless, once an economic evaluation study is complete – whether it is focused on efficiency or is a new technique focused on equity – the decision about what to do in the light of economic evidence will still have to be made. Making policy decisions encompasses many issues of organization, hierarchies, networks (Williamson 1975), the ideological thrust of the government of the day and the money in the kitty.

Conclusion

It is unlikely that health economists will be able to prioritize equity over efficiency in techniques they propagate for use in public health evaluation.

However, the time is right for the framework of economic evaluation within the arena of public health research and practice to develop further. In particular, the involvement of service users, their families and carers should be sought at both the problem definition and equity assessment stages of evaluation. (See Chapters 8 and 9 for more about involvement of the public in health care decisions.)

Public health interventions have numerous outcomes, many levels and objectives that are not always clear. In view of these features, cost–consequences analysis seems to be the best placed of the family of economic evaluation techniques for further development and application at a local level.

More effort should be made to ensure greater scientific validity of evaluations in public health research. However, the complexity of many public health interventions may require non-standard modifications to study designs or a greater role for qualitative methods in the practice of economic evaluation. Health economists should learn to take a more pragmatic view of data and to find ways of measuring the interactive elements of public health interventions.

17

STUART HASHAGEN
Frameworks for measuring community health and well being

Editors' introduction

Community health and well being work is a core area of 21st century public health. Complex programmes are implemented by a range of professionals working in partnership for health and well being, linking with communities themselves who are one of driving forces.

A feature of the government modernization agenda for public health is a renewed focus on the *outcomes* of public health interventions that seek to improve health and well being in communities. But evaluation of complex, context specific health and well being programmes is difficult; outcomes do not readily lend themselves to the established 'hierarchy of evidence' that has dominated traditional evidence-based public health practice.

In this chapter, all public health workers involved in community health and well being programmes will find something useful in the mix of theory and practical advice for 'measuring' outcomes in terms of community health and well being.

The author starts by discussing what is meant by community health and well being and the core values that inform policy and practice. He outlines the Achieving Better Community Development (ABCD) framework of indicators developed by the Scottish Community Development Centre to evaluate community development. He suggests ways in which the outputs and outcomes of health and well being work might be measured and public health programmes evaluated, discussing the inherent tensions with traditional evidence-based public health approaches.

A model of health and well being developed by Labonte is used to inform a model for planning and evaluation called the Learning Evaluation and Planning model (LEAP), which focuses on the three core elements of healthy people, strong communities and good quality of life.

The author concludes that the current emphasis on evidence-based practice challenges public health workers to establish approaches to planning and evaluation that are informed by social principles, shifting the culture towards a more participative and empowering ethos.

Introduction

This chapter is concerned with approaches to planning and evaluation for the new public health. Its focus is mainly to review tools for planning and evaluating community development work created by the Scottish Community Development Centre between 1996 and 2002. The development of these tools is traced and their use is discussed with reference to policy in Scotland and more widespread issues in the evaluation and validation of what I shall call 'community health and well being action'.

Community health and well being action

Community health and well being action is characterized by:

- a concern with health inequalities: a recognition that unacceptable inequalities in health persist, that they affect the whole of society, and that they can be identified at all stages of the life course from birth to old age;
- a focus on community development: drawing on the experience of a large number of community health projects and initiatives that have adopted a community development approach, working to support communities to take action on needs and issues that they identify as critical;
- adoption of a social model of health: recognizing that good health is a product of social, economic and psychological factors, and not simply a medical or physiological matter;
- recognition of policy and organizational change: the health and quality of life in communities is affected as much by the policies and practices of the NHS and other organizations, as by the nature of the communities themselves;
- an emphasis on partnerships: acknowledging that effective strategies for change often require a partnership approach – drawing on the knowledge, skills and resources of the community and service agencies, working to a shared vision for change; and
- clear and explicit value systems: these help to shape and frame planning, action and evaluation of practice; these values are, of course, subject to review and debate.

Value systems to inform policy and practice

There is a broad agreement in the literature of community development on the core values that should inform policy and practice (SCDC 2001). Participants in community health and well being action should be supported and empowered to enhance their ability to exercise influence over their individual, group or community circumstances. Empowered people participate in the process of their own development and exercise citizenship in working towards community and individual change. For example, black and minority ethnic groups, disabled groups and children have more restricted opportunities and influence in communities and should therefore be given particular attention to ensure there is equity and justice in community health and well being development.

The persistence of inequalities in health is a primary motivator of community health and well being action (Wilkinson 1996; Blamey *et al.* 2002), so practice must be explicitly anti-discriminatory and challenge direct or indirect discrimination within a community. However, while the right of people to make their own self-determined choices must be respected, it is important to recognize the limits of self-determination and the value of people working together in their common interest. Many different agencies (statutory, voluntary and community) can contribute to personal develop-ment and building community capacity, and should work together to maximize the value of their resources in partnership with each other. Finally, positive development and change only occur when all participants are prepared to be open and to learn from each other.

Fields of community health and well being and 21st century public health

The characteristics and value system described above locate 'community health and well being action' in Scotland firmly within 21st century public health as defined in the Introduction to this book. The term 'community health and well being action' is adopted in this chapter because of problems in definition of this territory.

The term 'community health' has been used to describe the field, but is problematic because it is also used, as is 'public health', to refer to the health status of a whole population. It also refers to the activities of community health practitioners who deliver services. 'Community health' does not convey the ideas of process and participation that are required of this term in current public health practice. The term 'community development and health' is also widely applied; for example, the network of community health projects and practitioners in Northern Ireland is the Community Development and Health Network.

In many ways 'community development and health' describes the field correctly. However, some policy makers and practitioners understand community development in quite restricted terms as essentially the relationship between community workers and community groups. Where such a view is held there is a danger that key players may exclude themselves from efforts to improve the health of communities. We need a broader term to ensure that all relevant partners are included.

The term 'well being' is used for two reasons in the definition of community health and well being action. First, the outcome of new public health interventions is to improve the health and well being of a community. This distinguishes new public health interventions from 'health' interventions by the medical emphasis that links them to the outcome of control or absence of illness (Jones 1999). Second, in new Scottish legislation for local government, the power to promote 'well being' has been introduced and local authorities are set to lead interagency community planning partnerships to realize this goal. Similar terminology is in use in other parts of the UK.

In Northern Ireland, the 1997–2002 *Regional Strategy for Health and Social Well-being* (Northern Ireland Department of Health and Social Services 1995) was in many ways a radical document, setting out principles that were to be adopted later in England and Scotland. This strategy recognized the role of the health and personal social services to provide care, but also that 'other government departments and agencies have an important contribution to make to health and social gain', and crucially went on to emphasize the 'need to develop strong alliances for health and social gain with communities themselves. A community . . . has a right to be involved in making choices about how health and social care is delivered to respond to its needs' (Northern Ireland Department of Health and Social Services 1995: 5).

This strategy was based on four underlying principles:

- encouraging public policy which supports health and social welfare;
- *supporting community development;*
- enhancing primary care; and
- placing increased emphasis on effectiveness and measuring outcomes.

The strategy report went on to make important observations about the role of community development:

> The strength of community development lies in its diversity; it has the potential to make a major impact on a wide range of policies and programmes . . . It has a particularly important role to play within the health and personal social services . . . enhancing the ability of the public and voluntary sectors to reach and involve people in need . . . [encouraging] active participation by communities in needs assessment and [maximising] the participation of service users in the decision making process . . . to make services more responsive to user's needs and to generate a sense of local ownership and control over those matters which affect the lives of the people involved.
> (Northern Ireland Department of Health and Social Services 1995: 6)

Having given community development a central role in its strategy, the Department of Health and Social Services then needed to develop the capacity of the health and social services boards to deliver services based on community development principles. To do this, a framework for monitoring and evaluation was required, both to define what was actually meant by community development and to provide a set of indicators with which progress in community development could be measured. The Scottish Community Development Centre (a partnership of the Community Development Foundation and the University of Glasgow) was engaged to undertake this work, and was particularly enthusiastic because its recently completed study by Barr *et al.* (1996) of the relationship between community education and community development had concluded that there was a need for 'a set of specific community development evaluation tools and criteria'. The next section describes their development.

Achieving Better Community Development (ABCD)

Developing the indicators for ABCD involved consultations with community workers, health workers and researchers in England, Scotland and the Irish Republic as well as in Northern Ireland. The resulting report was published by the Northern Ireland Voluntary Activity Unit (Northern Ireland Department of Health and Social Services Voluntary Activity Unit 1996) and later published in a revised form as the *Achieving Better Community Development* handbook and support materials (Barr and Hashagen 2000).

Principles of ABCD

Planning and evaluation

ABCD establishes several basic principles about planning and evaluation for community and social action. First, community development cannot be effective unless planning and evaluation are built in, so intended objectives and outcomes must be clearly specified in order to examine change. Second, planning and evaluation are linked integrally as community development operates in a complex world in which communities vary enormously. No two contexts will be the same, so it is essential that all those involved share an understanding of the issues and problems and the shape of possible solutions. It is only with this understanding of what will be evaluated that planning can commence to build strategy to achieve outcomes.

Empowerment

In order that community health and well being and the wider field of public health can justify public health action, its impact on the quality of life in communities, social inclusion and building social capital has to be identified with evidence of such changes (Wallerstein 1993). Ultimately, those involved in community health and well being action need to win the argument that participation and empowerment can be defined and measured, and that investment in these areas is of equivalent or greater value to investment in, for example, medical technology or health education.

Learning organizations

Community health and well being are complex concepts and they interact with an infinite variety of social, economic, technical, cultural and political factors. These factors operate locally as well as at wider levels. Because of this complexity, it is important that organizations seeking change, for example, community groups, public health practitioners or wider partnerships, see themselves as learning organizations. A learning organization interacts with its environment, is flexible and open, proactive and participative, and responds rapidly to change.

Learning organizations have to be able to evaluate their actions in order to learn from experience. The link between learning and evaluation is reinforced in community health and well being action because of the difficulty of establishing direct connections between causes and effects in this field. Learning organizations need to be able to monitor the environment in order to be able to identify critical change rapidly and accurately and be able to base their future action on such evidence.

Participative evaluation

If the aim of community health and well being action is to increase participation and ownership, it follows that the evaluation process should be consistent with this. Thus, the community must be included as partners in the process of evaluation. Community development action seeks to develop agendas for change from within communities and to draw on the resources of the community to lead them towards change. It follows that community development cannot be evaluated appropriately using externally imposed, cost-based or output quantifying models or measures. This is not to suggest that having clear goals and considering the costs involved are unimportant, but these should be established collaboratively by the community and other partners in consultation with funders or policy makers and not simply imposed by the latter (Hancock *et al.* 1999). A lack of clarity or agreement about what is expected from community health and well being practice is a major issue in the field.

Measurable outcomes from community health and well being action

Key to addressing this lack of clarity is recognizing that community development has outputs and outcomes that can be isolated and measured. In the past the field of community development has been weak in defining, explaining and taking ownership of these ideas and has not been sufficiently clear about understanding or communicating how the things it does (actions) have effects (outcomes) which may be described as 'empowering communities'. But there are ways in which 'empowering communities' can be defined and measured, provided that those involved in community health and well being action take the trouble to specify both outcomes and outputs and how they are linked (Hashagen 1998).

For example, an after school club might provide a certain number of places, a homework group and a programme of games or physical activity. All these things are outputs and all can be measured as such. But their presence may also contribute to wider outcomes of benefit to the well being of children, their families and the wider community. So:

- if the provision of places allows parents to work when they could not otherwise have done so there will be gains to family (and community) income;
- a homework group might support the children to fare better at school;
- the physical activity may bring gains in fitness; and
- taken together, the children may be more connected to community and more skilled, and these things all contribute to health and well being.

Each of these outcomes can be measured using quantitative or qualitative information.

To evaluate such a community initiative we can look directly at the outputs: How many places are available? How well run is the homework group? How many children attend the games programme? Many approaches to evaluation ask for little more. But what we should really be interested in is the wider impact of the club on the children and the community. It may be harder to assess this, but ways can be found. In the example above, additional income to families can be calculated readily and any changes in school performance can be assessed from school records. The children's feeling of fitness and confidence can be observed or self-reported. It is important to define possible outcomes in order to know where to look for the evidence of change. While many other factors may impinge on school performance, fitness or family income, it is nevertheless important to recognize that the club may have an impact and to be able to assess its value.

Stakeholder owned indicators of change

This discussion leads to the next observation that community development needs indicative rather than prescriptive approaches to evaluation. The ABCD model and the related LEAP framework both argue that the stakeholders in any community development initiative must develop and agree the measures and indicators of change that they intend to use, and these will be unique to the particular situation and context of the work. While the indicators chosen may reflect national targets or may use examples set elsewhere, the actual choice should be made by the stakeholders in the initiative so that the things that are assessed are those that are of key significance to that initiative and owned by all the participants (Dixon 1995).

Level of action and participative evaluation

Community development generally operates at policy, programme and project levels. In other words, most community development work is implemented through community projects or by providing support to community organizations. However, such support is usually a component of a wider programme, for example, the programme of a social inclusion partnership to encourage community involvement or of a local authority to promote community learning and development. In turn, these programmes are in most cases a response to wider policy initiatives. The examples above would be reflections of Scottish Executive policy on social inclusion and community learning (Taylor 2002).

Two observations flow from this. First, the politics of evaluation in community development often lead to the lowest and most local of these levels being the most closely monitored. Yet this is unfair: the programmes and policies within which projects operate should be equally open to scrutiny. Second, in approaching evaluation in community development we should be able to ask questions at each of the three levels and be able to make the connections between all three.

Public health programme evaluation

Whenever work with people and communities is undertaken basic questions should spring to mind; the following checklist sets them out. Such considerations will almost certainly be in the mind of the bodies that fund the work.

A checklist for community development programme evaluation (Barr 2002)

- Are we gaining a new understanding of community needs and issues?
- Are we being effective in tackling them?
- Are we being inclusive?
- Are the participants achieving their personal goals?
- Are we building community assets and resources?
- Is our work empowering people?
- Are we building a culture of collaboration, participation and sustainable change?
- Are we learning from our experience?
- Are we contributing to health and well being?
- Are we making the best possible use of the resources we have?
- Do we have the evidence we need to influence future decisions?

Good planning and evaluation helps to answer these questions and to improve practice. It provides evidence that action is making the best use of limited resources and thus provides partners and communities with confidence that they are benefiting from the action. Put simply, good practice requires that all participants in action for community development have:

- a clear view of what they are trying to achieve *(vision)*;
- agreement on how they intend to get there *(planning)*;
- evidence to show whether they have done what they said they would do *(monitoring)*; and
- evidence to tell them whether they achieved what was intended, whether anything else happened and whether these things were helpful or not *(evaluation)*.

Evaluation of impact in community development practice

One of the major problems for evaluating community development is measuring change satisfactorily. Approaches to current public health action can be contentious and one of the main battlefields is that of evaluation of public health action. It is here that the workers and agencies that adopt what may broadly be described as a community health and well being approach may find themselves having to account for what they do and what it achieves against criteria and assumptions that they do not necessarily own or share. The dominant approach to programme evaluation is:

- quantitative: encompassing concrete, measurable activities or end points;
- target focused: primarily interested in the long term in the impact on national targets for social justice or health (Scottish Executive Health Department 2001); and
- output led: mainly looking at what happens rather than on the impact it has.

By contrast, the community well being approach tends to concentrate on:

- qualitative influences: being interested in the extent to which an activity is felt to have an effect on the way people feel or experience their lives;

- outcomes: having an interest in the impact of what is done on the quality of life, and seeking to understand and learn from it;

- process variables: recognizing that the way things are done can be as important – or more so – than what is achieved. This is a crucial point if we seek to work in empowering ways;

- behavioural factors: emphasizing behaviour – in the field of health and well being the emphasis is often on the ways individuals change their behaviour, for example, by smoking less, taking more exercise or practising safer sex; and

- holistic factors: recognizing the complexity of factors that impinge on health and well being, and recognizing that change occurs through development work with individuals, communities and with the policies and services of the organizations that impact on them.

Thus, the field of community health and well being brings together two very different traditions of evaluation and it is essential that the basis for evaluation of a given initiative is established and agreed from the start. Traditionally the field of health has invested heavily in evaluation, with medical practitioners needing to know as much as possible concerning the impact and possible side effects of a particular course of action. This has led to an emphasis on calls for epidemiological and quantitative evidence and, in the field of community well being, evidence that community activities are having a demonstrable impact on rates of illness or on behaviours such as people's diets, their exercise or smoking habits. Needless to say, such connections are almost impossible to substantiate and alternative approaches to evaluation are needed if, in the longer term, the health impacts of well being work are to be acknowledged. (This reflects the tensions inherent in an evidence-based approach to health care and public health discussed in Chapter 14.)

The tradition of evaluation in community participation is rather different. It has often emphasized process over outcome, looking at the quality of people's experience rather than the impact of the work (East End Health Action 2000; Partners in Change 2001). Until recently, community development has not been good at establishing or 'owning' the criteria on which it can be evaluated. In these circumstances, participants and practitioners in community health and well being have criticized funders for:

- imposing agendas that may have little to do with local views of needs and issues;

- emphasizing value for money above all else;

- giving more weight to the quantity of the outputs than the quality of the outcomes; and

- giving too little attention to understanding the processes of achieving change.

Funders and policy makers have conversely criticized community health initiatives for being unable to specify the impact of what they do, and for emphasizing process above outputs.

The emergence of 21st century public health encourages us to ask whether there may be alternative approaches to evaluation that might satisfy people, rooted in both the medical and social models of health. Such approaches would have to deal with the complexities of what 'well being' actually means, and how practitioners and partnerships can go about working towards it.

A third way

A very useful paper by Labonte (1998) encourages us to take a fresh look at health and well being and to consider how those interested in promoting good health might understand their task. For people working in the NHS and other settings where the impact of well being activity has to demonstrate an impact on the health status of individual participants, it is important to be able to make the connection between actions and impacts.

To help with this task, Labonte provides a valuable framework, arguing that good health for the individual is a product of physical, mental and social factors, as expressed in Figure 17.1.

Labonte suggests that to experience health and well being, three things need to be in place: physical capability, including vitality and energy; mental health, essentially described as having meaning and purpose in life; and a social context of connection to family and others in a community. Labonte's model theorizes that people need energy and connection to others to enjoy good social relationships, connection to community and a sense of purpose to feel some control over life, and both energy and a sense of purpose to be able to live enjoyable lives. It should be clear from this

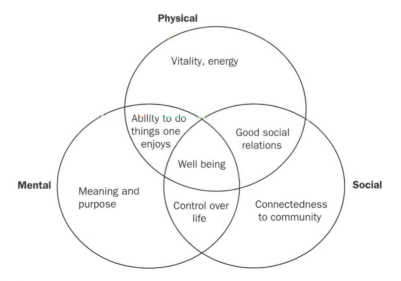

Figure 17.1 Labonte's model

interpretation that well being is essentially a psycho-social phenomenon and one that is considerably more complex than simply addressing behavioural issues or medical practices.

Labonte's model encourages those involved in community health and well being action to question what actions can facilitate outcomes for health and well being for people and communities. Labonte goes on to describe the risk factors that prevent people from enjoying health and well being and these risk factors are identified in Figure 17.2.

The application of the model in Figure 17.2 helps to understand the connection between well being action and its impact on people's health. By focusing on the way people relate to communities and services, well being action is particularly concerned with psycho-social factors and risk conditions described therein. Where community empowerment leads to people in communities having more skills and confidence, better networks, more control and influence over their lives, the psycho-social risk factors are addressed. Similarly, engagement in well being activity to improve the quality of community life will have an impact on risk conditions such as poverty, pollution and low socio-economic status.

Turning to behavioural factors a number of points can be made. First, the educational and publicity strategies of much traditional health promotion practice do not fit comfortably into a well being approach to action. People are generally aware of factors that contribute to a healthy lifestyle, but the motives for smoking or drinking may outweigh the case against them. Such behaviour can be an attempt to exercise some power and control over negative or chaotic circumstances. Second, concern with issues of diet, drugs and alcohol may not figure highly in self-defined community

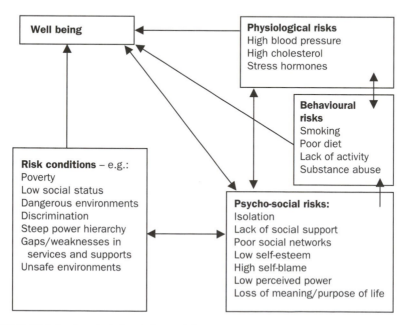

Figure 17.2 Risk factors in Labonte's model

definitions of need. Thus it can be difficult to establish such issues as high on the list of a community's priorities. Without such priority, there is unlikely to be active community participation in planning for action.

From a community well being practice perspective it is perhaps more helpful to understand behavioural factors as consequential to changes in psycho-social factors and risk conditions. Thus, if people feel better about themselves and if they are less exposed to external risk conditions, they are more likely to pay attention to their behaviour patterns and be more prepared to take action. If we can accept this approach a chain of actions and impacts can be established and built into our evaluation frameworks.

Learning Evaluation and Planning model (LEAP)

All this leads us towards establishing a model for both planning and evaluation. Work completed by the Scottish Community Development Centre, based on the ABCD framework that has already been discussed, developed a model for planning and evaluating community development-based learning, including promoting personal development and building community capacity. The model is called LEAP – Learning Evaluation and Planning (Barr 2002). Originally written for the field of community learning, a version of LEAP is now being written for the community health field (Atherton *et al.* 2003) and has the following features:

- *Needs, problems and issues*: the first principle is that community health and well being work must start with a clear understanding of the needs, problems and issues experienced by the people, groups or communities in question. This is in contrast to the idea of resource led planning, in which agencies start with a known level of resources, staff, equipment and budgets, and decide how those resources will be applied. Such an approach is unlikely to be accepted by the recipients. A need led approach implies that time and energy can be wisely invested in reaching a clear understanding of issues that can be owned and shared by the community.

- *Participative learning*: community health and well being learning requires a different sort of culture to the 'experts on top' model. It thrives within an 'experts on tap' environment. To do this, and to establish ways of working that are based on the empowering approaches discussed at the beginning of this chapter, we need to move towards a culture where people, whether patients, local groups or community organizations, are engaged in defining needs and developing solutions, drawing on the expertise of others where appropriate. This means moving to a culture based on dialogue, equality and involvement. The effectiveness of moving towards this can itself be planned for and evaluated.

- *Partnership based*: the earlier discussion about the complexity of health and well being, and the importance of physical, mental, community and policy factors in experiencing well being, leads to the inevitable conclusion that no single agency or interest can promote well being alone. Partnerships are needed both to bring a range of perspectives to bear on a problem or issue and to work to find solutions that are likely to work. Partnerships are also vehicles for securing participative practice and a need led approach, assuming that the partnerships are themselves effective in engaging the interest and commitment of the agencies and communities concerned. It has been widely recognized that development of community partnerships is a process that should be developed and managed according to community development principles and some useful tools have been developed to support this (Low 2001; Yorkshire Forward 2001). (Partnerships are discussed in detail in Chapters 4 and 9.)

LEAP framework – outcome areas

The *LEAP for Health* framework suggests that there are three broad areas in which outcomes can be sought and that each of these can be divided into several major 'dimensions' on which plans and evaluation can be framed. These dimensions are expressed in Figure 17.3.

Quality of life
This outcome area is intended to express the flavour of community health and well being practice in working towards outcomes that impact upon people's physical

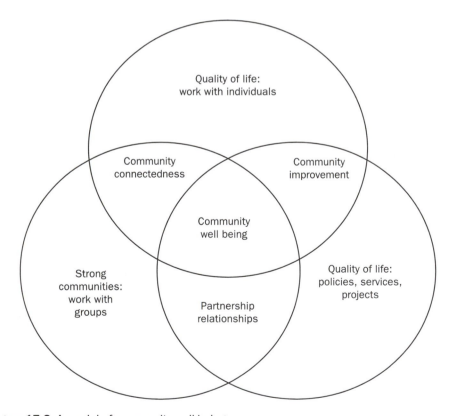

Figure 17.3 A model of community well being

and mental health and their connection to community, as expressed in the work of Labonte (1998). *LEAP for Health* proposes four main areas within which the idea of 'healthy people' can be defined and others into an analytical framework. These are:

- Awareness and knowledge: the extent to which people have the knowledge they need to be able to exercise informed choices about the way they live. This is an important factor in mental well being and a prerequisite for the other factors.

- Confidence, choice and control: the extent to which people are able to make informed decisions in their own interests and are able to assert themselves in social situations and in their dealings with public agencies.

- Self-reliance and independence: which suggests that 'community health' is where people are able to lead and control their own lives relatively autonomously, drawing on services and supports where necessary, but not being over dependent on them.

- Connection to community: responding to the idea that well being is a social idea; the way in which people contribute to and draw from their relationship to others is crucial.

It is important to emphasize that, if it can be agreed that these things are indeed core aspects of 'well being', the activities of partners can be directed towards achieving them, and that they can in some way be measured. For some agencies in the NHS it can be a considerable paradigm shift to accept that such outcomes should be recognized and measured, and that it is an important part of well being practice to encourage such a shift. To reach a clear understanding of what outcomes can be expected and how these might be measured is a central part of this debate. The LEAP model is intended to facilitate this process.

LEAP for Health does not provide ready made indicators. Its approach is to say that each situation is unique and indicators need to be developed by those involved in a given piece of work. In this area some indicators that have been established and agreed in specific projects include:

- women from asylum seeking families having the confidence to go shopping; and
- young people in a young offenders institution making eye contact with workers.

Strong communities

The second main area of well being practice is in the area of communities. The culture and structure of communities is a significant part of the context in which people, especially excluded people, live their lives. Community well being practitioners should therefore be interested in the way communities work and organize themselves, how they contribute to well being, and how they interact with the wider political and economic environment. The ABCD model discussed earlier explores this in some detail, and establishes a set of dimensions in this area as follows:

- *Community skills*: the knowledge, skills and confidence of people in the community have a direct relationship to the 'connection to community' dimension discussed above. Communities do need community skills to be successful and the idea of a 'learning community' encapsulates this idea.

- *Equalities*: given that inequality and exclusion are key factors in poor health, work in communities should reflect an explicit equalities and justice agenda. This principle is core to community development work and must consequently be built into its evaluation. As with the rest of the ABCD approach it is possible to define equalities and develop indicators or measure to assess progress and change.

- *Community organization*: in simple tasks such as sharing childcare or helping a housebound neighbour, or major initiatives like a healthy living centre, people in communities can organize to meet needs, solve problems or make good use of common assets. Communities can also develop strong networks of care and support, and can also establish networks between communities, or between groups of people confronting similar issues (see Chapter 9 for a detailed look at networking for health).

- *Community involvement*: the fourth area is the nature of the interaction between a community and the social, economic and political forces that shape its experience. The term 'community' refers not only to communities of place (villages, streets and housing estates) but also to communities of common interest. It is important to note that community as a term extends to people with diabetes, parents with pre-school children, or senior citizens, members of the same church or social club.

Participation is a crucial component of well being, as argued throughout this chapter and consequently those involved in community health and well being practice should attend to the ways in which communities are encouraged to participate. This will include consideration of practical and financial barriers, the response of public agencies or the availability of information, advice and support. As noted earlier, indicators for all these areas of community strength can be developed. The *ABCD* handbook already mentioned does so, and a more recent publication by Skinner and Wilson (2001) gives useful guidance on how these factors may be assessed and evaluated. (See also Chapters 4, 8 and 9 for more about participation.)

Quality of life

The third broad area of interest for community health and well being is the quality of the environment in which people and communities live and work. Again it is possible to recognize that some environments will tend to promote well being, while others will have an opposite effect. Labonte (1998) explores this area in his discussion of 'risk conditions'. Individuals and communities are of course interested in quality of life; partnerships have a central role in helping identify visions for change and strategies for shared action. Outcomes in this area are very much specific to a given context, but are likely to be concerned with one or more of the issues in Table 17.1.

Indicators can be established for all the outcomes identified in Table 17.1 and progress can be measured in their achievement (Chanan 2002).

Table 17.1 Quality of life

Dimension	Health related outcomes
Community economy	Increased community income
	Reduced community expenditure
	Enhanced community assets
	Elimination of waste and wasteful practices
	Beneficial external investment decisions
Community service	Good networks of care and support
	Accessible services
	Responsive services
	Community involved in service decisions and priorities
Community health and safety	Safe routes and spaces
	Environmental pollution control
	Energy efficient housing and community buildings
	Knowledge and awareness of healthy behaviours and choices
Community culture	A sense of identity and culture
	Celebration of difference
	Opportunities for recreation, physical activity, self-expression
	Freedom of religious expressions
Local democracy	Elected representatives and policy makers engage with the community
	Organizations adopt democratic and participative practices
	Community institutions are open, accountable and democratic

As Figure 17.3 illustrates, community well being brings together the ideas of healthy people, strong communities and quality of life. Where people engage with their communities, this can be described as 'community connectedness'. The relationship between strong communities and the quality of life is normally addressed through participative partnership work, hence the use of the term 'partnership relationships'; while the term 'community improvement' is used to describe the relationship between the quality of community life and people's enjoyment of it.

Action planning

The discussion above should have helped to establish that health and well being are broad concepts that must be tackled robustly and in partnerships involving communities as well as agencies. In addition, health and well being is about the outcomes from practice, not simply the outputs. It may be difficult, but it is possible to find and agree ways to measure well being and the process of change in community

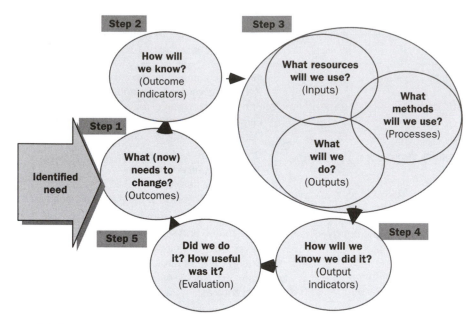

Figure 17.4 Action planning and evaluation framework

development. Figure 17.4 summarizes an integrated action planning and evaluation framework.

LEAP materials go into detail about the way in which this model may be applied in practice. The key points are that:

- It is need led: as discussed earlier, practitioners must know and agree what problems need to be addressed before commencement of planning or evaluation.

- At step 1, What needs to change? and at step 2, How will the impact of change be reflected? must be questioned.

- Step 3 asks those involved in partnerships to consider the resources they have; the methods they intend to use; and what actions they will implement. It also asks people to consider whether and why they think that what they intend to do will have an impact on the outcomes they seek.

- In step 4, partners are simply asked to monitor whether what they intended actually took place.

- In step 5 the relationship between the outputs (what was actually done) and the outcomes (the effect of what was done) is examined in order to learn and shape future action.

- The cycle iterates and step 1 then asks, What now needs to change?

The LEAP model provides a framework within which both the quantity and the quality of the inputs, processes and outputs can be measured, as well as the impact. In assessing impact, considerations of effectiveness, equity and efficiency can be included. By integrating planning and evaluation, emphasizing process and qualitative factors, and by attempting to specify the types of outcomes that can emerge from community development-based work, the model provides an alternative to medically dominated approaches.

Conclusions

The new approach to 21st century public health is in its infancy (although many have been arguing its value for some time). The encouragement in policy to adopt innovative approaches, to engage communities and to work in partnership provides new challenges and opportunities. Equally, the emphasis on evidence-based practice challenges those of us committed to a social model of practice to propose and establish approaches to planning and evaluation that are informed by social principles. Working to give such approaches a weight equal to traditional methods is an effective strategy in shifting the culture towards a more participative and empowering ethos.

18

JACK DOWIE

Health impact: its estimation, assessment and analysis

Editors' introduction

Health impact assessment is a relatively new approach which accepts that social, economic and environmental factors as well as genetic make up and health care, make a difference to people's health. It is a systematic way of assessing what difference a policy, programme or project (often about social, economic or environment factors) makes to people's health. For example, it has been used when public sector organizations and partnerships have wanted to understand the effect on people's health of a new policy on transport or housing.

This chapter provides a critical appraisal of health impact assessment, pointing out that health impact assessment, estimation and analysis are three separate techniques, at different points within the 'hierarchy of evidence', for measuring the impact of public health action on populations. It provides much food for thought by exploring how health impact can be approached from a conceptual rather than practical perspective. It raises many generic questions and issues that are also applicable to the use and application of evidence in 21st century public health practice.

These techniques discussed in this chapter are useful for all public health professionals, policy makers and evaluators at national and local level concerned with assessment, estimation and analysis of the effects of specified actions on the health of a defined population. Users must ensure that each 'health impact' technique is matched to its relevant public health objective, as each health impact technique has a different method and is based upon a different value system or philosophy.

In the first section, the author explores the position and usefulness of health impact assessment; he characterizes it as a technique formed from a melange of multidisciplinary and multiprofessional working. The second section outlines the conceptual basis of health impact estimation and health impact analysis, introducing a critique of health impact techniques and an examination of the separateness of the 'hierarchy of evidence' and the 'modes of cognition' in the 'hierarchy for decisions'. The author concludes with a summary of his arguments.

Introduction

The term 'health impact' has become a prominent feature of public health discourse over the last decade, nationally and globally, largely in connection with the burgeoning activity called 'health impact assessment'. The innocent reader first encountering the term 'health impact' could be forgiven for asking whether it relates to the impact of something on *health* or to the impact of health on *something else*. Going on to read about what happens in health impact assessment they would find that, as in 'environmental impact assessment', it relates to the former – the 'assessment' is of the impact on *health* of projects, programmes or policies and, more specifically, ones not primarily aimed at promoting health. The impact of health sector programmes explicitly targeted at health has, and continues to be, the focus of health economics and less comprehensive forms of evaluation, such as clinical trials. (See Chapter 16 for more about health economics and public health.)

This chapter has a limited purpose. It is to establish that three very different activities can be carried out in relation to health impact and that treating the two – health impact *estimation* and health impact *analysis* – as sub-sets of, or adjuncts to the third, health impact *assessment*, means masking crucial differences in methodology and objective as well as in underlying value judgements about processes. The first two activities should be regarded as independent disciplines and always carefully distinguished from health impact assessment.

Health impact assessment

There is insufficient space here to give a thorough account of health impact assessment as expounded by its various exponents and proponents, but there is an introductory description in Box 18.1.

Interested readers will have read, or be moved to read, one or more of the summary papers (Scott-Samuel 1998; Lock 2000; Scott-Samuel *et al.* 2001; Taylor and Blair-Stevens 2002). It is, however, useful to start with some reflections on the key points from the excellent introductory paper by Lock (2000: 1396–8).

- health impact assessment is a structured method for assessing and improving the health consequences of projects and policies in the non-health sector;
- it is a multidisciplinary process combining a range of qualitative and quantitative evidence in a decision-making framework;
- applications include national policy appraisal, local urban planning, transport, and water and agricultural projects;
- benefits include improved interagency collaboration and public participation; and
- limitations include a lack of agreed methods and gaps in the evidence base for health impacts.

To discuss the first point, health impact assessment is indeed a 'structured method' in the sense that it sets out a series of broadly defined tasks that need to be

---

Box 18.1 Introducing health impact assessment

Health impact assessment has been defined as the estimation of the effects of a specified action on the health of a defined population (Scott-Samuel 1998).

Health impact assessment is a relatively new approach which accepts that social, economic and environmental factors, as well as genetic make up and health care, make a difference to people's health. It is a systematic way of assessing what difference a policy, programme or project (often about social, economic or environment factors) makes to people's health. For example, it has been used when public sector organizations and partnerships have wanted to understand the effect on people's health of policies on transport, air quality, economic development, regeneration or housing.

The assessment can be carried out before, during or after a policy is implemented, but ideally it is done before so that the findings can inform decisions about whether and how to implement the policy. Key steps are to:

- select and analyse policies, programmes or projects for assessment;
- profile the affected population – who is likely to be affected and their characteristics;
- identify the potential health impacts by getting information from the range of people who have an interest in the policy or who are likely to be affected by it;
- evaluate the importance, scale and likelihood of the potential impacts; and
- report on the impacts and make recommendations for managing the impacts.

Health impact assessment is a tool for bringing public health issues into the foreground when organizations and partnerships are making policies and decisions. Public health workers may find it useful if they are considering new policies on, for example, transport or regenerating areas of social deprivation.

(Ewles and Simnett 2003: 141)

---

tackled – such as screening, scoping, assessment and appraisal, reporting, monitoring, and evaluation (see *The Merseyside Guidelines*, Scott-Samuel *et al.* 2001). However, when one comes to the details of what is to be done within each of these tasks the 'structure' remains essentially *procedural* rather than becoming *analytical*. Commitment to serious analysis is very low in the central task of assessment and appraisal, which is particularly unfortunate since this is by far the most significant task. Of course it must be preceded, as it is in both health impact estimation and health impact analysis, by the sub-tasks of deciding the limits of the exercise. It must be followed by the sub-tasks of reporting the results and – if it is possible that the original decision may be modified or changed – deciding what research and monitoring should be undertaken *ex post* that decision. But no matter how well these sub-tasks are undertaken, their performance cannot compensate for deficiencies in the central task.

Second, we turn to issues about a multidisciplinary process, interagency collaboration and public participation. The equation of methods for assessment and appraisal with procedures (such as profiling of communities, interviewing of stakeholders and key informants, identification of health determinants affected and assessment of evidence) rather than with analytical techniques, arises in large part from the underlying commitment in health impact assessment to the goals of improved interagency collaboration and public participation. Without denying the possible benefits of these, such gains are bought at a very high cost if, in the pursuit of 'inclusiveness' and 'partnership working', the appraisal stage of health impact assessment has to be reduced to the lowest common denominator, analytically speaking.

It is easy to picture something as 'a *multidisciplinary* process *combining* a range of qualitative and quantitative evidence in a decision making framework' (Lock 2000: 1396–8, my italics). The much harder thing is to explain, with any precision and conviction, how the multiple disciplines are to be brought together, as *disciplines* and not just as *people*, and how the qualitative and quantitative evidence are actually to be combined. We argue below that these syntheses of disciplines and integrations of evidence can happen in a coherent and transparent way only at a mode of cognition that is substantially more analytical than most proponents of health impact assessment are willing to contemplate.

Finally, what about the acknowledged current 'lack of agreed methods' – the final point in the list above? This will come as no surprise in view of what we have said above, and Lock admits:

> Those looking for an established analytical framework for considering health impacts will be disappointed. Currently there is neither an accepted gold standard nor even a simple, reliable, and evaluated method for carrying out health impact assessment. Only a few assessments have been completed and these used several approaches . . . Many methodological problems have still to be overcome.
>
> (Lock 2000: 1396–7)

But this lack of agreed methods, where method is defined as something more than a series of procedural steps, is not something that health impact assessment will be able to overcome in time, which is the implication of Lock's use of the word 'currently'. The absence of agreed methods is endemic in the activity as presently conceptualized, but these are, indeed, absolutely essential to the accomplishment of the many benefits it seeks, especially inclusiveness and public participation. There is a clear tension between treating health impact assessment as a single activity and as a useful umbrella label for a heterogeneous collection of activities. This latent tension is amply manifested in the adjoining sentences in the following passage:

> Health impact assessment should be thought of as a group of research activities being developed to identify the health impact of projects and policies both prospectively and retrospectively. It is a structured way of bringing together evaluation, partnership working, public consultation, and available evidence for more explicit decision making.
>
> (Lock 2000: 1396–7)

Paradigms and disciplines

Many of the methodological problems referred to as still to be overcome have, in fact, already been substantially solved elsewhere, notably within the specialist disciplines of epidemiology and decision analysis (in its economic evaluation form). (See Chapter 15 on epidemiology.) It is their solutions that are rejected by leading health impact assessors.

The rejection is partly on simple paradigmatic grounds. In a volume produced jointly by the British Medical Association and Liverpool Public Health Observatory (British Medical Association 1998) the Department of Health (1995b) document, *Policy Appraisal and Health*, is castigated for suggesting that:

> Health Impact Assessments can and should be conducted using techniques some of which are untried, untested, contentious and contested. The guidance which the document provides begs a complex set of conceptual and methodological issues without detailed comment or justification. In particular the following issues of concern need to be addressed: the issue of establishing causality, the use of QALYs to quantify the health effects of policies, attaching monetary values to QALYs . . . [The document] pretends that all aspects of health impacts can be evaluated using one single consolidating monetary measure.
>
> (British Medical Association 1998: 139–41)

Ironically, this dismissal of most of the accomplishments of health economics in relation to policy evaluation precedes a section headed 'Health impact assessment and health economics: scope for interdisciplinary collaboration'! (Chapter 16 discusses health economics and public health; it includes explanation of QALYs.)

But the rejection is not just paradigmatic. It is partly because the disciplines of epidemiology and economics – and indeed *all* true disciplines – are necessarily 'excluding'. Health impact assessment is particularly proud of its flexibility and adaptability and, above all, its inclusiveness. But the reverse side of these virtues is an almost total lack of disciplinary and analytical grounding for the activity. The precise way one integrates evidence from sources of differing credibility (for example, interventional studies and expert opinion) and an originating paradigm (for example, qualitative and quantitative studies) and the precise way one 'takes into account' the views of stakeholders and partners, is not a matter of having the politically correct attitudes and being willing to make sustained efforts to engage with others in a series of workshops and meetings. This lack of foundations is currently masked by a concentration on establishing sets of procedures and guidelines for both carrying out health impact assessments and training others to carry them out, almost as if following the recommended process is itself the product.

It is also masked by repetitively insisting that the exercise is 'multidisciplinary'. Multidisciplinarity of the extent and type called for in health impact assessment, however much of a 'new sound' it may appear to create, is barely distinguishable from non-disciplinarity. The resulting penalty is huge. Rewarding and involving as the process may have been for the people involved, the final product can provide little or no added value to decision makers seeking to arrive at decisions that are analytically coherent as well as transparent and looking for some indication of the direction and magnitude of the differences in health impact between the options under their consideration. So far, the output being offered up to those decision makers from health impact assessments are little more than the public health equivalents of 'motherhood and apple pie'.

The limitations of health impact assessment are perfectly exemplified in a recently published paper (Fleeman and Scott-Samuel 2000). To characterize what is self-reported in this paper as 'a new approach' seems wildly optimistic. What has been done – and in most of the studies carried out under the Merseyside guidelines – is to undertake a largely qualitative literature review plus a series of lengthy interviews with people who are termed 'key stakeholders' and 'key informants'. But the product emerging from this research and consultation is hardly different from what would have been produced in a few hours' reflection on the possible interactions between transport and health, using (as all of us would agree is appropriate) a model of health determinants that is broad, multilevel and extends to 'upstream' socio-economic determinants. Often, as in the large Table 3 of the Fleeman and Scott-Samuel paper, there is not even any suggestion as to the sign (positive or negative) of the impact, let along any indication of the strength. Certainly no attempt is made to aggregate the impacts across the multiple dimensions in the way decision making requires.

The reader will need to consult this and other examples in order to make up their own mind about whether health impact assessment of this sort makes any contribution apart from vaguely 'getting health on the agenda' – something which could surely be achieved with much less effort. It may be that the some decision makers are pleased to be able to point to a largely qualitative and ambiguous health impact assessment as support for what they have decided to do, or will decide to do, on other grounds. But that is hardly what is needed from a societal point of view and certainly not at any public expense.

In view of the harshness of this criticism it is vital to establish that we are not arguing that it is easy to produce analyses of health impact that are not vague and ambiguous, we are simply pointing out that to pursue an activity that is inherently incapable of doing this is of highly questionable worth. There are analytical methods which offer a serious chance of something substantially more, notably the simulation modelling and stochastic cost–effectiveness analysis that are the methodological foundations of decision analysis and (hence) health impact analysis.

The retreat from analysis

In the light of this assessment of health impact assessment, its increasing prominence is very interesting. The retreat from serious analysis involved is captured brilliantly in the contrast between two public documents, the first produced in 1995 (Department of Health 1995), the second by the Health Development Agency in 2002 (Taylor and Blair-Stevens 2002).

Policy Appraisal and Health produced by the Department of Health (1995b) was designed to give practical advice to public sector bodies on how to assess the anticipated impact of their policies on health, and specifically on 'how to incorporate health impacts consistently throughout the public sector into the wider assessment of costs and benefits required for policy development' (p. 1). While showing some signs of being restrained in its commitment to its underlying principles this document was nevertheless a serious attempt to introduce a methodologically sound and discipline-based approach to what we would now call health impact analysis. It has since, regrettably, disappeared without trace (according to the Department of Health search engine), partly, no doubt, because of the hostile reaction from the health impact assessment community.

Compare it with the methodologically ungrounded document, *Introducing Health Impact Assessment*, produced by the Health Development Agency seven years later. Any serious attempt at discipline-based analysis has now disappeared in the desire to ensure that everyone can have their say in whatever way they want, with no concern about the underlying coherence or transparency of the resulting contributions, either singly or jointly. All 'validation' is purely procedural.

> One of the basic principles of [health impact assessment] is that the views of all those affected need to be acknowledged and valued. Much of the value and creativity of the assessment lies in bringing different voices together and creating a 'new sound', with an enhanced understanding of the range of different perspectives about the potential or actual impact of a proposal or area of activity . . . [health impact assessment] should not be viewed as the domain of the expert – all those involved can offer incisive insights and important opinions, experiences and expectations.
>
> (Taylor and Blair-Stevens 2002: 17)

The analytically challenging tasks of accepting and recognizing the existence of different forms of expertise and then tackling their coherent integration are to be avoided in health impact assessment, effectively by pretending that they are not needed. But if health impact assessment is to have any long-term future it needs to be very clear on what it can and what it cannot be. It needs to recognize and accept, rather than decry, activities that seek not to produce a collage or mélange of views, opinions and beliefs from virtually anyone and everyone, but aim to bring together well specified inputs of two simple sorts – assessments of probability and assessments of desirability – in a well specified way. These conceptually distinct assessments should be made by those most competent and most entitled to make them – and these will usually be *different* people.

Unfortunately, once we introduce the 'well specified' requirement and make the basic conceptual distinction between knowledge claims and value judgements, much of the 'social lubrication' provided by vagueness and fuzziness disappears and the relevance of current capacity differences among people (as well as differences in their values and interests) becomes much more transparent. Disciplines are, by definition, arenas of expertise and are necessarily, by their nature, discriminatory and excluding. It is not irrational to trade off the benefits of drawing on disciplinary expertise against the benefits from pursuing other goals (such as inclusiveness), but it *is* irrational to deny that there are opportunity costs involved.

Health impact estimation and health impact analysis

Health impact estimation and health impact analysis are grounded in the disciplines of epidemiology and decision analysis respectively and should not be confused with health impact assessment. They are entitled to reject evaluative judgements that are more reflections of paradigmatic prejudice than of 'level playing field' comparisons. We can note that the BMA volume cited above implies that policy makers can *intuitively* overcome all the issues that health economists have purportedly failed to resolve; that indeed they can do so without 'begging any questions'; and that they can 'add everything up' without measuring anything. This is all simply unacceptable. Health economists and health impact analysts would agree that they haven't solved the big (technical) issues definitively, and probably never will. But the ethics of comparative evaluation requires others to say explicitly and transparently how they have solved or will solve them, not merely implicitly claim that they, or by assumption others, are able to do so.

The cognitive continuum framework

Most of what has been said above reflects an underlying framework in which alternative activities are characterized by the differing balances of intuition and analysis they embody as modes of cognition. Modes of cognition are located on a 'cognitive continuum', a continuum of changing balances between two fundamentally different ways of thinking – the intuitive and the analytical (Hammond 1996; Dowie 2001c). While imposing internal divisions on this continuum is in many respects arbitrary, it is useful to identify six broad ranges (or modes) within it (see Figure 18.1). These

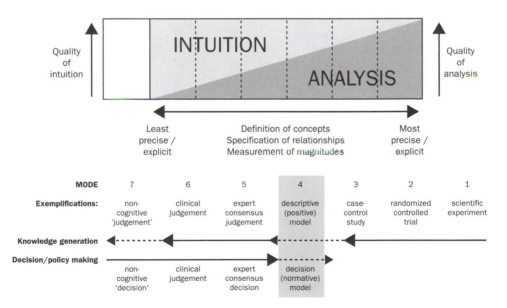

Figure 18.1 The cognitive continuum framework

are numbered from 6 (the most intuitive, least analytical) to 1 (the most analytical, least intuitive) as the analysis to intuition ratio increases, but this is for convenience only and has no other significance.

Most activities involving any cognition *can* be instantiated at alternative modes, though it will instantly be obvious that individuals and groups take very different views as to the validity of some of these instantiations and many wish to impose restrictions on what mode is acceptable or legitimate, depending on the task. For example, many will argue that mode 1, 'science', is the only legitimate way of generating true knowledge, others that 'choice' at mode 6 is the only truly human way of making decisions.

We can now locate two of our three activities by applying this cognitive continuum framework to the fundamentally distinct tasks of knowledge generation and decision making. (The diagram is rotated through 90 degrees for simplicity.)

Health impact estimation emerges as a knowledge generating and evaluating activity located in the more analytical modes 1–3 (see Figure 18.2). It is a quantitative discipline exemplified in risk assessment and attributable risk epidemiology, for example, estimating the number of excess winter deaths or establishing the exposure–response relationships for chemical pollutants. (Occasionally (WHO 2000) the term health impact assessment is used for this activity but this is a very different usage from the dominant one we are concerned with in this paper.) As mode 2/3 epidemiology, health impact estimation therefore employs criteria that are entirely appropriate for science – but not for decision making.

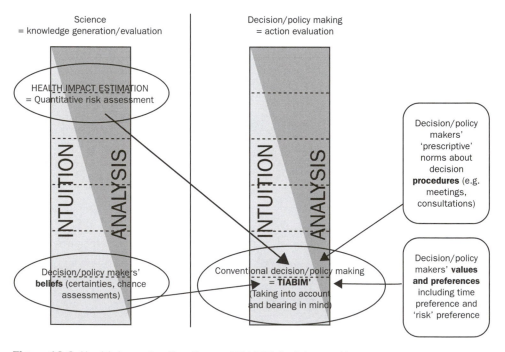

Figure 18.2 Health impact estimation and TIABIM decision making

The more ambitious exercises involved in measuring the global or national burden of disease(s), both in total and as arising from various conditions (such as cancer) and/or risk factors (such as smoking), necessarily involve breaching these scientific standards. While they may therefore be called 'health impact estimation' we take the view that such breaching can only be justified by their production specifically for use in option evaluation. Documenting the size of the problem (the health impact burden estimation) has no necessary implications for the allocation of resources and use of such estimates is likely to lead to divergences from equitably efficient allocation (Williams 1999).

Health impact estimation typically sees itself as feeding into the discursive mode 5, decision-making, process that we are all familiar with and which is here labelled 'taking into account and bearing in mind'.

By comparison, health impact analysis is a decision focused activity, based at mode 4 (see Figure 18.3). It draws on all modes of knowledge generation. In so doing it respects the hierarchy of evidence (as symbolized by the narrowing of the bars) but rejects any science-based cut off for data quality because of its necessary commitment to use the *best available* evidence. Health impact analysis incorporates a mode 4 elicitation of values using techniques such as time trade-off or standard gamble and mode 4 integration of the resulting preferences or 'utilities' with knowledge inputs in order to identify optimal actions. It is a quantitative discipline which involves the modelling of the health components of a decision analysis-based cost–effectiveness approach to non-health sector policy evaluation. It is no more nor less than the application of health economic evaluation principles in non-health

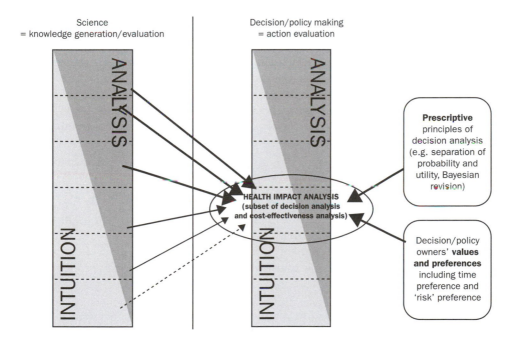

Figure 18.3 Health impact analysis

service contexts in order to establish the health related elements of a decision analysis of the programme, policy or project concerned (Edwards 2001).

Health impact analysis is committed to the explicit identification and processing of the manifold uncertainties in this modelling and in this regard *stochastic* modelling is increasingly replacing *deterministic* modelling (accompanied by restricted sensitivity analyses) as best practice (Briggs *et al.* 2002).

Where is the equivalent diagram for health impact assessment? We are unable to draw one for all the reasons touched on earlier. Different varieties of health impact assessment could be located simultaneously on most modes of the knowledge generation continuum (with a concentration of mode 2–3 and mode 5–6), and on the decision-making continuum at modes 6 and (especially) 5. The two things we can say clearly are that:

- the 'broad church' does not extend to embrace any activity at mode 4 on the decision-making continuum and there is a fairly general distaste for mode 4 modelling activity on the knowledge continuum;

- as a participatory, politically engaged activity it seeks to straddle, or override, the fundamental dividing line between knowledge generation and decision making. The division between these, the respecting of which is central to the activity of health impact estimation (as epidemiology-based knowledge generation) and health impact analysis (as decision focused action evaluation), is lost.

In adopting as its home base the particular balance of intuition and analysis that we refer to as mode 5, health impact assessment does represents a step forward. Its desire to introduce greater clarity and structure produces a significant quality improvement compared both with previous activity *within* that mode and particularly compared with the traditional 'political judgement' process whose home base is at the almost entirely non-analytical mode 6. However, we argue that in relation to the sort of public decisions in which it seeks to play an important role health impact assessment represents no more than a transitional step towards the minimum analytical level necessary to cope with the task in a coherent – and *transparently* coherent – way. That minimum level is that of mode 4, the home base of health impact analysis.

'Robust quantitative health impact assessment'

In order to clinch the difference between health impact assessment, and health impact analysis and health impact estimation it is worth looking briefly at a paper on 'robust quantitative health impact assessment' (Mindell *et al.* 2001). This presents the most formalized and disciplined conceptualization of the activity so far produced and implicitly seeks to distinguish it from the sort of health impact assessment we have concentrated on earlier.

However, as far as 'quantitative health impact assessment' is concerned, it rapidly becomes clear that this is actually only epidemiology-based health impact estimation. Mindell and colleagues write confidently that

First, not everything that can be quantified is important. Second, not everything that is being quantified at present should be, if this cannot be done robustly. Finally not everything that is important can be quantified: rigorous qualitative [health impact assessment] will still be needed for a thorough assessment.

(Mindell *et al.* 2001: 173)

But our framework enables us to see that what they are arguing for is the use of different modes of cognition for different parts of a health impact assessment exercise – and almost all is going to be at mode 5. There is no indication that the authors are willing to address values in anything but a discursive way, in fact there is every indication that they would strongly resist a move to a mode 4 elicitation and processing of values. Moreover, they suggest that while cost–effectiveness analyses of options to mitigate harm or enhance benefits can be useful, there are several difficulties with the economic approach. These difficulties turn out to be much the same as those presented in the British Medical Association volume, which either misrepresent what health economists say and do or (more importantly) imply that tasks that cannot (in their view) be satisfactory tackled analytically – for example, combining diverse impacts into a single metric – can somehow be tackled satisfactorily at modes 5 and 6.

There is no evidence for the implicit assumption that decision makers are competent to deal with such problems and complexities better than an analyst. That is a non-evidence-based *faith* which is universally used to support the mode 5 decision making that is preferred on other grounds. A democracy can clearly choose to act on the basis of non-evidence-based faith. But in terms of public accountability and informed choice it needs to be recognized for what it is and not implied that it has been shown to be 'better' on the basis of the sort of level playing field evaluation required for all technologies other than decision technologies (Dowie 2001a, b).

It is vital not to be distracted by the use of the word 'economic'. What is being attacked here, as in the British Medical Association Merseyside volume, is essentially decision analysis – the systematic *analysis* of decisions in the form of option evaluation. Economic evaluation is simply another label for decision analysis in which costs are considered, as an outcome measure, as well as effects. The integration of multiple effect measures into a single metric has nothing to do with economics and everything to do with the need to arrive at a comprehensive comparative evaluation of competing options, whatever the discipline carrying this out is called.

It is of course no part of the role of the analyst, as analyst, to influence the decision maker's mode of decision making. But the responsible, accountable and indeed ethical decision maker would be well advised not to assume that they are able to outperform the recommendations emerging from a modelling exercise merely because they can point to flaws and limitations in the model. There is considerable evidence that the implicit decision models of human decision makers have flaws and limitations and so the real issue is the *comparative* imperfection of these alternative decision technologies. Failure to recognize and accept this leads to the endemic phenomenon of 'double standards' and the 'nirvana trap' which involve applying standards of perfection to technologies, particularly mode 4 technologies, that one has no intention of applying to oneself (at mode 6) or in collaboration with one's fellow decision makers (at mode 5). While it is socially acceptable and almost mandatory to stress that 'it is essential that the content of [a health impact assessment] is robust, that is, it can withstand critical scrutiny and possible challenge' (Mindell *et al.* 2001: 173), it is much less acceptable to rephrase this in terms of the content of decision makers' assessments.

The problems of living at mode 4 of the continuum

Mode 4 analysts and modellers suffer the perils of 'living in the middle' of the continuum. Historically, the universal desire for certainty has led to the privileging of the two poles of the A–I continuum, that is, mode 1, where we feel we can trust the process of *objective science* to yield the certainty we seek, and mode 6, where we feel we can trust the personal authority of the *individual expert* ('trust me I'm a consultant'). Recently, growing disaffection with and distrust of both these poles has led to greater willingness to move inwards at both ends, to high quality mode 2 research processed by expert groups at mode 5. (Evidence-based is the term now applied to this. See Chapter 14.)

But there is still great reluctance to move further inward to modes 4 and 3 which represent the most equal balancing of analysis and intuition. Why this reluctance? Because in the middle of the continuum one actually maximizes uncertainty by exposing all its sources as completely as possible and insisting that all the uncertainties be dealt with explicitly, transparently and quantitatively, rather than being denied or dealt with implicitly, covertly and qualitatively, as is still substantially the case at mode 5 – even though less so than at mode 6. Equally, at mode 4 one maximizes the extent to which one learns about and is confronted by the existence of *value differences* and *conflicts*. The inefficiencies and inequities arising from the failure to expose and deal with uncertainties and value differences as transparently and coherently as possible, particularly the longer-term ones, represent the price to be paid for the benefits of a discursive, mode 5 process.

Incidentally, those who are rightly concerned with power differentials in decision making would be well advised to note that they are much harder to combat at a transparent mode 4 than in a 'taking into account and bearing in mind' process at mode 5.

Summary

Health impact *analysis* is, like the decision analysis in which it is subsumed, focused on policy/decision making conceptualized as an action analysing/evaluating exercise and not a knowledge generating and evaluation exercise. It produces a model which can, among other things, establish the threshold for the non-health benefits – by definition the prime motivation of the policy/programme/project – necessary to offset any negative health impact. And it can do this using the beliefs and values of different parties to the decision, thereby helping identify and expose the precise location of any conflicts and disagreements.

Health impact *assessment*, as exemplified in the Merseyside approach and guidelines, is a qualitative activity emphasizing the participation and involvement of 'partners' and 'stakeholders' in a discursive process. While taking into account any existing rigorous health impact estimates (defined as those produced by science orientated epidemiology), it joins health impact analysis in recognizing the necessity to use different 'knowledge' standards for decision making than for science. However, it jumps mode 4 to modes 5 and 6, preferring to use key informants as a major sources. In all other respects, including the quantification of values and preferences and their integration with the best available evidence, it explicitly rejects health impact analysis and favours a 'taking into account and bearing in mind' decision practice at mode 5, a mode in which phrases such as 'bringing everything into the equation' and 'giving considerations due weight' are much heard, but no equations or weights are to be seen.

Glossary

The Glossary contains explanations of jargon and abbreviations used in this book and in public health generally. (Refer to the Index to find where terms are used in the text.)

Words in *italics* are also in this list as separate entries.

Advocacy Representing the interests of people who cannot speak up for themselves because of illness, disability or other disadvantage.

Aetiological explanations Explanations of causation, often to be carefully distinguished from associations by epidemiological elimination of bias, chance and confounding.

Agenda 21 A worldwide movement to address environmental concerns for the 21st century, focusing on *sustainable development*. All local authorities are required to develop a local Agenda 21 strategy.

Anti-urbanism A movement that fulfils a desire for people to move from city and town dwelling.

Average/unit cost The total cost of a treatment or programme divided by the total units of production.

Best value It replaced compulsory competitive tendering. It requires all local authority service providers, both internal and external, to justify the efficiency and effectiveness of their services. It aims to ensure that local councils get the best service provider to deliver each local service whether this is the council, voluntary or private sector. It emphasizes quality and service user involvement as well as cost. Councils must carry out best value reviews on all their services.

Boards Governing bodies of many organizations including the *NHS trusts* and *primary care trusts*. A board decides on the overall strategic direction of the organization and ensures that it meets its statutory financial and legal obligations. Boards are usually made up of executive and non-executive directors. The board is answerable for the actions of the organization.

Care Standards Act 2001 Established for the first time a national regulatory body for both the independent and statutory sector. From April 2002 the National Care Standards Commission took over all the present functions of local authorities and health authorities on the registration and regulation of children's homes, independent hospitals, independent clinics, care homes, residential family centres, independent medical agencies, domiciliary care agencies, fostering agencies, childminding, nurses agencies and voluntary adoption agencies. The Act also set up the General Social Care Council to register social care workers, set standards in social care work and regulate the education and training of social care workers.

Care trusts New integrated trusts, formed by merging local authority social care services with NHS primary and *community health services*. The first care trust was launched in 2002 and works under one roof to provide seamless *health and social care services*, particularly for older people.

Case controlled study A research study that compares the characteristics of a group with a specific characteristic such as a disease ('cases') with a comparable group without that characteristic ('controls').

City Challenge A five year Government initiative, now completed, aimed at transforming specific run down inner-city areas and significantly improving the quality of life for local residents within its policy area.

Clinical governance A system for ensuring high quality NHS treatment and care services. It is the framework by which NHS organizations are accountable for continuously improving the quality of their services through a systematic process that is underpinned by a commitment to lifelong learning.

Clinical networks Networks of health professionals for treating patients by sharing information and resources.

Cohort study A research study that examines a whole group over time.

Commission for Health Improvement (CHI) A national body responsible for ensuring good quality services in the NHS. It does this by carrying out inspections.

Commissioning In the context of commissioning health services this means deciding what health services and programmes are needed to improve the health status of the local population and ensuring that they are provided.

Communicable diseases Diseases which can be transmitted from one person to another, often called infectious or contagious diseases.

Community action Activity carried out by people under their own control in order to improve their collective conditions. It may involve campaigning on negotiating with/ challenging authorities and those with power.

Community development Working with people to identify their concerns and support them in collective action for the good of the community as whole.

Community Health Council (CHC) An independent public watchdog which advised the local NHS until it was replaced in 2002 by *Patient Advice and Liaison Services (PALS)* and Patient Forums.

Community health project A programme of work organized by an agency or a local organization with the aim of improving health by some combination of community activity, self-help, *community action* and/or *community development*.

Community health services/community services Health services provided in people's homes or from premises in the community such as GP surgeries, health centres, clinics and small community hospitals (as distinct from services provided in major hospitals).

Community health work This is *community work* with a focus on health concerns, but generally health is defined broadly to include social and economic aspects, so that community health work may encompass almost as broad a range of activities as community work, which does not have a specific health remit.

Community safety partnerships Multiagency partnerships which work to create safer places for people to live and work in. They tackle problems such as anti-social behaviour, domestic violence and crime. They aim to reduce accidents and injuries.

Community strategy The *Local Government Act 2000* requires local authorities to prepare a community strategy to promote the social, economic and environmental well being of their communities. A community strategy should offer a ten year perspective. *Local strategic partnerships* will coordinate the community strategy.

Community work Working with community groups and organizations to overcome the community's problems and improve people's conditions of life. Community work aims to enhance the sense of solidarity and competence in the community.

Confidence interval The range of values above and below a statistic, such as an average or a percentage, within which the real value probably lies. Values outside these limits could have happened by chance. A reduced confidence interval means that we can be more certain that the result did not happen by chance.

Confounders Variables that affect the apparent strength of relationship between a risk factor and a health outcome due to their own relationship with both, for example, smoking confounds the strength of the relationship between exercise and heart disease because it is itself related to both exercise and heart disease. Only by controlling for the effects of confounders can the true relationship be determined.

Consequence Any change in the natural history of an illness or disease brought about by an intervention.

Cost–benefit analysis A type of economic study design that measures both costs and consequences of different interventions in monetary units and computes a net monetary gain/loss or cost/benefit ratio.

Cost–effectiveness analysis A type of economic evaluation study design in which the consequences of different interventions are measured in terms of a unidimensional outcome measure, for example, life years or blood pressure.

Cost minimization analysis A type of economic evaluation study that finds the least costly programme among those shown to be of equal benefit/consequence.

Cost–utility analysis A type of economic evaluation study that compares competing interventions in terms of cost per utility. Utility is an outcome measure comprising quantity and quality of life following an intervention and is usually expressed in quality adjusted life years (QALYs).

Cost/QALY (quality adjusted life years) gained The ratio used in *cost–utility analyses* to make comparisons between competing interventions programmes. The ratio for each intervention is expressed in terms of monetary cost per QALY gained.

Critical appraisal The process of assessing and interpreting evidence by systematically considering its validity, results and relevance to your own work.

Cross-sectoral Working across the boundaries of different sectors, for example, health services working together with businesses and voluntary organizations. Sometimes also called intersectoral.

Decile In describing distribution of a variable (such as income), a decile describes one-tenth of the total population.

Demography The study of the statistics about a population such as birth, death and age profile.

Department for Transport, Local Government and the Regions (DTLR) A government department also responsible for housing, regeneration and elections.

Downstream policy Tackling existing health problems.

Ecological fallacy The error in assuming that factors influencing the different incidences of disease between large populations (such as whole nations) are necessarily the same as those influencing individual variation in disease susceptibility within populations.

Economic evaluation A comparative analysis of two or more alternatives in terms of their costs and consequences.

Effectiveness The extent to which a programme, activity, service or treatment achieves the result it aimed for, for example, the effectiveness of a public health programme would mean the extent to which it had achieved objectives such as specified positive change in the population's health.

Efficiency A term applied to a programme or activity to denote how good the *process* (as distinct from the *outcome*) is in terms of, for example, value for money or use of time; it is about how results are achieved compared with other ways of achieving them.

Epidemiology The study of the distribution, determinants and control of disease in populations.

Evaluation The process of assessing what has been achieved (the *outcome*) and how it has been achieved (the *process*).

Evidence-based Based on reliable evidence that something works. For example, evidence-based health promotion means health promotion projects or programmes based on sound research which shows that they are likely to be successful in achieving their aims.

Gini coefficient An indicator of income inequality in a population. If income is distributed equally, the coefficient is equal to 0 and if a few people hold most of the wealth, the coefficient is closer to 1.

Green Paper A government policy document issued for consultation. Becomes a *White Paper* when it is finalized and formally agreed as government policy.

Health 21 A policy framework published by the World Health Organisation in 1999, which sets out 21 targets for improving health in the European region in the 21st century.

Health Act 1999 It gives powers to health and local authorities, *primary care trusts* and *NHS trusts* to make arrangements to pool funds, have a lead organization commission services and/or provide integrated services. The Act also allows health authorities and *PCTs* to transfer money to local authorities or the *voluntary sector* for any health related local authority function. Local authorities can transfer funds to health authorities and *PCTs* to improve the health of people in their areas.

Health Action Zones (HAZs) Established to provide a framework for the NHS, local authorities and other partners to work together in reducing local health inequalities. HAZs vary in size and type of area they cover. They are areas of high health need selected by the government for special funding and health programmes.

Health and social care services A wide range of services to meet people's health and social needs. Health care tends to mean services provided by the NHS, and social care usually refers to services provided by local authorities, especially social services departments. In many instances, services are provided by both. They may also be provided by the *voluntary sector*.

Health Authority The statutory NHS organization responsible for health services for a defined population until it was abolished in 2002, when its responsibilities were largely taken on (in England) by *primary care trusts* and *care trusts*.

Health Development Agency National public body established in 2000 as a resource for public health work in England. Its remit includes maintaining a database of research evidence about what works to improve health and providing information about the effectiveness of health improvement programmes. There are comparable bodies in Scotland (the Health Education Board for Scotland), Wales (the Health Promotion Division of the National Assembly for Wales) and Northern Ireland (the Health Promotion Agency for Northern Ireland).

Health education Planned opportunities for people to learn about health and to undertake voluntary changes in their behaviour.

Health For All A movement started in the 1980s by the World Health Organisation. It included *health targets* for year 2000 and stressed basic principles of promoting positive health through health promotion and disease prevention; reducing inequalities in health; community participation; cooperation between health authorities, local authorities and others with an impact on health; and a focus on *primary care* as the main basis of the health care system.

Health gain A measurable improvement in health status in an individual or population attributable to earlier intervention.

Health gap The difference between the overall health of the better off and the more deprived communities in a population.

Health impact assessment Systematic process to estimate the effects of a specified action – a programme, policy or project – on the health of a defined population, for example, what difference a new transport policy would have on the health of the population affected by it.

Health Improvement and Modernization Plan (HIMP) A three year local rolling plan of action to improve health and services for health and social care, led by local NHS organizations such as *primary care trusts*. (Formerly known as the health improvement programme.)

Health inequalities The gap between the health of different population groups. People who are better off have better health and are less likely to die under the age of 75 from all the main diseases that kill. Improving the health and life expectancy of the less well off to reduce this gap is a priority of the *NHS National Plan*.

Health promotion The process of enabling people to increase control over, and to improve, their health.

Health related behaviour What people habitually do in their daily life which affects their health. Usually refers to issues such as whether they smoke, whether they take exercise, what they eat, their sexual behaviour, how much alcohol they drink and whether they use drugs. Sometimes simply called 'health behaviour'.

Health target A quantified, measurable improvement in health status, by a given date, which achieves a health objective. It provides a yardstick against which progress can be monitored.

Healthy Cities A WHO initiative started in 1987 to improve health in urban areas. Involves collaborative work between local government, health services, local businesses, community organizations and citizens. The Health for All (UK) Network is the coordinating body for action on Healthy Cities within the UK.

Healthy Living Centres Centres or networks of activity which aim to promote good health, developed by partnerships with local participation. Funded from the National Lottery. Healthy Living Centres are more people centred than resource centred and are based on programmes of activities which can be held in existing premises. Examples are health and fitness screening in pubs and betting shops, health promotion in schools, linking the arts and health, and fitness for people with chronic conditions.

Healthy Universities A WHO initiative to promote health in university settings.

High risk approach A public health approach which prioritizes people who are particularly at risk of ill health (compare with the *whole population approach*).

Holistic In the health context (as in 'holistic approach to health') this means taking into account all aspects of a person – physical, mental, emotional and social – as well as their social, economic and physical environment. (As distinct from an approach which only focuses on, for example, the physical functioning of the body.)

Impact A term sometimes used to describe short-term *outcomes*, for example, the impact of a programme to encourage women to attend a breast cancer screening test (mammogram) might be assessed in terms of how many women attended; the long-term outcome could be a change in the rate of women who died of breast cancer.

Incidence The number of new episodes of illness arising in a population over a specified period of time.

Index of Deprivation (IOD) It ranks districts to show relative deprivation. It uses 12 indicators of deprivation, covering such things as income, housing, education, environment, crime and health, and measures how much a district is above or below the national average. The individual scores are then added together to produce an overall 'deprivation' score for each district.

Indirect costs Productivity losses (decreases in the output of the economy) that occur as a result of health care interventions, for example, a person will need to take time from work to attend hospital for an operation.

Infrastructure All the things and systems that are not directly involved in providing a service, but which have to be there for services to operate efficiently or consistently, like management and administration, or communications and distribution networks. In the voluntary sector, the word is often used to describe organizations, like local development agencies and umbrella groups, which help other *voluntary organizations* work better by providing them with things like information, advice, training, coordination and representation.

Input The resources that go into a programme or activity including money, time, staff and materials.

Lay members Members of the public who sit on the boards of public bodies such as NHS and *primary care trusts*. They are sometimes called non-executive directors. They are involved with the overall strategic direction of an organization rather than the day to day administration, which is done by paid staff. They are usually part-time. NHS lay members are usually recommended by the NHS locally from a regional register of potential members. The Secretary of State for Health makes the final decision. *Primary care trusts* also have lay representatives who can also be called lay members. The job of these lay representatives is to ensure the views of local people are taken into account and to help develop public participation.

Local Government Act 1999 It introduced *Best Value* and placed a duty on councils to improve their services continuously, and replaced the previous Conservative government's compulsory competitive tendering regime.

Local Government Act 2000 It requires all local authorities to introduce new ways of making decisions. All local authorities are required to choose between three different decision-making models, all of which involve separating powers between a decision-making function and a scrutinizing one. The three models are: directly elected mayor with cabinet, cabinet with leader and directly elected mayor with a council manager.

Local Public Service Agreement Agreements between individual local authorities and the government, setting out the authority's commitment to deliver specific improvements in performance, and the government's commitment to reward these improvements. The agreement also records what the government will do to help the authority achieve the improved performance. (see, http://www.local-regions.odpm.gov.uk/lpsa/index.htm).

Local Strategic Partnership (LSP) NHS, local authority and other agencies working together to develop and implement local strategies for *neighbourhood renewal.*

Modernization Agency Set up in the *NHS National Plan* to support local NHS clinicians and managers redesign services to make them more patient friendly, quicker and efficient, and to secure continuous service improvements across the NHS. It is responsible for the NHS leadership centre and the NHS beacon services programme.

Morbidity/morbidity rate Illness/incidence of illness in a population in a given period.

Mortality/mortality rate Death/incidence of death in a population in a given period.

Multidisciplinary Involving people from different professions (disciplines) and backgrounds.

Multivariate techniques Analytical and statistical methods that examine simultaneously the influence of many variables together on an outcome.

National Health Service and Community Care Act 1990 It gave local authorities the lead responsibility for the social care of older people and disabled people (including people with learning difficulties and mental health problems). It also acknowledged the role of carers.

National Health Service and Social Care Act 2001 It enables new integrated *care trusts* to be created, with health and social services working under one roof. It also made the NHS responsible for paying for nursing care in nursing homes but not personal care. It included proposals for major investment in GP surgeries; incentives to improve NHS performance; a new contract for GPs; and extending the scope of the direct payments scheme for disabled people. It also said that *patients' forums* and *patient advice and liaison services* would be set up in every *NHS trust.* It established local authority overview and scrutiny committees to monitor the NHS locally.

National Institute for Clinical Excellence (NICE) National body which provides patients, health professionals and the public with authoritative, robust and reliable guidance on 'best practice' in relation to drugs, treatments and services across the NHS.

National Service Framework National document which sets out the pattern and level of service (standards) which should be provided for a major care area or disease group such as mental health or heart disease.

National strategies for health Government strategies to improve the health of national populations. Strategies current in 2002:

- Northern Ireland: *Health and Wellbeing: Into the Millennium*
- England: *Saving Lives: Our Healthier Nation*
- Scotland: *Towards a Healthier Scotland*
- Wales: *Improving Health in Wales: A Summary Plan for the NHS with its Partners* and an action plan *Promoting Health and Wellbeing: Implementing the National Health Promotion Strategy.*

Neighbourhood management programme A way of encouraging stakeholders to work with service providers to help improve the quality of services delivered in deprived neighbourhoods.

Neighbourhood Renewal Community Chests A total of £50 million central government money in England over three years 2001–04 for small grants to community groups.

Neighbourhood Renewal Fund Provides public services and communities in the 88 poorest local authority districts with extra funds to tackle deprivation. The original £900 million pot has been extended for a further three years and has been increased by a further £975 million.

Neighbourhood Renewal Strategy Strategy developed by local agencies with a coordinated approach to tackle the social and economic conditions in the most deprived local authority areas.

Neighbourhood Support Fund Government grants of £10,000 upwards to community groups to enable them to re-engage disaffected young people.

Network A group of people who exchange information, contacts and experience for mutual benefit.

New Deal for Communities Government funding for deprived communities to support plans that bring together local people, community and voluntary organizations, public agencies and local business in an attempt to make improvements in health, employment, education and the physical environment.

New Public Health An approach to public health which emerged in the 1980s. It shifted emphasis from a lifestyle approach focused on people's individual health behaviour to a new focus on political and social action to address underlying issues which affect health such as poverty, employment, discrimination and the environment people live in.

New Deal for Regeneration It provides money through the *regional development agencies* to regenerate urban areas in England. Bids should be from partnerships of local authorities, learning and skills councils, other public bodies, the private sector, the *voluntary sector* and local communities. Another strand of this is the *New Deal for Communities* which operates in areas with the highest levels of disadvantage and aims to tackle *social exclusion*.

New NHS: Modern Dependable A government's *White Paper* published in December 1997 which outlined the government's plans for modernizing the NHS. It introduced *primary care groups* and health improvement programmes and announced the end of fund holding.

NHS Direct A national NHS telephone help line staffed by specially trained nurses.

NHS Reform and Health Care Professions A bill that was published in November 2001. The functions and commissioning budgets of health authorities were transferred to *primary care trusts*. It established the Commission for Patient and Public Involvement in Health which will encourage the public to get more involved with their local health trusts.

NHS National Plan It was published in July 2000, and is the government's strategy for reforming and modernizing the NHS over ten years. The plan says that the NHS has to be redesigned around the needs of the patient with fast, convenient care delivered to a consistently high standard. It acknowledges that the NHS cannot tackle health inequalities alone and calls for a new partnership between health and local government. Local government will be given power to scrutinize the NHS locally and *best value* will be extended to health.

NHS trust An independent body within the NHS which provides health services in hospitals. Some NHS trusts provide specialized services such as ambulance services or mental health services.

Nominal variable A variable composed of categories with qualitatively different values, for example, occupation or gender.

Non-governmental organization (NGO) An organization which is independent of government control.

Non-statutory sector Anybody who is not part of the statutory sector. This includes voluntary and community organizations, private sector organizations, service users and carers.

Null hypothesis The hypothesis that no association exists between two variables or no difference exists between two groups. Conventional statistics only test the probability that the observed data are consistent with the Null hypothesis.

Opportunity costs Potential benefits which will not be realized if one thing is done instead of another. For example, if there is only enough time and money for one health programme, A or B, and it is spent on A, the opportunity costs are the potential benefits of spending on B which will be foregone or sacrificed.

Ordinal A variable composed of categories with quantitatively ordered values, for example, council tax bands.

OECD Organization for Economic Cooperation and Development. This numbers 30 member nations including Australia, Canada, Germany, Japan, Spain, the UK and the USA.

Ottawa Charter A document launched in 1986 at an international World Health Organisation conference in Ottawa, Canada, which identified key themes for health promotion practice.

Our Healthier Nation A government *Green Paper* published in 1998. It was the first government health strategy document in recent years to acknowledge the link between poverty and ill health and the need to do something about the social causes of ill health. Key aims were to improve the health of the population as a whole, to improve the health of the worst off and to narrow the health gap. It introduced health improvement (now *health improvement and modernization*) programmes and the idea of local authorities having a new duty to promote economic, social and environmental well being in their areas.

Outcome The end product of a health programme or activity, expressed in whatever terms are appropriate, for example, changes in people's attitudes or knowledge, changes in health policy, changes in the uptake of services or changes in the rate of illness.

Partnership Different organizations such as social services, health and the *voluntary sector* working together to achieve a common aim. The partnership ideal is one of independent and equal partners who work closely within a common framework. Partnership is a key word for New Labour. All their policies stress the importance of departments and sectors working together to provide better and more seamless services.

Partnership boards/forums There is a partnership board/forum in each of the local authority areas. They have wide representation with representatives from local authority (a range of departments) *primary care organizations* and *NHS trusts*, as well as the *voluntary sector*, service users and carers. Partnership boards aim to work together to develop a joint understanding of the needs within each area and to plan services from different agencies.

Patient advice and liaison services (PALS) Established from April 2002 within NHS trusts to help patients, families and carers to resolve problems or air concerns. They, together with patient forums, replaced *community health councils*.

Patients' forums Independent statutory bodies being established within every *NHS and primary care trust* to provide direct input from patients into how local NHS services are run. They will be expected to find out what patients and their carers think about the services they use. They will also monitor the quality of local services from the patient perspective and to work with the local NHS trust to bring about improvements.

Performance management Systematic management practices and monitoring systems which monitor and support people so that they can achieve their work objectives.

Policy A broad statement of the principles of how to proceed in relation to a specific issue, such as a national policy on transport, a local authority policy on housing or a policy on how to deal with alcohol issues in a workplace.

Pooled budgets The *Health Act 1999* enabled *health authorities, primary care trusts*, and local authorities to pool budgets. This means that they can each agree to put in funding to be used to meet the needs of a specific group of people, for example, people with learning difficulties. Once the money is pooled it loses its identity as health or social services so that the expenditure will be based on the needs of the people who use the services and not on the level of contribution of each partner. Each partner still has statutory responsibility for functions carried out using the pooled fund.

Primary care organization A term used to describe *care trusts, primary care groups* and *primary care trusts*. Since 1997 there have been different initiatives in England, Northern Ireland, Scotland and Wales. In England the development of primary care has been focused on *primary care groups* and *trusts* who have gradually taken on the majority of health care services and public health functions. In Northern Ireland health boards currently retain most commissioning and public health functions although there are proposals to develop English type *primary care trusts*. In Scotland non-commissioning *primary care trusts* have been developed with health boards retaining commissioning and strategic public health roles. In Wales there are local health groups that have a wider *voluntary sector* and local authority representation than in England with the Welsh Assembly playing a strong strategic public health role.

Prevalence Measure of how much illness there is in a population at a particular point in time or over a specified period of time.

Primary care Services which are people's first point of contact with the NHS, for example, services provided by GPs, practice nurses, district nurses, health visitors, opticians, dentists and pharmacists (as distinct from *secondary care* provided in hospitals).

Primary care group (PCG) An NHS body which was first set up around 1999, formed from groups of GP practices in a locality. In the early 2000s primary care groups became *primary care trusts* and were given more responsibilities.

Primary care trust (PCT) An NHS body whose main tasks are to assess local health needs, develop and implement *health improvement and modernization plans*, provide *primary care* services and commission *secondary care* services from hospitals and specialized services run by *NHS trusts*.

Primary health care team Health workers usually based at a GP surgery or health centre who together provide local *community health services*. They include GPs, district nurses, practice nurses and health visitors.

Primary prevention Stopping ill health arising in the first place. For example, eating a healthy diet, not smoking and taking enough exercise are factors in the primary prevention of heart disease.

Process All the implementation stages of a health programme or activity which happen between *input* and *outcome*.

Proximal mechanisms Pathways of influence that most immediately lead to the *outcome*. Poor diet may be the proximal effect on the health of low income families.

Public health Preventing disease, prolonging life and promoting health through work focused on the population as a whole.

Public sector A collective term for organizations which are controlled by the state and are publicly funded, such as the NHS, local authorities, and the police, fire, probation and prison services. Often also called statutory sector/services because they are governed by laws (statutes).

Qualitative Concerned with quality – how good or bad something is according to specified criteria, usually expressed as a description in words rather than numbers. For example, qualitative data about the outcome of a breast screening programme could include users' descriptions of how they felt about it: whether they found it painful, embarrassing, well organized, etc. (Compare with *quantitative*.)

Quality How 'good' something (such as health service) is when judged against a number of criteria.

Quality Protects Services for children in need, including vulnerable children in local authority care.

Quality standard An agreed level of performance negotiated within available resources.

Quantitative Concerned with measurable quantity, usually expressed in numbers. For example, quantitative data about the outcome of a breast screening programme could include the percentage of the women invited who actually attended, the percentage called back for further assessment and (ultimately) the decrease in rates of illness and death from breast cancer. (Compare with *qualitative*.)

Randomized controlled trial (RCT) An experimental method whereby subjects are allocated randomly between an experimental group which receives an intervention and a control group which does not, so that the two groups can be fairly compared to see the effect of the intervention.

Recall bias A bias affected by differences in obtaining accurate information on historical events or exposures between groups of subjects with different characteristics, irrespective of their true exposures. For example, women experiencing a miscarriage are more likely to remember and report specific events early in their pregnancy than those who had uneventful pregnancies.

Regeneration The revitalization and renewal of deprived areas, often inner-city urban areas. It involves reviving local economies and communities and improving services. It is about improving the quality of life and promoting equality of opportunity for all communities. It involves tackling *social exclusion*, unemployment and training.

Regional Development Agencies (RDAs) The government has established regional development agencies to promote sustainable economic development and social and physical regeneration, and to coordinate the work of regional and local partners in areas such as training, investment, regeneration and business support. Regional development agencies are quangos. They each have a board which is mainly made up of business people and four local authority members. A high priority for regional development agencies will be the development of regional strategies, to improve economic performance and enhance their region's competitiveness and to provide a framework for regional economic decision taking.

Saving Lives: Our Healthier Nation a *national strategy for health* in England published in 1999, which sets out priority areas (cancer, heart disease and strokes, accidents and mental health) and sets national targets.

Screening The application of a special test for everyone at risk of a particular disease to detect whether the disease is present at an early stage. It is used for diseases where early detection makes treatment more successful.

Secondary care Specialized health care services provided by hospital inpatient and outpatient services.

Secondary prevention Intervention during the early stages of a disease so that further damage can be prevented.

Selection bias A bias effected in a sample by systematically choosing certain subject types in preference to others. For example, selecting a sample of persons from a football crowd is unlikely to give you a study group representative of the whole population.

Service user An individual who uses health or local authority services. They may also be referred to as a client, patient or consumer.

Single Regeneration Budget A major source of government funding since 1994. The funding concentrates on specific local areas, usually with high levels of deprivation. It aims to help them improve by developing more economic and social activities. It is linked to job creation, training opportunities and partnerships between the statutory, private and *voluntary sectors*. It brought *City Challenge* and a number of other urban funding programmes into a single budget. It is distributed annually by the Department of the Environment who choose the most successful bids across a large region.

Social capital Investment in the social fabric of society to encourage communities to develop high levels of trust and supportive networks for the exchange of information, ideas and practical help.

Social inclusion/exclusion A sense of belonging to/feeling alienated from the community in which a person lives.

Stages of change A cycle of stages a person usually goes through when they change a health related behaviour such as when they stop smoking. Stages are: (1) not yet thinking about it; (2) thinking about changing; (3) being ready to change; (4) action – making changes; (5) maintaining change; then either maintaining the changed behaviour permanently; or (6) relapsing – often then repeating the cycle by thinking about changing again (2).

Standard gamble A method of eliciting from individuals values for health states. Respondents are asked to make a choice between the certainty of living in a health state below full health (the health state to be valued) and a gamble involving the possibility of full health and the risk of death.

Standardized mortality ratio A way of comparing death rates in which allowances have been made for the different age structures of populations. This means that fair comparisons can be made between populations with, for example, different proportions of children or older people.

Statutory organizations/agencies *Public sector* organizations or agencies such as local authorities and NHS organizations.

Statutory sector Another term for the *public sector*.

Strategy A broad plan of action that specifies what is to be achieved, how and by when; it provides a framework for more detailed planning.

Strategic Health Authority From 2002, 30 new strategic health authorities replaced the 95 *health authorities* in England. They aim to be a bridge between the Department of Health and local NHS services and to provide strategic leadership to ensure the delivery of improvements in health, well being and health services locally.

Sure Start Part of the government's drive to eradicate child poverty in 20 years and to halve it by 2010. It aims to improve the health and well being of families and children from birth so they can flourish when they go to school. Government schemes are targeted in areas of high health need and aim to support parents and children under the age of 4. This initiative is aimed at improving services for expectant parents and for children aged 0–3 in deprived areas. It is a partnership of local parents and *statutory* and *voluntary organizations*. It aims to promote the physical, intellectual and social development of babies and young children breaking the cycle of disadvantage.

Sustainable development Development which meets the needs of the present without damaging the health or environment of future generations.

Target group The people who are intended to benefit from a public health or health promotion activity.

Targets Quantified and measurable achievements for which to aim by specified dates, which provide yardsticks against which progress can be monitored. (See also *health target*.)

Tertiary care services Very specialized NHS services which cannot be provided within every health authority area, for example, a unit for treating eating disorders or specialist cancer clinic. Access is through GPs or local hospital consultants.

Third sector *Voluntary organizations*, community groups and other non-profit organizations are sometimes called the third sector because they are not part of the public or private sector. The phrase is sometimes used instead of the *voluntary sector* because people think 'voluntary sector' is misleading as it implies that the sector is only about volunteers.

Time trade-off A method of eliciting health state values from individuals. Respondents are asked to rate periods of time in various health states in terms of years of full health.

Trilateralism The interconnections between Europe, North America and East Asia which accounts for 85 percent of world trade. Connected terms are regionalization and triadization.

Upstream policy Tackling the fundamental causes of ill health through national, social and economic policy thus preventing many problems.

Urbanization Movement of people to live in cities and towns.

User involvement People who use services are involved in making decisions about, and planning those services. *Service users* could be asked for their views on a particular subject or may join a working group which decides how a service will develop.

Voluntary organizations Not-for-profit organizations, ranging from large national organizations to small groups of local people, run by volunteers but possibly employing paid staff. Small local voluntary organizations are often called community groups.

Voluntary sector A collective term for *voluntary organizations*, community groups and charities.

White Paper Government policy, often accompanied by legislation. Usually follows a *Green Paper*.

Whole population approach Public health approach which focuses on a whole community rather than individuals who are identified as being in particular need. (Compare with *high risk approach*.)

World Health Organisation (WHO) An intergovernmental organization within the United Nations system whose purpose is to help all people attain the highest possible level of health through public health programmes. Its headquarters are in Geneva, Switzerland.

Note

Website glossaries and other sources used: http://www.thecareforum.org.uk;
http://www.neighbourhood.gov.uk/glossary.asp?pageid=10#n; Ewles and Simnett (2003).

References

Abbott, S., Florin, D., Fulop, N. and Gillam, S. (2001) *Primary Care Groups and Trusts: Improving Health.* London: King's Fund.

Acheson, D. (1988) *Public Health in England. Report of the Committee of Inquiry into the Future of the Public Health Function,* Cm289. London: HMSO.

Acheson, D. (1998) *Independent Inquiry into Inequalities in Health.* London: The Stationery Office.

Active Community Unit (ACU) (2001) *Funding Community Groups – A Consultation Document Issued by ACU on Behalf of the Inter-Departmental Working Group on Resourcing Community Capacity Building.* London: ACU, Home Office.

Ahmad, Y. and Broussine, M. (2003 forthcoming) The public sector modernisation agenda – reconciliation or renewal? *Public Management Review.*

Allen, T. (2000) Housing Renewal – doesn't it make you sick? *Housing Studies,* 15(3):443–63.

Allen, P. (2001) Health promotion, environmental health and local authorities, in A. Scriven and J. Orme (eds) *Health Promotion: Professional Perspectives.* Basingstoke: Palgrave.

Altmann, D.G. (2001) Systematic reviews of evaluations of prognostic variables, in M. Egger, G. Davey Smith and D.G. Altmann (eds) *Systematic Reviews in Health Care: Metanalysis in Context.* London: BMJ Books.

Andersen, H. and Munck, R. (1999) *Neighbourhood Images in Liverpool.* JRF Area Regeneration Series. York: York Publishing Services.

Annandale, E. (1998) *The Sociology of Health and Medicine: A Critical Introduction.* Cambridge: Polity Press.

Arblaster, L., Entwistle, V., Lambert, M. *et al.* (1995) *Review of the Research on the Effectiveness of Health Service Interventions to Reduce Variations in Health,* CRD Report 3. York: NHS Centre for Reviews and Dissemination, The University of York.

Arblaster, L., Lambert, M., Entwistle, V. *et al.* (1996) A systematic review of the effectiveness of health service interventions aimed at reducing inequalities in health, *Journal of Health Services Research and Policy,* 1(2): 93–103.

Argyle, M. (1989) *The Psychology of Happiness.* London: Routledge.

Argyle, M. (1996a) The effects of relationships on well-being, in N. Baker (ed) *Building a Relational Society: New Priorities for Public Policy.* Aldershot: Arena.

Argyle, M. (1996b) *The Social Psychology of Leisure.* Harmondsworth: Penguin.

Ashby, D. and Smith, A.F. (2000) Evidence-based medicine in Bayesian decision-making, *Statistics in Medicine,* 19: 3291–305.

Ashton, J. (1992) The origin of healthy cities, in J. Ashton (ed.) *Healthy Cities*. Milton Keynes: Open University Press.

Ashton, J.R. (2000) Public health observatories – the key to timely public health intelligence in the new century, *Journal of Epidemiology and Community Health*, 54: 724–5.

Ashton, J. and Seymour, H. (1988) *The New Public Health*. Buckingham: Open University Press.

Aspinall, J. (1999) Ethnic groups and our healthier nation: whither the information base? *Journal of Public Health Medicine*, 21: 125–32.

Atherton, G. and Hashagen, S. with Chanan, G., Garratt, C. and West, A. (2003) *Including Local People in Community Planning in Scotland*. London: Community Development Foundation.

Atkinson, R. (1999) Discourses of partnership and empowerment in contemporary British urban policy, *Urban Studies*, 36(1): 59–77.

Audit Commission (1998) *A Fruitful Partnership: Effective Partnership Working*. London: Audit Commission.

Audit Commission (2002) *Neighbourhood Renewal: Policy Focus*. London: Audit Commission.

Bachrach, P. and Baratz, M.S. (1970) *Power and Poverty*. New York: Oxford University Press.

Baggot, R. (2000) *Public Health: Policy and Politics*. Basingstoke: Macmillan Press.

Ball, R., Heafey, M. and King, D. (2001) Private finance initiative – a good deal for the public or a drain on future generations? *Policy and Politics*, 29(1): 95–108.

Barker, D.P. (1998) *Mothers, Babies and Health in Late Life*. Edinburgh: Churchill Livingstone.

Barnes, M. (1997) *Care Communities and Citizens*. London: Longman.

Barnes, M. (1999) Users as citizens: collective action and the local governance of welfare, *Social Policy and Administration*, March, 33(1): 73–90.

Barnes, M. and Sullivan, H. (2002) Building capacity for collaboration in English health action zones, in C. Glendinning, M. Powell and K. Rummery (eds) *Partnerships, New Labour and the Governance of Welfare*. Bristol: Policy Press.

Barnes, M., Harrison, S., Mort, M. and Shardlow, P. (1999) *Unequal Partners: User Groups and Community Care*. Bristol: Policy Press.

Barnes, M., Matka, E. and Sullivan, H. (2003 forthcoming) *Evaluation*.

Barr, A. (2002) *Learning Evaluation and Planning*. London: Community Development Foundation.

Barr, A. and Hashagen, S. (2000) *Achieving Better Community Development*. London: Community Development Foundation.

Barr, A., Hamilton, R. and Purcell, R. (1996) *Learning for Change*. London: Community Development Foundation.

Bartley, M., Blane, D. and Montgomery, S. (1997) Health and the lifecourse: why safety nets matter, *British Medical Journal*, 314: 1194–6.

Bauld, L., Mackinnon, J. and Judge, K. (2001a) *Community Health Initiatives: Recent Policy Developments and the Emerging Evidence Base*. Glasgow: University of Glasgow.

Bauld, L., Judge, K., Lawson, L. *et al.* (2001b) *Health Action Zones in Transition: Progress in 2000*. Glasgow: University of Glasgow.

Baum, F. (2000) Social capital, economic capital and power: further issues for a public health agenda, *Journal of Epidemiology and Community Health*, 53: 195–6.

Baum, F. (2001) Health, equity, justice and globalisation: some lessons from the People's Health Assembly, *Journal of Epidemiology and Community Health*, 55: 613–16.

Beaglehole, R. and Bonita, R. (1997) *Public Health at the Crossroads*. Cambridge: Cambridge University Press.

Beattie, A. (1991) *Success and Failure in Community Development Initiatives in National Health Service Settings: Eight Case Studies*. Milton Keynes: Open University Press.

Beck, U. (1992) *Risk Society: Towards a New Modernity*. London: Sage.

Beck, U. (1999) *World Risk Society*. Boston, MA: Blackwell.

Beck, U. (2000a) *What is Globalisation?* Cambridge: Polity Press.

Beck, U. (2000b) *The Brave New World of Work*. Cambridge: Polity Press.

Beecham, J. (2000) *Unit Costs not Exactly Child's Play: A Guide to Estimating Unit Costs for Children's Social Care*. London: Department of Health.

Bennett, P. and Calman, K. (eds) (1999) *Risk Communication and Public Health*. Oxford: Oxford University Press.

Bennis, W. (1988) *On Becoming a Leader*. New York: Addison-Wesley.

Ben-Shlomo, Y. and Chaturvedi, N. (1995) Assessing equity in access to health care provision in the UK: does where you live affect your chances of getting a coronary artery bypass graft? *Journal of Epidemiology and Community Health*, 49: 200–4.

Ben-Schlomo, Y. and Kuh, D. (2002) A life course approach to chronic disease epidemiology: conceptual models, empirical challenges and interdisciplinary perspectives, *International Journal of Epidemiology*, 31: 285–93.

Ben-Shlomo, Y., White, I.R. and Marmot, M. (1996) Does the variation in the socio-economic characteristics of an area affect mortality? *British Medical Journal*, 312: 1013–14.

Bentham, J. (1834) *Deontology: Or, the Science of Morality*, J. Bowring (ed.), 2 volumes. London: Longman.

Benzeval, M., Judge, K. and Whitehead, M. (eds.) (1995) *Tackling Inequalities in Health: An Agenda for Action*. London: King's Fund.

Benzeval, M., Taylor, J. and Judge, K. (2000) Evidence on the relationship between low income and poor health: is the government doing enough? *Fiscal Studies*, 21(3): 375–99.

Beresford, P. (2001) Service users, social policy and the future of welfare, *Critical Social Policy*, 21(4): 494–512.

Beresford, P. and Croft, S. (1993) *Citizen Involvement*. Basingstoke: Macmillan.

Beresford, P. and Trevillion, S. (1995) *Developing Skills for Community Care: A Collaborative Approach*. Aldershot: Arena.

Bergrund, L. (1994) Eco-balancing: A Göteborg Example, in UNCED, *Agenda 21, Report to the Manchester Conference*, pp. 199–59.

Bergson, A. (1938) A reformulation of certain aspects of welfare economics, *Quarterly Journal of Economics*, 98: 371–400.

Berridge, V. (1999) *Health and Society in Britain Since 1939*. Cambridge: Cambridge University Press.

Bettcher, D.W. and Wipfli, H. (2001) Towards a more sustainable globalisation: the role of the public health community, *Journal of Epidemiology and Community Health*, 55: 617–18.

Beveridge, W. (1942) *The Beveridge Report*, CMND 6404. London: HMSO.

Biles, A., Mornement, A. and Palmer, H. (2001) From the ballot box to the real world, *Regeneration and Renewal*, 8 June, pp. 14–15.

Blackstone, T. and Plowden, W. (1988) *Inside the Think Tank*. London: Heinemann.

Blair, T. (1996) *New Britain: My Vision of a Young Country*. London: Fourth Estate.

Blair, T. (1998a) *Leading the Way: A New Vision for Local Government*. London: Institute for Public Policy Research.

Blair, T. (1998b), *Compact on Relations between Government and the Voluntary and Community Sector in England*, Cm 4100. London: HMSO.

Blair, T. (2002) *The Courage of our Convictions: Why Reform of the Public Services is the Route to Social Justice*. London: Fabian Society.

Blamey, A., Hanlon, P., Judge, K. and Murie, J. (eds) (2002) *Health Inequalities in the New Scotland*. Glasgow: Public Health Institute Scotland.

Bland, M. (2001) *Cluster Designs: A Personal View*. Talk given on 11 October 2001 at The Contributions of Statistics to Public Health meeting at the Public Health Laboratory Service Communicable Disease Centre, Colindale, London. www.sghms.ac.uk/depts/phs/staff/jmb/clustalk.htm (accessed 1 January 2003).

Bland, J.M. and Altmann, D.G. (1998) Bayesians and frequentists, *British Medical Journal*, 317: 1151.

Blane, D., Brunner, E. and Wilkinson, R. (eds) (1996) *Health and Social Organization: Towards a Health Policy for the 21st Century*. London: Routledge.

Blaxter, M. (1990) *Health and Lifestyles*. London: Routledge.

Blaxter, M. (1995) *Consumers and Research in the NHS: Consumer Issues within the NHS*. London: Department of Health.

Blaxter, M. and Poland, F. (2002) Moving beyond the survey in exploring social capital, in C. Swann and A. Morgan (eds) *Social Capital for Health: Insights from Qualitative Research*. London: Health Development Agency.

Blears, H. (2002) *The Challenges Facing Public Health*. Speech by Hazel Blears, Minister for Public Health. Annual Scientific Conference of Faculty of Public Health Medicine, 27 June. London: Department of Health.

Book, G.R. and Whelan, J. (eds) (1991) *The Childhood Environment and Adult Disease*, CIBA Foundation Symposium 156. Chichester: John Wiley and Sons.

Booth, C. (1902) *Life and Labour of the People in London*. London: Macmillan.

Bourdieu, P. (1993) *Sociology in Question*. London: Sage.

Bovaird, T. and Halachmi, A. (2001) Learning from international approaches to best value, *Policy and Politics*, 29(4): 451–63.

Bowling, A. (2001) *Measuring Disease*, 2nd edn. Buckingham: Open University Press.

Boyd Orr, J. (1936) *Food, Health and Income*. London: Macmillan.

Braveman, P. and Tarimo, E. (2002) Social inequalities in health within countries: not only an issue for affluent nations, *Social Science and Medicine*, 54: 1621–35.

Brenton, M. (1985) *The Voluntary Sector in British Social Services*. London: Longman.

Briggs, A.H., O'Brien, B.J. and Blackhouse, G. (2002) Thinking outside the box: recent advances in the analysis and presentation of uncertainty in cost-effectiveness studies, *Annual Review of Public Health*, 23: 377–401.

British Medical Association (1998) *Health and Environmental Impact Assessment: An Integrated Approach*. Earthscan: London.

British Thoracic Society (2000) The Joint Committee of the British Thoracic Society: control and prevention of tuberculosis in the UK, code of practice, *Thorax*, 55: 887–901.

Brown, G. and Harris, T. (1978) *Social Origins of Depression*. London: Routledge.

Brown, P. (2001) Return of malaria feared as climate warms, *Guardian*, 10 February.

Brundtland, G. (ed.) (1987) *Our Common Future: World Commission on Environment and Development*. Oxford: Oxford University Press.

Brunner, E., White, I., Thorogood, M. *et al.* (1997) Can dietary interventions change diet and cardiovascular risk factors? A meta-analysis of randomized controlled trials, *American Journal of Public Health*, 87(9): 1415–22.

Bryson, J.M. and Crosby, B.C. (1992) *Leadership for the Common Good*. San Francisco: Jossey-Bass.

Buchan, J. (2002) Rallying the troops, *Health Service Journal*, 30 May, pp. 24–6.

Buckland, S., Lupton, C. and Moon, G. (1994) *An Evaluation of the Role and Impact of Community Health Councils*. Portsmouth: Social Services Research and Information Unit, Portsmouth University.

Bull, J. and Hamer, L. (2002) *Closing the Gap: Setting Local Targets to Reduce Health Inequalities*. London: Health Development Agency.

Bulmer, M. (1987) *The Social Basis of Community Care*. London: Unwin Hyman.

Bunton, R. and Macdonald, G. (eds) (1992) *Health Promotion: Disciplines and Diversity*. London: Routledge.

Bush, J., Fanshel, S. and Chen, M. (1972) Analysis of a tuberculin-testing program using a health status index, *Socio-Economic Planning in Science*, 6: 49–68.

C2 Steering Group and Secretariat (2001) *The Campbell Collaboration: Concept, Status and Plans* (revision date 6/01/01) http://econ.dur.ac.uk/eb2003/proceedings.htm (paper under Boruch, Robert F. *et al.*)

Cabinet Office (1999) *Modernising Government*, Cm4310. London: HMSO.

Cabinet Office (2000a) *Wiring It Up*. London: Performance and Innovation Unit, The Stationery Office.

Cabinet Office (2000b) *Reaching Out: The Role of Central Government at Regional and Local Level*. London: Performance and Innovation Unit, The Stationery Office.

Cabinet Office (2001a) *Better Policy Delivery and Design*, discussion paper. London: Performance and Innovation Unit, The Stationery Office.

Cabinet Office (2001b) *Strengthening Leadership in the Public Sector*, a research study by the Performance and Innovation Unit. London: Performance and Innovation Unit, The Stationery Office.

Cabinet Office (2001c) *HAZMOD Intranet Pilot – Summary Report of Results*. London. Civil Contingencies Secretariat, The Stationery Office. www.ukresilience.info/contingencies/cont hazmod.htm (accessed 24 January 2003).

Cabinet Office (2001d) *The Future of Emergency Planning in England and Wales: Results of the Consultation*. London: UK Resilience Unit, The Stationery Office. www.ukresilience.info.epr/eprconsltres.pdf (accessed 23 January 2003).

Cabinet Office (2002) *Roles of Lead Government Departments on Planning and Managing Crises*. London: UK Resilience Unit, The Stationery Office.

Campaign Against Racism and Facism (2000) *Dispersal and the New Racism*. www.carf.demon.co.uk/feat35.html (accessed 2 August 2002).

Campbell, C. and Jovchelovitch, S. (2000) Health and community development: towards a social psychology of participation, *Journal of Applied and Community Social Psychology*, 10: 255–70.

Campbell, C., Wood, R. and Kelly, M. (1999) *Social Capital and Health*. London: Health Education Authority.

Carr-Hill, R. (1989) Assumptions of the QALY procedure, *Social Science and Medicine*, 29(3): 469–77.

Cartwright, A. (1979) *The Dignity of Labour?* London: Tavistock.

Cattell, V. and Evans, M. (1999) *Neighbourhood Images in East London*, Joseph Rowntree Foundation Area Regeneration Series. York: York Publishing Services.

Cattell, V. and Herring, R. (2002) Social capital, generations and health in East London, in C. Swann and A. Morgan (eds) *Social Capital for Health: Insights from Qualitative Research*. London: Health Development Agency.

Centre for the Advancement of Interprofessional Education (CAIPE) (1997) *Interprofessional Education – A Definition*, Bulletin 13. London: CAIPE.

Challis, L., Fuller, M., Henwood, M. *et al.* (1988) *Joint Approaches to Social Policy: Rationality and Practice*. Cambridge: Cambridge University Press.

Chanan, G. (2002) *Measures of Community*. London: Community Development Foundation.

Chapman, S. (2001) Using media advocacy to shape policy, in D. Pencheon, C. Gust, D. Melzer and J. Muir Gray (eds) *Oxford Handbook of Public Health Practice*. Oxford: Oxford University Press.

Chapman, J. (2002) *System Failure: Why Governments Must Learn to Think Differently*. London: DEMOS.

Chief Medical Officer (CMO) (1997) *Avian (H5N1) Influenza in Hong Kong*, PL/CMO/97/3, Department of Health. London: The Stationery Office.

Chief Medical Officer (CMO) (1998) *Antenatal Testing for HIV*, PL/CMO (98) 4, PL/CMO (98) 10, Department of Health. London: The Stationery Office.

CHMRC (Chemical and Hazard Management Research Centre) (2002) *IPPC: A Practical Guide for Health Authorities*. Birmingham: University of Birmingham, (www.doh.gov.uk/pdfs/ippchag.pdf).

CIEH (Chartered Institute of Environmental Health) (1997) *Agendas for Change*. London: CIEH.

Clarence, E. and Painter, C. (1998) Public services under new Labour: collaborative discourses and local networking, *Public Policy and Administration*, 13(3): 8–22.

Clarke, M. and Newman, J. (1997) *The Managerial State*. London: Sage.

Coe, R., Fitz-Gibbon, C. and Tymms, P. (2000) *Promoting Evidence-based Education: The Role of Practitioners*. Durham: Durham University Curriculum, Evaluation and Management Centre, Mountjoy Research Center.

Cohen, D.R. and Henderson, J.B. (1988) *Health Prevention and Economics*. Oxford: Oxford Medical Publications.

Coker, N. (2001) Asylum seekers' and refugees' health experience, *Health Care UK*, autumn, pp. 34–40.

Colborn, T., Myers, J.P. and Dumanoski, D. (1997). *Our Stolen Future – Are We Threatening Fertility, Intelligence and Survival – A Scientific Detective Story*. London: Abacus.

Colver, A., Hutchinson, P. and Judson, E. (1982) Promoting children's home safety, *British Medical Journal*, 285: 1177–80.

COMAH (Control of Major Accident Hazard Regulations) (1999) *Control of Major Accident Hazard Regulations 1999*. London: The Stationery Office.

Commission on Environmental Health (1997) *Agendas for Change Environmental Health Commission*. London: Chadwick House Group.

Commission of the European Communities (1990) *Green Paper on the Urban Environment*, COM(90) 218. Luxembourg: OOPEC.

Commission of the European Communities (1994a) *Community Initiative Concerning Urban Areas*. (URBAN) COM(94) 61 Final, 2 March. Brussels: Commission of European Communities.

Commission of the European Communities (1994b) *European Sustainable Cities*, Part One. Luxembourg: OOPEC.

Commission of the European Communities (1994c) *State of Europe's Environment*. Brussels: Commission of European Communities.

Commission of the European Communities (1996) *European Sustainable Cities*. Luxembourg: OOPEC.

Commission of the European Communities (1997) *Towards an Urban Agenda in the European Union*, COM (97) 197 Final. Luxembourg: OOPEC.

Commission of the European Communities (1998) *Sustainable Urban Development in the European Union: A Framework for Action*, COM (98) 605 Final. Luxembourg: OOPEC.

Commission of the European Communities (2001) *Amended Proposal for a Decision of the European Parliament and of the Council Adopting a Programme of Community Action in the Field of Public Health (2001–2006)*, COM(2001)302. Brussels: Commission of the European Communities.

Commission for Health Improvement (2002) *Nothing About Us Without Us*. London: The Stationery Office.

Connell, J.P. and Kubisch, A.C. (1998) Applying a theory of change approach to the evaluation of comprehensive community initiatives: progress, prospects and problems, in K. Fulbright-Anderson (ed.) *New Approaches to Evaluating Community Initiatives. Volume 2. Theory, Measurement and Analysis.* Washington, DC: Aspen Institute.

Connett, J. and Stamler, J. (1984) Responses of black and white males to the special intervention programme of the Multiple Risk Factor Intervention Trial, *American Heart Journal*, 108: 839–49.

Cooke, S. and Yarrow, D. (1993) Culture and organisational learning, *Journal of Management Inquiry*, 2.

Cooper, H., Arber, S., Fee, L. and Ginn, J. (1999) *The Influence of Social Support and Social Capital on Health.* London: Health Education Authority.

Cornwall, J. (1984) *Hard Earned Lives: Accounts of Health and Illness from East London.* London: Tavistock.

Corrigan, P. and Joyce, P. (1997) Reconstructing public management, *International Journal of Public Sector Management*, 10: 417–32.

Countryside Commission (1995) *State of the Countryside – Environmental Indicators.* Cheltenham: Countryside Commission.

Cowe, R. (2000) Swap shop, *Guardian*, 30 August.

Craig, P. and Lindsay, G. (2000) *Nursing for Public Health: Population Based Care.* London: Churchill Livingstone.

Curtis, S., Cave, B. and Coutts, A. (2002) Is urban regeneration good for health? Perceptions and theories of the health impacts of urban change, *Environment and Planning Government and Policy*, 20(4): 517–34.

Cutler, T. and Waine, B. (2000) Managerialism reformed? New Labour and public sector management, *Social Policy and Administration*, September 34(3): 318–32.

Dahlgren, G. and Whitehead, M. (1992) Policies and strategies to promote equity in health. (unpublished). Geneva: World Health Organisation.

Dalziel, Y. (2000) Community development as a strategy for public health, in P. Craig and G.M. Lindsay (eds) *Nursing for Public Health. Population-based Care.* London: Churchill Livingstone.

Davey Smith, G. and Ebrahim, S. (1998) Commentary: dietary change, cholesterol reduction, and the public health: what does meta-analysis add? *British Medical Journal*, 316: 1120.

Davey Smith, G. and Ebrahim, S. (2001) Epidemiology – is it time to call it a day? *International Journal of Epidemiology*, 30: 1–11.

Davey Smith, G. and Egger, M. (1999) Meta-analysis of observational data should be done with due care, *British Medical Journal*, 318: 56.

Davey Smith, G., Dorling, D., Gordon, D. and Shaw, M. (1999) The widening health gap: what are the solutions? *Critical Public Health*, 9(2): 151–70.

Davey Smith, G., Chaturvedi, N., Harding, S., Nazroo, J. and Williams, R. (2000a) Ethnic inequalities in health: a review of UK epidemiological evidence, *Critical Public Health*, 10(4): 375–408.

Davey Smith, G., Harding, S. and Rosato, M. (2000b) Relation between infants' birthweight and mothers' mortality: prospective observational study, *British Medical Journal*, 320: 839–40.

Davey Smith, G., Dorling, D. and Shaw, M. (2001a) *Poverty, Inequality and Health in Britain: A Reader.* Bristol: Policy Press.

Davey Smith, G., Ebrahim, S. and Frankel, S. (2001b) How policy informs the evidence: 'Evidence based' thinking can lead to debased policy making, *British Medical Journal*, 322: 184–5.

Davey Smith, G., Gunnell, D. and Ben-Shlomo, Y. (2001c) Life-course approaches to socio-economic differentials in cause-specific adult mortality, in D. Leon and G. Walt (eds) *Poverty, Inequality and Health*. Oxford: Oxford University Press.

Davey Smith, G., Dorling, D., Mitchell, R. and Shaw, M. (2002) Health inequalities in Britain: continuing increases up to the end of the 20th century, *Journal of Epidemiology and Community Health*, 56: 434–5.

Davies, A. (1993) Who needs user research? Service users as subjects or participants, in M. Barnes and G. Wistow (eds) *Researching User Involvement*. Leeds: Nuffield Institute for Health Service Studies.

Davies, J.K. and Kelly, M.P. (1992) *Healthy Cities: Research and Practice*. London: Routledge.

Davies, H.T.O., Nutley, S.M. and Smith, P.C. (eds) (2000) *What Works? Evidence-based Policy and Practice in the Public Services*. Bristol: Policy Press.

Day, P. and Klein, R. (1987) *Accountabilities: Five Public Services*. London: Tavistock.

Daykin, N. and Doyal, L. (eds) (1999) *Work and Health*. London: Palgrave.

D'Cruze, S. (2000) Don't reject asylum seekers, *Nursing Standard*, 15(7): 28.

Deacon, A. (2000) Learning from the US? The influence of American ideas upon 'new Labour' thinking on welfare reform, *Policy and Politics*, 28(1): 5–18.

DEFRA (Department of Environment, Food and Rural Affairs) (2002) *Farming and Food. A Sustainable Future*, policy commission report. London: The Stationery Office.

Dennis, N., Henriques, F.M. and Slaughter, C. (1957) *Coal is Our Life*. London: Eyre and Spottiswoode.

Department of the Environment, Transport and the Regions (DETR) (1997) *The UK National Air Quality Strategy*. London: The Stationery Office.

Department of the Environment, Transport and the Regions (DETR) (1998) *Modern Local Government – In Touch with the People*, Cm 4014. London: DETR.

Department of the Environment, Transport and the Regions (DETR) (2000a) *Preparing Community Strategies: Guidance to Local Authorities*. London: DETR.

Department of the Environment, Transport and the Regions (DETR) (2000b) *Our Towns and Cities: the Future: Delivering an Urban Renaissance*. London: DETR.

Department of the Environment, Transport and the Regions (DETR) (2000c) *Modernising Local Government*. London: DETR.

Department of the Environment, Transport and the Regions (DETR) (2000d) *Joining It Up Locally*. Report of policy Action Team 17. London: DETR.

Department of the Environment, Transport and the Regions (DETR) (2000e) *Social Exclusion and the Provision and Availability of Public Transport*. TraC at the University of North London for DETR. London: DETR.

Department of the Environment, Transport and the Regions (DETR) (2000f) *Indices of Deprivation 2000*. London: DETR.

Department of the Environment, Transport and the Regions (DETR) (2001a) *Strong Local Leadership – Quality Public Services*. London: DETR.

Department of the Environment, Transport and the Regions (DETR) (2001b) *Local Strategic Partnerships – Government Guidance*. London: DETR.

Department of the Environment/Welsh Office (1993) *Integrated Pollution Control, A Practical Guide*. London: The Stationery Office.

Department of Health (1995a) *The Health of the Nation: Variations in Health. What Can the Department of Health and the NHS Do?* London: HMSO.

Department of Health (1995b) *Policy Appraisal and Health: A Guide from the Department of Health*. London: The Stationery Office.

Department of Health (1997a) *The New NHS: Modern, Dependable*, Cm 3807. London: The Stationery Office.

Department of Health (1997b) *Communications about Risk to the Public Health – Pointers to Good Practice*. London: The Stationery Office.

Department of Health (1998a) *Screening of Pregnant Women for Hepatitis B and Immunisation of Babies at Risk*, HSC (98) 127. London: The Stationery Office.

Department of Health (1998b) *A First Class Service: Quality in the New NHS*, a consultation paper. London: The Stationery Office.

Department of Health (1998c) *The Health of the Nation – A Policy Assessed*. London: The Stationery Office.

Department of Health (1999a) *Reducing Health Inequalities: An Action Report*. London: The Stationery Office.

Department of Health (1999b) *Health Impact Assessment: Report of a Methodological Seminar*. London: The Stationery Office.

Department of Health (1999c) *Reducing Mother to Baby Transmission of HIV*, HSC, 1999/183. London: The Stationery Office.

Department of Health (2000a) *The Expert Patient: A New Approach to Chronic Disease Management for the 21st Century*. London: Department of Health.

Department of Health (2000b) *Asylum Seekers – Access to National Health Service Treatment*. www.doh.gov.uk/hsd/asylumseekers.htm (accessed 21 June 2002).

Department of Health (2001a) *Shifting the Balance of Power: Securing Delivery*. London: The Stationery Office.

Department of Health (2001b) *The Report of the Chief Medical Officer's Project to Strengthen the Public Health Function*. London: The Stationery Office.

Department of Health (2001c) *Tackling Health Inequalities: Consultation on a Plan for Delivery*. London: The Stationery Office.

Department of Health (2001d) *Vision to Reality*. London: The Stationery Office.

Department of Health (2001e) *Involving Patients and the Public in Healthcare*. London: The Stationery Office.

Department of Health (2001f) *A Research and Development Strategy for Public Health*. www.doh.gov.uk

Department of Health (2001g) *Health Effects of Climate Change: An Expert Review*. London: The Stationery Office.

Department of Health (2002a) *Tackling Health Inequalities*, the results of the consultation exercise. London: The Stationery Office.

Department of Health (2002b) *Shifting the Balance of Power: Next Steps*. London: The Stationery Office.

Department of Health (2002c) *Getting Ahead of the Curve – A Strategy for Infectious Diseases (Including Other Aspects of Health Protection)*, Chief Medical Officer's report. London: The Stationery Office.

Department of Health (2002d) *Foot and Mouth: An Update on Risks to Health From Pyres and other Methods of Burning Used for Disposal of Animals*. www.doh.gov.uk/fmguidance (accessed 12 January 2003).

Department of Health (2003) *The Social Amplication of Risk – The Media and the Public*, summary of commissioned risk research. www.doh.gov/risk/riskampl.htm (accessed 12 January 2003).

Department of Health COMEAP (Committee on the Medical Effects of Air Pollutants) (1995) *Non Biological Particles and Health*. London: The Stationery Office.

Department of Health COMEAP (Committee on the Medical Effects of Air Pollutants) (1997) *Handbook on Air Pollution and Health*. London: The Stationery Office.

Department of Health EPCU (Emergency Planning Coordination Unit) (2002a) *Emergency Planning and Response to Major Incidents: Summary of Roles and Responsibilities*. London: The Stationery Office (www.doh.gov.uk/epcu accessed 24 January 2003).

Department of Health EPCU (Emergency Planning Coordination Unit) (2002b) *Planning for Major Incidents: Updated NHS Guidance.* London: The Stationery Office (www.doh.gov.uk/epcu accessed 24 January 2003).

Department of Health/Neighbourhood Renewal Unit (DoH/NRU)(2002) *Health and Neighbourhood Renewal: Guidance from the Department of Health and the Neighbourhoood Renewal Unit.* London: DoH/NRU.

Department of Health/Welsh Office (2002) *Health Protection: A Consultation Document on Creating a Health Protection Agency.* London: The Stationery Office.

Department of Transport, Local Government and the Regions (DTLR) (2001) *Strong Local Leadership: Quality Public Services.* London: DTLR.

Department of Transport, Local Government and the Regions (DTLR) (2002) *Collaboration and Co-ordination in Area based Initiatives.* London: NRU/RCU.

Department of Transport, Local Government and the Regions/Cabinet Office (2002) *Your Region, Your Choice: Revitalising the English Regions.* Cm 5511. London: The Stationery Office.

Detsky, A.S. (1985) Using economic analysis to determine the resource consequences of choices made in planning clinical trials, *Journal of Chronic Diseases,* 38: 753–65.

DHSS (1980) *Inequalities in Health: Report of a Research Working Party.* London: DHSS.

DHSS (1986) *Primary Health Care: An Agenda for Discussion,* Cmnd. 9771. London: HMSO.

DHSS (1987) *Promoting Better Health: The Government's Programme for Improving Primary Health Care,* Cmnd. 249. London: HMSO.

Dickson, D. (1997) UK policy learns about risk the hard way, *Nature,* 385: 8–9.

Dixon, J. (1995) Community stories and indicators for evaluating community development, *Community Development Journal,* 30: 327–36.

Dixon, D.O. and Simon, R. (1992) Bayesian subset analysis in a colorectal cancer trial, *Statistics in Medicine,* 11: 13–22.

Dixon, J., Kouzmin, A. and Korac-Kokabadse, N. (1998) Managerialism – something old, something borrowed, little new, *International Journal of Public Sector Management,* 11(2/3): 164–87.

Dolan, P. (1998) The measurement of individual utility and social welfare, *Journal of Health Economics,* 17: 39–52.

Dolan, P. (2001) Output measures and valuation in health, in M. Drummond and A. McGuire *Economic Evaluation in Health Care: Merging Theory with Practice.* Oxford: Oxford University Press.

Donner, A. and Klar, N. (1994) Cluster randomization trials in epidemiology: theory and application, *Journal of Statistical Planning and Inference,* 42: 37–56.

Donner, A. and Klar, N. (2000) *Design and Analysis of Cluster Randomization Trials in Health Research.* London: Arnold.

Douglas, I. (1995) Private communication.

Dowie, J. (1996) The research–practice gap and the role of decision analysis in closing it, *Health Care Analysis,* 4: 5–18.

Dowie, J. (2001a) Decision analysis and the evaluation of decision technologies, *Quality in Health Care,* 10: 1–2.

Dowie, J. (2001b) Decision technologies and the independent professional: the future's challenge to learning and leadership, *Quality in Health Care,* 10: ii59–ii63.

Dowie, J. (2001c) *Towards Value-based, Science-informed Public Health Policy: Conceptual Framework and Practical Guidelines.* Consultation on risks to health: better management for decision making. Geneva: WHO/Department of Health.

Driver, S. and Martell, L. (1998) *New Labour: Politics after Thatcherism.* Cambridge: Polity Press.

Drummond, M. and McGuire, A. (2001) *Economic Evaluation in Health Care: Merging Theory with Practice*. Oxford: Oxford University Press.

Drummond, M., O'Brien, B., Stoddart, G.L. and Torrance, G.W. (1997) *Methods for the Economic Evaluation of Health Care Programmes*, 2nd edn. Oxford: Oxford Medical Publications.

Duck, S. (1992) *Human Relationships*. London: Sage.

Duggan, M. (2001) *Healthy Living: The Role of Modern Local Authorities in Creating Healthy Communities*. Birmingham: Society of Local Authority Chief Executives.

Duggan, M. (2002) Social exclusion, discrimination and the promotion of health, in L. Adams, M. Amos and J. Munro (eds) *Promoting Health: Politics and Practice*. London: Sage.

Earl, P. (1995) *Microeconomics for Business and Marketing*. Hampshire: Edward Elgar.

East End Health Action (2000) *Report of Participatory Appraisal Workshops*. Glasgow: East End Health Action.

Easterby-Smith, M. (1997) Disciplines of organisational learning: contributions and critiques, *Human Relations*, 50(9): 1085–113.

Easterlow, D., Smith, S.J. and Mallinson, S. (2000) Housing for health: the role of owner occupation, *Housing Studies*, 15(3): 443–63.

Ebrahim, S. and Davey Smith, G. (1997) Systematic review of randomised controlled trials of multiple risk factor interventions for preventing coronary heart disease, *British Medical Journal*, 314: 1666–74.

Eddy, D.M., Hasselblad, V. and Shachter, R. (1990) A Bayesian method for synthesising evidence: the confidence profile method, *International Journal for Technological Assessment in Health Care*, 6: 31–55.

Edwards, R.T. (2001) Paradigms and research programmes: is it time to move from health care economics to health economics? *Health Economics*, 10: 635–49.

Egger, M., Davey Smith, G. and Schneider, M. (2001) Systematic reviews of observational studies, in M. Egger, G. Davey Smith and D.G. Altmann (eds) *Systematic Reviews in Health Care: Metanalysis in Context*. London: BMJ Books.

Ekstrøm, A.M., Serafini, M., Nyren, O. *et al.* (2000) Dietary antioxidant intake and the risk of cardia cancer and non-cardia cancer of the intestinal and diffuse types: a population-based case control study in Sweden, *International Journal of Cancer*, 87: 133–40.

El Ansari, W., Phillips, C.J. and Hammick, M. (2001) Collaboration and partnerships: developing the evidence base, *Health and Social Care in the Community*, 9(4): 215–27.

El Din, E.Z. (2000) Buy organic – local or global? *Health Matters*, 41: 16.

El-Omar, E.M., Carrington, M., Chow, W.H. *et al.* (2000) Interleukin-1 polymorphisms associated with increased risk of gastric cancer, *Nature*, 404: 398–402.

Elixhauser, A., Halpern, M., Schmier, J. and Luce, B. (1998) Health care CBA and CEA from 1991 to 1996: an updated bibliography, *Medical Care*, 31: 7 (suppl).

Environment Agency (2000) *Environmental Impact of the Foot and Mouth Outbreak – an Interim Assessment*. www.environment-agency.gov.uk (accessed 14 January 2003).

European Commission (1996) *European Sustainable Cities Report*. Brussels: Expert Group on the Urban Environment. http://europa.eu.int

European Commission (1998) Setting up a network for epidemiological surveillance and control of communicable diseases in the Community, *Official Journal of the European Community*, OJL 268, 3 October, p. 1.

European Commission Air Pollution and Health European Environmental Information System (APHEIS) (2002) *Report of the Investigation of Premature Deaths from Exposure to PM10 Particulates*. Brussels: EC APHEIS.

European Community (1999) *Fourth Report on the Integration of Health Protection Requirements in Community Policies*, V/99/408-EN. Brussels: European Community.

European Community (2001) A *Programme of Action in the Field of Public Health 2001–2006*, COM 302. Brussels: European Community.

European Community (2002) Environment 2010: our future, our choice. the sixth environment action programme of the European Community. *Official Journal of the European Community*, OJL 242, 10 September.

European Sustainable Cities and Towns Campaign (1996) The Lisbon Action Plan, *Brussels Eurosurveillance Weekly*, European communicable disease surveillance network and reports. www.eurosurveillance.org

Evans, D. and Killoran, A. (2000) Tackling health inequalities through partnership working: learning from a realistic evaluation, *Critical Public Health*, 10(2): 125–40.

Ewles, L. and Simnett, I. (2003) *Promoting Health: A Practical Guide* (5th edn). Edinburgh: Baillière Tindall.

Exworthy, M. and Powell, M. (2000) Variations on a theme: new Labour, health inequalities and policy failure, in A. Hann (ed) *Analysing Health Policy*. Aldershot: Ashgate.

Exworthy, M., Berney, L. and Powell, M. (2002) How great expectations in Westminster may be dashed locally: the local implementation of national policy on health inequalities, *Policy and Politics*, 30(1): 79–96.

Faculty of Public Health Medicine (2002) *Statement on Managed Public Health Networks*. www.fphm.org.uk/Policy/Policy_frame.htm

Faculty of Public Health Medicine and Health Development Agency (2001) *Statement on Managed Public Health Networks*. London: Faculty of Public Health Medicine.

Farmer, P. (1997) Social Scientists and the New Tuberculosis, *Social Science and Medicine*, 44(3): 347–58.

Fassil, Y. (2000) Looking after the health of refugees, *British Medical Journal*, 321: 59.

Feachem, R.G.A. (2001) Globalisation is good for your health, mostly, *British Medical Journal*, September, 323: 504–6.

Fehr, R. (1999) Environmental Impact Assessment: Evaluation of Ten-step Model, *Epidemiology*, 10(5): 618–25.

Fernie, K. and McCarthy, J. (2001) Partnership and community involvement: institutional morphing in Dundee, *Local Economy*, 16(4): 299–311.

Finch, J. and Groves, D. (1983) *A Labour of Love: Women, Work and Caring*. London: Routledge and Kegan Paul.

Fine, B. (1999) The developmental state is dead – long live social capital? *Development and Change*, 30: 1–19.

Fitzpatrick, M. (2001) *The Tyranny of Health. Doctors and the Regulation of Lifestyle*. London: Routledge.

Fleeman, N. and Scott-Samuel, A. (2000) A prospective health impact assessment of the Merseyside Integrated Transport Strategy (MerITS), *Journal of Public Health Medicine*, 22: 268–74.

Florey, C. du V. (1988) Weak associations in epidemiological research: some examples and their interpretation, *International Journal of Epidemiology*, 17(4): 950–4.

Flyvbjerg, B. (2001) *Making Social Science Matter. Why Social Inquiry Fails and How it Can Succeed Again*. Cambridge; Cambridge University Press.

Forbes, J. and Sashidharan, S. (1997) User involvement in services – incorporation or challenge? *British Journal of Social Work*, 27(4): 481–98.

Forrest, R. and Kearns, A. (1999) *Joined Up Places? Social Cohesion and Neighbourhood Regeneration*. York: York Publishing Services.

Foucault, M. (1979) Governmentality, *Ideology and Consciousness*, 6: 5–22.

Frankel, S., Davidson, C. and Davey Smith, G. (1991) Lay epidemiology and the rationality of responses to health education, *British Journal of General Practice*, 41: 428–30.

Frankenberg, R. (1957) *Village on the Border*. London: Cohen and West.

Freedman, L. (1996) Bayesian statistical methods: a natural way to assess clinical evidence, *British Medical Journal*, 313(7057): 569–70.

Freidson, E. (1986) *Professional Power: A Study of the Institutionalisation of Formal Knowledge*. Chicago: University of Chicago Press.

Freiman, J.A., Chalmers, T.C., Smith, H. and Kuebler, R.R. (1992) The importance of beta, the type II error, and sample size in the design and interpretation of the randomized controlled trial: survey of two sets of 'negative' trials, in J.C. Bailar and F. Mosteller (eds) *Medical Uses of Statistics*, 2nd edn. Boston, MA: NEJM Books.

Frenk, J. (1992) The new public health, in Pan American Health Organization, *The Crisis of Public Health: Reflections for Debate*. Washington: PAHO/WHO.

Fry, J. and Hodder, J.P. (1994) *Primary Health Care in an International Context*. London: Nuffield Provincial Hospitals Trust.

Fudge, C. (1995) *International Healthy and Ecological Cities Congress: Our City, Our Future*, Rapporteur's Report. Copenhagen: WHO.

Fudge, C. and Rowe, J. (1997) *Urban Environment and Sustainability: Developing the Agenda for Socio-Economic Environmental Research*, research report for DG XII. Bristol: University of the West of England, Bristol.

Fudge, C. and Rowe, J. (2000) *Implementing Sustainable Futures in Sweden*. Stockholm: BFR.

Fudge, C. and Rowe, J. (2001) Ecological modernisation as a framework for sustainable development: a case study in Sweden, *Environment and Planning A*, 33: 527–1546.

Fudge, C. and Antrobus, J. (2002) *Climate Change Research: Scoping Exercise*, MISTRA Research Programme, June. Bristol: University of the West of England, Bristol.

Fulop, N. and Hunter, D.J. (1999) Saving lives or sustaining the public's health? *British Medical Journal*, 319: 139–40.

Fussler, C. and James, P. (1996) *Driving Eco-Innovation: A Breakthrough Discipline for Innovation and Sustainability*. London: Pitman Publishing.

Gabarino, J. (1983) Social support networks for the helping professions, in J. Whittaker and J. Gabarino (eds) *Social Support Networks: Informal Helping in the Human Services*. Hawthorne, NY: Aldine DeGruyter.

Gaster, L. and Deakin, N. (1998) Quality and citizens, in A. Coulson (ed.) *Trust and Contracts: Relationships in local government, health and public services*. Bristol: Policy Press.

Geddes, M. (1997) *Partnership Against Poverty and Exclusion: Local Regeneration Strategies and Excluded Communities in the UK*. Bristol: Policy Press.

Giddens, A. (1990) *The Consequences of Modernity*. Cambridge: Polity Press.

Giddens, A. (1994) *Beyond Left and Right: The Future of Radical Politics*. Cambridge: Polity Press.

Giddens, A. (1999) *Reith Lecture on 'Globalisation'*. London: BBC. http://news.bbc.co.uk/hi/english/static/events/reith_99/week1/week1.htm

Giesecke, J. and Weinberg, J. (1998) A European centre for infectious disease? *Lancet*, 352: 1308.

Gilchrist, A. (1998) Connectors and catalysts, *SCCD News*, 18: 18–20.

Gilchrist, A. (2001) Strength through diversity: networking for community development. Unpublished PhD thesis. Bristol: University of Bristol.

Gilchrist, A. (2003) Partnerships and networks, in S. Banks, H. Butcher, P. Henderson and J. Robertson (eds) *Managing Community Practice*. Bristol: Policy Press.

Gill, O., Tanner, C. and Bland, L. (2000) *Family Support; Strengths and Pressures in a 'High Risk' Neighbourhood*. Ilford: Barnardo's.

Gillam, S. and Smith, K. (2002) in Wilkin *et al.* (eds) *The National Tracker Survey of Primary*

Care Groups and Trusts 2001/2002: Taking Responsibility? Manchester: National Primary Care Research and Development Centre, University of Manchester.

Gillam, S., Abbott, S. and Banks-Smith, J. (2001) Can primary care groups and trusts improve health? *British Medical Journal*, 323: 89–92.

Gilliatt, S., Fenwick, J., and Alford, D. (2000) Public services and the consumer: empowerment or control? *Social Policy and Administration*, 34(3) September, pp. 333–49.

Gillies, P. (1998a) Effectiveness of alliances and partnerships for health promotion, *Health Promotion International*, 13(2): 1–21.

Gillies, P. (1998b) Effectiveness of alliances and partnerships for health promotion, *Health Promotion International*, 13: 99–120.

Gillies, P. (1998c) Social capital and its contribution to public health, *Forum*, 8.2(5): 47–51.

Gillman, M.W. (2002) Epidemiological challenges in studying the fetal origins of adult chronic disease, *International Journal of Epidemiology*, 31: 294–9.

Ginnety, P. (2001) *Tools of the Trade – A Toolkit for Those Using Community Development Approaches to Health and Social Wellbeing*. Newry: Community Development and Health Network Northern Ireland.

Gladstone, F. (1979) *Voluntary Action in a Changing World*. London: The Bedford Square Press.

Glass, R. (1955) Urban sociology in Great Britain, *Current Sociology*, 4: 5–19.

Glendinning, C. (2002) Partnerships between health and social services: developing a framework for evaluation, *Policy and Politics*, 30(1): 115–27.

Glendinning, C., Powell, M. and Rummery, K. (eds) (2002) *Partnerships, New Labour and the Governance of Welfare*. Bristol: Policy Press.

Golding, J., Pembrey, M. and Jones, R. (2001) ALSPAC – the Avon longitudinal study of parents and children. I. Study Methodology, *Paediatric and Perinatal Epidemiology*, 15: 74–87.

Goss, S. and Kent, C. (1995) *Health and Housing: Working Together? A Review of the Extent of Inter-agency Working*. Bristol: Policy Press.

Gowman, N. and Coote, A. (2000) *Evidence and Public Health. Towards a Common Framework*. London: King's Fund.

Graham, H. (1993) *When Life's a Drag: Women, Smoking and Disadvantage*. London: HMSO.

Granovetter, M. (1973) The strength of weak ties, *American Journal of Sociology*, 78: 1360–80.

Green Alliance (1997) *Making Environmental Decisions: Cost Benefit Analysis, Contingent Valuation and Alternatives*, proceedings of a conference, Green Alliance/Centre for the Study of Environmental Change, January. London: Green Alliance.

Green, G. and Grimsley, M. (2002) *4 Capitals for Neighbourhood Sustainability*. Paper presented to the Health Development Agency conference Social Action for Health and Wellbeing: Experiences from Policy, Research and Practice, 20–1 June. London: Health Development Agency.

Greenland, S. and Robins, J. (1994) Ecologic studies; biases, misconceptions and counter-examples, *American Journal of Epidemiology*, 139: 747–71.

Greer, S. (2001) *Divergence and Devolution*. London: Nuffield Trust.

Grossdkurth, H., Mosha, F. and Todd, J. (1995) Improved treatment of sexually transmitted diseases on HIV infection in rural Tanzania: randomised controlled trial, *Lancet*, 346: 530–6.

Guinchard, C-G. (1997) Swedish planning: towards sustainable development, special edition of PLAN, *Swedish Journal of Planning*, Stockholm.

Gwatkin, D.R., Guillot, M. and Heuveline, P. (1999) The burden of disease among the global poor, *Lancet*, 354: 586–9.

Halpern, D. (2003 forthcoming) *Social Capital*. Cambridge: Polity Press.

Hamer, L. and Easton, N. (2002) *Community Strategies and Health Improvement: A Review of Policy and Practice.* London: I&DeA/DTLR/HDA.

Hamer, L. and Smithies, J. (2002) *Planning Across the Local Strategic Partnership: Case Studies of Integrating Community Strategies and Health Improvement.* London: HDA/LGA/DTLR.

Hammarby Sjöstad (undated) Stockholm City Council, Stockholm, Sweden.

Hammond, K.R. (1996) *Human Judgment and Social Policy: Irreducible Uncertainty, Inevitable Error, Unavoidable Injustice.* New York: Oxford University Press.

Hampshire, M. (2001) Out of reach, *Nursing Standard*, 15(51): 16–17.

Hancock, T., Labonte, R. and Edwards, R. (1999) Indicators that count! Measuring population health at the community level, *Canadian Journal of Public Health*, 90: 522–6.

Hannerz, U. (1996) *Transnational Connections: Culture, People, Places.* London: Routledge.

Harding, A. (1998) Public–private partnerships in the UK, in J. Pierre (ed) *Partnerships in Urban Governance.* Basingstoke: Macmillan.

Harifan, L.J. (1916) The rural school community centre, *Annals of the American Academy of Political and Social Science*, 67: 130–8.

Harris, A. (1995) Fresh fields: the relationship between public health medicine and general medical practice, *Primary Care Management*, 5(7): 3–9.

Harrison, A. (2000) Urban policy: addressing wicked issues, in H. Davies, S. Nutley and P. Smith (eds) *Evidence Based Policy and Practice in Public Services.* Bristol: Policy Press.

Harrison, S. and Mort, M. (1998) Which champions, which people? Public and user involvement in health care as a technology of legitimation, *Social Policy and Administration*, 32(1): 60–70.

Harvey, D. (1996) *Justice, Nature and the Geography of Difference.* Oxford: Blackwell.

Hashagen, S. (1998) *Strengthening Communities.* Edinburgh: Health Education Board for Scotland.

Hashagen, S. (ed) (forthcoming) *LEAP for Health.* Edinburgh: Health Education Board for Scotland.

Hastings, A. (1996) Unravelling the process of partnership in urban regeneration policy, *Urban Studies*, 33: 2.

Hastings, A., McArthur, A. and McGregor, A. (1996) *Less than Equal: Community Organizations and Estate Regeneration Partnerships.* Bristol: Policy Press.

Hawe, P. and Shiell, A. (2000) Social capital and health promotion: a review, *Social Science and Medicine*, 51: 871–85.

HDA (Health Development Agency)/CIEH (Chartered Institute of Environmental Health) (2002) *Environmental Health 2012: A Key Partner in Developing the Public Health Agenda*, September. London: HDA.

Health Education Unit and Open University (1991) *Roots and Branches: Papers from the Open University / Health Education Authority 1990 Winter School on Community Development and Health.* Milton Keynes: Open University.

Health Promotion Policy Unit (2002) *An Analysis of the Health Domain of the Delivery Plans.* London: New Deal for Communities National Evaluation.

Healthwork UK (2001) *National Standards for Specialist Practice in Public Health.* Dorset: Healthwork UK.

Held, D. and McGrew, A. (eds) (2000) *The Global Transformations Reader: An Introduction to the Globalization Debate.* Cambridge: Polity Press.

Held, D., McGrew, A.G., Goldblatt, D. and Perraton, J. (eds) (1999) *Global Transformations: Politics, Economics and Culture.* Cambridge: Polity Press.

Heller, D. (2002) *How can Primary Care Trusts Develop and Implement their Public Health Roles to Help Reduce Health Inequalities?* Paper to the HDA seminar on tackling health inequalities, June. London: Health Development Agency.

Heller, R.F. and Page, J. (2002) A population perspective to evidence-based medicine: evidence for population health, *Journal of Epidemiology and Community Health*, 56: 45–7.

Henning, C. and Leiberg, M. (1996) Strong ties or weak ties? Neighbourhood networks in a new perspective, *Scandinavian Housing and Planning Research*, 13: 3–26.

Hine, J. and Mitchell, F. (2001) Better for everyone? Travel experiences and transport exclusion, *Urban Studies*, 38(2): 319–32.

HM Treasury (2000a) *Government Interventions in Deprived Areas*. London: The Stationery Office.

HM Treasury (2000b) *Public Private Partnerships: The Government's Approach*. London: The Stationery Office.

HM Treasury and Department of Health (2002) *Tackling Health Inequalities: Summary of the 2002 Cross-Cutting Review*. London: HM Treasury and Department of Health.

Hogg, C. (1999) *Patients, Power and Politics: From Patients to Citizens*. London: Sage.

Hoggett, P. (1997) (ed.) *Contested Communities: Experiences, Struggles, Policies*. Bristol: Policy Press.

Home Office (1998) *Compact: Getting it Right Together – Compact on Relations Between Government and the Voluntary and Community Sector in England*, Cm 4100, November. London: The Stationery Office.

Home Office (1999) *Standards for Civil Protection in England and Wales*. London: The Stationery Office.

Home Office (2001) *Secure Borders, Safe Haven: Integration with Diversity in Modern Britain February 2002*. London: The Stationery Office.

Hornby, S. (1993) *Collaborative Care*. Oxford: Blackwell.

Horton, S. and Farnham, D. (2000) New Labour and the management of public services: legacies, impact and prospects, in S. Horton and D. Farnham (eds) *Public Management in Britain*. Basingstoke: Macmillan.

House of Commons Defence Committee (2001/02) *Report of the Proceedings of the House of Commons Defence Committee, Defence and Security in the UK*. Sixth report, session 2001–02, vol. 1. London: The Stationery Office.

House of Commons Health Select Committee (2001a) *Public Health*. Second report, volume I report and proceedings of the committee, session 2000–01, HC30-I. London: The Stationery Office.

House of Commons Health Select Committee (2001b) *Public Health*. Second report, volume II minutes of evidence and appendices, session 2000–01, HC30-II. London: The Stationery Office.

House of Commons Health Select Committee (2001c) *Second Report for the Session 2000–2001*. www.parliament.the-stationery-office.co.uk/pa/cm200001/cmselect/cmhealth/30/3002.htm (accessed 2 December 2002).

House of Lords (1995) *Report from the Select Committee on Sustainable Development*, session 1994–95, June. London: HMSO.

Howson, C.P., Fineberg, H.V. and Bloom, B.R. (1998) The pursuit of global health: the relevance of engagement for developed countries, *Lancet*, 351: 586–90.

HSC/DETR (Health and Safety Commission and Department of Environment, Transport and the Regions) (1999) *Revitalising Health and Safety*. London: The Stationery Office.

Hudson, B. (1987) Collaboration in social welfare: a framework for analysis, *Policy and Politics*, 15(3): 175–82.

Hudson, B. (1999) Dismantling the Berlin Wall: developments at the health–social care interface, in H. Dean and R. Woods (eds) *Social Policy Review 11*. Luton: SPA.

Hudson, B. and Hardy, B. (2001) Localization and partnership in the New National Health Service: England and Scotland compared, *Public Administration*, 79(2): 315–25.

Hudson, B., Hardy, B., Henwood, M. and Wistow, G. (1997) *Inter-agency Collaboration: Primary Health Care Sub-study*, final report. University of Leeds: Nuffield Institute for Health.

Hudson, B., Callaghan, G., Exworthy, M. and Peckham, S. (1999) *Locality Partnerships: The Early PCG Experience*, report to Northern and Yorkshire NHS Executive Research and Development. Luton: Social Policy Association.

Hunt, S. (1987) Evaluating a community development project, *British Journal of Social Work*, 17: 661–7.

Hunter, D. (1997) Managing the public health, in G. Scally (ed.) *Progress in Public Health*. London: RSM Press.

Hunter, D. (1998) *The Health of the Nation – A Policy Assessed*. Leeds: University of Leeds, University of Glamorgan and London School of Hygiene and Tropical Medicine.

Hunter, D.J. (2002) Wanless with a pinch of salt, *Health Service Journal*, 10 January.

Hunter, D.J. (2003) *Public Health Policy*. Oxford: Polity Press.

Hurrell, A. and Woods, N. (eds) (1999) *Inequality, Globalization, and World Politics*. Oxford: Oxford University Press.

Huxham, C. (ed.) (1996) *Creating Collaborative Advantage*. London: Sage.

Huxham, C. and Macdonald, D. ([1882] 1999) Introducing Collaborative Advantage, in H. Ibsen *An Enemy of the People*. Oxford: Oxford Paperbacks.

IEH (Institute for Environment and Health) (1995) *Environmental Oestrogens – Consequences for Human Health and Wildlife*. Leicester: University of Leicester.

Institute of Medicine (1988) *The Future of Public Health*. Washington: National Aacdemy Press.

International Union for the Conservation of Nature (IUCN) (1980) *World Conservation Strategy: Resource Conservation for Sustainable Development*. Geneva: IUCN.

Isaacs, W. (1993) Taking flight: dialogue, collective thinking, and organisational learning, *Organisational Dynamics*, 22(2) autumn, pp. 24–39.

Jacobs, J. (1961) *The Death and Life of Great American Cities*. New York: Random House.

Jaffe, M. and Mindell, J. (2002) A framework for the evidence base to support health impact assessment, *Journal of Epidemiology and Community Health*, 56: 132–8.

Jan, S. (1998) A holistic approach to the economic evaluation of health programs using institutionalist methodology, *Social Science and Medicine*, 47(10): 1565–72.

Jones, J. (1999) *Private Troubles and Public Issues: A Community Development Approach to Health*. Edinburgh: Community Learning Scotland.

Jones, D. and Gill, P.S. (1998) Refugees and primary care: tackling the inequalities, *British Medical Journal*, 317(7170): 1444–6.

Jonsen, A.R. and Hellegers, A.E. (1987) Conceptual foundations for an ethics of medical care, in L.R. Tancredi (ed) *Ethics of Health Care*. Washington, DC: National Academy of Sciences.

Kavanagh, D. and Richards, D. (2001) Departmentalism and joined-up government: back to the future, *Parliamentary Affairs*, 54: 1–18.

Kawachi, I. (1997) A prospective study of social networks in relation to total mortality and cardiovascular disease in the USA, *Journal of Epidemiology and Community Health*, 50: 245–91.

Kawachi, I., Kennedy, B.P., Lochner, K. and Prothrow-Stith, D. (1997). Social capital, income and inequality, *American Journal of Public Health*, 89(9): 1491–8.

Kearns, A., Hiscock, R., Ellaway, A. and Macintyre, S. (2000) Beyond four walls: the psycho-social benefits of home: evidence from west-central Scotland, *Housing Studies*, 15(3): 443–63.

Kerrison, S. and MacFarlane, A. (eds) (2000) *Official Health Statistics: An Unofficial Guide*. London: Arnold.

Kibble, A.J. and Saunders, P. (eds) (2001) *Integrated Pollution Prevention and Control – A Practical Guide for Health Authorities, Version 1.* Birmingham: University of Birmingham.

Klandermans, B. (1997) *The Social Psychology of Protest.* Oxford: Blackwell.

Klein, R. (1996) The NHS and the new scientism: solution or delusion? *Quarterly Journal of Medicine,* 89: 85–7.

Klein, R. (1998) *The New Politics of the NHS,* 4th edn. London: Longman.

Knoke, D. (1990) *Political Networks: The Structural Perspective.* Cambridge: Cambridge University Press.

Labonte, R. (1998) *A Community Development Approach to Health Promotion.* Edinburgh: Health Education Board for Scotland and RUHBC, University of Edinburgh.

Labonte, R. (2001) Liberalisation, health and the World Trade Organisation, *Journal of Epidemiology and Community Health,* 55: 620–1.

Labonte, R. (2002) International governance and World Trade Organisation (WTO) reform, *Critical Public Health,* 12(1): 65–86.

Lancet (1997) Putting public health back into epidemiology, *Lancet,* 350(907): 229.

Lancet (2002) Who has the power over tobacco control? *Lancet,* 360: 267.

LaPorte, R.E., Akazawa, S., Hellmonds, P. *et al.* (1994) Global public health and the information superhighway, *British Medical Journal,* 308: 1651–2.

LaPorte, R.E., Bavinas, E., Chang, Y-F. and Libman, I. (1996) Global epidemiology and public health in the 21st century: applications of new technologies, *Annals of Epidemiology,* 6: 162–7.

Larson, M. (1977) *The Rise of Professionalism: A Sociological Analysis.* Berkeley: University of California Press.

Last, J. (1995) *A Dictionary of Epidemiology.* Oxford: Oxford University Press.

Laumann, E. and Pappi, F. (1976) *Networks of Collective Action: A Perspective on Community Influence Systems.* New York: Academic Press.

Lawless, P., Dabinett, G., Rhodes, J. and Tyler, P. (2000) *The Evidence Base for Regeneration Policy and Practice,* DETR Regeneration Research 39. London: DETR.

Leadbetter, D. (ed.) (2000) *Harnessing Official Statistics,* Harnessing Health Information Series No. 3. Oxford: Radcliffe Medical Press.

Lee, K. (2000a) Global sneezes spread diseases, *Health Matters,* 41: 14–15.

Lee, K. (2000b) The impact of globalisation on public health: implications for the Faculty of Public Health Medicine, *Journal of Public Health Medicine,* 22(3): 253–62.

Lee, K. (2001) A dialogue of the deaf: the health impacts of globalisation, *Journal of Epidemiology and Community Health,* 55: 619.

Le Grand, J., Mays, N. and Mulligan, J.A. (eds) (1998) *Learning from the NHS Internal Market: A Review of Evidence.* London: King's Fund.

Leifler, D. (1999) Giving refuge to those in need, *Nursing Standard,* 13(43): 16–17.

Leon, D. and Walt, G. (eds.) (2000) *Poverty, Inequality and Health.* Oxford: Oxford University Press.

Levitas, R. (1998) *The Inclusive Society?* Basingstoke: Macmillan.

Levitt, I. (1988) *Poverty and Welfare in Scotland.* Edinburgh: Edinburgh University Press.

Lewis, J. (1991) The public's health: philosophy and practice in Britain in the twentieth century, in E. Fee and R. Acheson (eds) *A History of Education in Public Health.* Oxford: Oxford University Press.

Lewis, M. and Hartley, J. (2001) Evolving forms of quality management in local government: lessons from the best value pilot programme, *Policy and Politics,* 29(4): 477–96.

Lilford, R.J. and Braunholtz, D. (1996) The statistical basis of public policy: a paradigm shift is overdue, *British Medical Journal,* 313: 603–7.

Lilford, R.J. and Braunholtz, D. (2000) Who's afraid of Thomas Bayes? *Journal of Epidemiology and Community Health*, 54: 731–9.

Lindow, V. (1993) *User Participation in Community Care*. London: Department of Health, Community Care Support Unit.

Ling, T. (2000) Unpacking partnership: the case of health care, in J. Clarke, S. Gerwitz and E. McLuaghlin (eds) *New Managerialism, New Welfare?* London: Sage.

Lister, R. (2001) New Labour: a study in ambiguity from a position of ambivalence, *Critical Social Policy*, 21(4): 425–47.

Local Government Association and UK Public Health Association (2000) *Joint Response to the Public Health White Paper: Saving Lives: Our Healthier Nation*. London: Local Government Association.

Local Government Management Board (LGMB) (1994a) *Local Agenda 21: Principles and Process. A Step-by-Step Guide*. London: LGMB

Local Government Management Board (LGMB) (1994b) *Sustainability Indicators Research Project: Report of Phase One*. London: LGMB.

Lock, K. (2000) Health impact assessment, *British Medical Journal*, 320: 1395–8.

Longford, E. (2001) *Wellington*. London: Abbacus.

Low, J. (ed.) (2001) *Regeneration in the 21st century*. London: Policy Press.

Lowey, H., Fullard, B., Tocque, K. and Bellis, M. (2002) *Are Smoking Cessation Services Reducing Inequalities in Health?* Liverpool: North West Public Health Observatory.

Lowndes, V. and Skelcher, C. (1998) The dynamics of multi-organisational partnership: an analysis of changing modes of governance, *Public Administration*, 76(2).

Lucas, K., Grosvenor, T. and Simpson, R. (2001) *Transport, the Environment and social exclusion*. York: York Publishing Services.

Lupton, D. (1995) *The Imperative of Health: Public Health and the Regulated Body*. London: Sage.

Lupton, R. and Power, A. (2002) Social exclusion and neighbourhoods, in J. Hills and J. Le Grand (eds) *Understanding Social Exclusion*. Oxford: Oxford University Press.

Lupton, C. and Taylor, P. (1994) *Consumer Involvement in Healthcare Commissioning*. Portsmouth: Social Services Research and Information Unit, University of Portsmouth.

Lupton, C., Peckham, S. and Taylor, P. (1998) *Managing Public Involvement in Healthcare Purchasing*. Buckingham: Open University Press.

Lynch, M.A. and Cuninghame, C. (2000) Understanding the needs of young asylum seekers, *Archives of Disease in Childhood*, 38(5): 384–7.

Macdonald, J. (1992) *Primary Health Care: Medicine in its Place*. London: Earthscan.

MacDonald, G. (1998) Promoting evidence-based practice in child protection, *Clinical Child Psychology and Psychiatry*, 3(1): 71–85.

Macdonald, G.M., Sheldon, B. and Gillespie, J. (1992) Contemporary studies of the effectiveness of social work, *British Journal of Social Work*, 22(6): 5–43.

Macintyre, S. (1997) The Black report and beyond: what are the issues? *Social Science and Medicine*, 44(6): 723–45.

Macintyre, S. (2001) Memorandum, in House of Commons Health Select Committee, *Second Report for the Session 2000–2001*. London: The Stationery Office.

Macintyre, S., Maciver, S. and Soomans, A. (1998) Area, class and health: should we be focussing on places or people? *Journal of Social Policy*, 22(2): 213–34.

Macintyre, S., Chalmers, I., Horton, R. and Smith, R. (2001) Using evidence to inform health policy: case study, *British Medical Journal*, 322: 222–5.

Mackenbach, J.P. (1995) Public health epidemiology, *Journal of Epidemiology and Community Health*, 49: 333–4.

Mackenbach, J. and Bakker, M. (eds.) (2002) *Reducing Inequalities in Health: A European Perspective*. London: Routledge.

Mackintosh, M. (1993) Partnership: Issues of Policy and Negotiation, *Local Economy*, 7(3).

Maclennan, D. and More, A. (1999) Evidence, what evidence? The foundations for housing policy, *Public Policy and Management*, January–March.

MacMahon, B., Pugh, T.F. and Ipsen, J. (1960) *Epidemiological Methods*. Boston: Little, Brown and Co.

Macpherson, W. (1998) *Report of the Inquiry into the Death of Stephen Lawrence*. London: Home Office.

Maddock, S. and Morgan, G. (1997) *Barriers to Professional Collaboration and Inter-agency Working Within Health and Social Care*. Paper presented at the Public Services Research Unit Conference, May.

Maes, H.M., Neale, M.C. and Eaves, L.J. (1997) Genetic and environmental factors in relative body weight and human adiposity, *Behavior Genetics*, 27: 325–51.

MAFF (1998) *The Food Standards Agency; A Force for Change*. London: The Stationery Office.

Malmö Högskolen (1998) Utbildningskatalog 1998/99, Malmö, Sweden, *Management Decision*, 30(3): 50–6.

Marmot, M.G., Shipley, M.J. and Rose, G. (1984) Inequalities in death: specific explanations of a general pattern, *Lancet*, 1: 1003–6.

Marsh, A., Gordon, D., Heslop, P. and Pantazis, C. (2000) Housing deprivation and health: a longitudinal analysis, *Housing Studies*, 15(3): 411–29.

Martell, R. and Murray, K. (2001) Carers who cross a chasm, *Nursing Standard*, 16(4): 12.

Marwell, G. and Oliver, P. (1993) *The Critical Mass in Collective Action: A Micro-social Theory*. Cambridge: Cambridge University Press.

Matka, E., Barnes, M. and Sullivan, H. (2002) Health action zones: creating alliances to achieve change, *Policy Studies*, 23(2): 97–106.

Mayes, L.C., Horwitz, R.I., Feinstein, A.R. (1989) A collection of 56 topics with contradictory results in case-control research, *International Journal of Epidemiology*, 3: 725–7.

Mayo, M. (1997) Partnerships for regeneration and community development, *Critical Social Policy*, 52, 17(3), August.

McArthur, A. (1996) The active involvement of local residents in strategic community partnerships, *Policy and Politics*, 23(1): 61–71.

McCol, N.P. and Kruse, P. (2002) National radiological protection, technical handbook: *The National Arrangements for Incidents involving Radioactivity* (NAIR). London: NRPB.

McCormick, A., Fleming, D. and Charlton, J. (1995) *Morbidity Statistics from General Practice: Fourth National Study 1991–92*, Series MB5, No. 3. London: HMSO.

McIver, S. (1991) *Obtaining Views of Users of the Health Services*. London: King's Fund.

McKee, M. (2001) Epidemiology in the 21st century: the challenges ahead, *European Journal of Public Health*, 11: 241–2.

McKee, M., Stott, R. and Garner, P. (2001) *International Co-operation and Health*. Oxford: Oxford University Press.

McKeown, T. (1976) *The Modern Rise of Population*. London: Edward Arnold.

McMichael, M. (1999) Prisoners of the proximate: loosening the constraints on epidemiology in an age of change, *American Journal of Epidemiology*, 149: 887–97.

McMichael, A.J. and Beaglehole, R. (2000) The changing global context of public health, *Lancet*, 356: 495–9.

McPherson, K. (2001) Are disease prevention initiatives working? *Lancet*, 357: 1790–2.

McPherson, K. and Fox, J. (1997) Public health: an organized multidisciplinary effort, in G. Scally (ed) *Progress in Public Health*. London: Royal Society of Medicine Press.

McQueen, D.V. (2002) The evidence debate, *Journal of Epidemiology and Community Health*, 56: 83–4.

Meads, G., Killoran, A., Ashcroft, J. and Cornish, Y. (1999) *Mixing Oil and Water: How can Primary Care Organizations Improve Health as Well as Deliver Effective Health Care?* London: Health Education Authority.

Means, R., Brenton, M., Harrison, L. and Heywood, F. (1997) *Making Partnerships Work in Community Care: A Guide for Practitioners in Housing, Health and Social Services*. Bristol: Policy Press.

Medical Research Council (2000) *A Framework for Development and Evaluation of RCTs for Complex Interventions to Improve Health*. London: Medical Research Council.

Merkel, B. and Hubel, M. (1999) Public health policy in the European Community, in W. Holland and E. Mossialos (eds) *Public Health Policies in the European Union*. Aldershot: Ashgate.

Middleton, J. (2002) Doctors in public health. Who needs them? in A. Watterson (ed) *Public Health in Practice*. Basingstoke: Palgrave.

Milburn, A. (2000) *A Healthier Nation and a Healthier Economy: The Contribution of a Modern NHS*. LSE Health Annual Lecture, 8 March, London.

Milburn, A. (2002) *Tackling Health Inequalities, Improving Public Health*, Speech to the Faculty of Public Health Medicine, 20 November, London.

Milewa, T., Harrison, S., Ahmad, W. and Tovey, P. (2002) Citizens' participation in primary healthcare planning: innovative citizenship practice in empirical perspective, *Critical Public Health*, 12(1).

Miller, A. B. (1996) Review of extant community based epidemiological studies on health effects of hazardous wastes, *Toxicology and Industrial Health*, 12(2): 225–33.

Mindell, J., Hansell, A., Morrison, D., Douglas, M. and Joffe, M. (2001) What do we need for robust, quantitative health impact assessment (HIA)? *Journal of Public Health Medicine*, 23: 173–8.

Ministry of the Environment and Natural Resources (1992) *Eco Cycles: The Basis of Sustainable Urban Development*, SOU, 43. Stockholm: Ministry of the Environment and Natural Resources.

Mokdad, A.H., Serdula, M.N., Dietz, W.H. *et al.* (2000) The continuing epidemic of obesity in the United States, *Journal of the American Medical Association*, 284: 1650–1.

Molyneux, P. and Palmer, J. (2000) *A Partnership Approach to Health and Housing. A Good Practice Briefing for Primary Care Practitioners*. London: Health and Housing Network and UKPHA.

Mondros, A. and Wilson, S. (1994) *Organizing for Power and Empowerment*. New York: Columbia University Press.

Moon, G., Myles, G. and colleagues (2000) *Epidemiology: An Introduction*. Buckingham: Open University Press.

Mooney, G. (1989) QALYs: are they enough? A health economist's perspective, *Journal of Medical Ethics*, 15: 148–52.

Mooney, G.H. (1992) *Economics, Medicine and Healthcare*. Brighton: Wheatsheaf.

Morris, J.N. (1975) *Uses of Epidemiology*. Edinburgh: Churchill Livingstone.

Morris, J. (1991) *Pride Against Prejudice: Transforming Attitudes to Disability*. London: The Women's Press.

Morrow, V. (2002) Children's experiences of 'community': implications of social capital discourses, *Social Capital: Insights From Research*. London: Health Development Agency.

Mossialos, E. and McKee, M. (2002) Health care and the European Union, *British Medical Journal*, 324: 991–2.

Muir Gray, J. (2001) The public health professional as political activist, in D. Pencheon, C. Gust, D. Melzer and J. Muir Gray (eds) *Oxford Handbook of Public Health Practice*. Oxford: Oxford University Press.

Mulrow, C.D. (1995) Rationale for systematic reviews, in I. Chalmers and D.G. Altman (eds) *Systematic Reviews*. London: BMJ Publishing Group.

Murkerjee, M. (1995) Toxins abounding – despite the lessons of Bhopal chemical accidents are on the rise, *Scientific American*, June, pp. 15–16.

Mykhalovskiy, E. and McCoy, L. (2002) Troubling ruling discourses of health: using institutional ethnography in community – based research, *Critical Public Health*, 12(1): 17–37.

Naidoo, J. and Wills, J. (1998) *Practising Health Promotion: Dilemmas and Challenges*. London: Baillière Tindall.

Nash, V. (2002) *Reclaiming Community*. London: Institute for Public Policy Research.

National Assembly for Wales (NAW) (1999) *Developing a Health Impact Assessment Toolkit in Wales*. Cardiff: NAW.

National Association of County and City Health Officials (2002) *National Public Health Performance Standards Program* www.naccho.org/project48.cfm (accessed 2 December 2002).

National Audit Office (2002) *Facing the Challenge: NHS Emergency Planning in England*. Report by the Comptroller and Auditor General, HC 36 Session 2002–03, 15 November. www.nao.gov.uk/publications/nao_reports/02–03/020336es.pdf (accessed 24 January 2003).

National Health Services Management Executive (NHSME) (1992) *Local Voices: The Views of Local People in Purchasing for Health*. London: NHSME.

Navarro, V. (1998) Comment: Whose Globalization? *American Journal of Public Health*, 88(5): 742.

Nazroo, J. (1997) *The Health of Britain's Ethnic Minorities*. London: Policy Studies Institute.

Neighbourhood Renewal Unit (2001) *Accreditation Guidance for Local Strategic Partnerships*. London: Department of Transport, Local Government and the Regions.

Neighbourhood Renewal Unit (2002) *The Learning Curve: Developing Skills and Knowledge for Neighbourhood Renewal*. London: Neighbourhood Renewal Unit, Office of the Deputy Prime Minister.

Nettleton, S. (1998) Women and the new paradigm of medicine, *Critical Social Policy*, 18(2).

NHS Centre for Reviews and Dissemination (1995) *Review of the Research on the Effectiveness of Health Service Interventions to reduce Variations in Health*. York: University of York.

NHS Centre for Reviews and Dissemination (2000a) *Evidence from Systematic Reviews of Research Relevant to Implementing the Wider Public Health Agenda*. York: University of York.

NHS Centre for Reviews and Dissemination (2000b) Promoting the initiation of breast-feeding, *Effective Healthcare Bulletin*, 6(2). York: NHS Centre for Reviews and Dissemination, University of York.

NHS Executive (1998a) *Establishing Primary Care Groups*, HSC 1998/065. Leeds: NHS Executive.

NHS Executive (1998b) Department of Health NHS executive guidance, *Planning for a Major Incident*. London: The Stationery Office.

NHS Executive (1999) *Quality and Performance in the NHS: High Level Performance Indicators*. Leeds: NHS Executive.

Nord, E. (1990) Unjustified use of the quality of well being scale in priority-setting in Oregon, *Health Policy*, 24(1): 943–4.

Nord, E. (1999) *Cost-value Analysis in Health Care* http://assets.cambridge.org/0521643082/sample/0521643082WSN01.pdf (accessed 30 August 2002).

North, D. (1990) *Institutions, Institutional Change and Economic Performance*. Cambridge: Cambridge University Press.

North, N. (1991) Neighbourhoods: the local population as health care consumers, citizens or providers? *Critical Public Health*, 4: 8–15.

Northern Ireland Department of Health and Social Services (1995) *Regional Strategy for Health and Social Well-being 1997–2002*. Belfast: Northern Ireland Department of Health and Social Services.

Northern Ireland Department of Health and Social Services Voluntary Activity Unit (1996) *Monitoring and Evaluating Community Development in Northern Ireland*. Belfast: Northern Ireland Department of Health and Social Services.

Northern Ireland Executive (2002) *Investing for Health*. Belfast: Department of Health Social Services and Public Safety.

Nutbeam, D. (2002) Unpublished address to UK Public Health Alliance Conference, March, Glasgow.

Nutbeam, B. and Wise, M. (2002) Structures and strategies for public health intervention, in R. Detels, J. McEwen, R. Beaglehole and H. Tanaka (eds) *Oxford Textbook of Public Health Volume 3. The Practice of Public Health*. (4th edn). Oxford: Oxford University Press.

Nutley, S., Davies, H. and Walter, I. (2002) *Evidence Based Policy and Practice: Cross Sector Lessons from the UK*. Working paper 9. London: ESRC Centre for Evidence Based Policy and Practice, University of London.

O'Brien, M. (2000) Have lessons been learned from the UK bovine spongiform encephalopathy (BSE) epidemic? *International Journal of Epidemiology*, 29: 730–3.

O'Keefe, E. (2000) Equity, democracy and globalisation, *Critical Public Health*, 10(2): 167–77.

O'Neill, J. (1996) Cost benefit analysis: rationality and the plurality of values, *The Ecologist*, 16(3): 98–103.

Oakley, A., Rajan, L. and Grant, A. (1990) Social support and pregnancy outcome, *British Journal of Obstetrics and Gynaecology*, 97: 155–62.

Oliver, M. (1996) *Understanding Disability: From Theory to Practice*. London: Macmillan.

Oliver, M. and Barnes, C. (1998) *Disabled People and Social Policy: From Exclusion to Inclusion*. London: Longman.

Organisation for Economic Cooperation and Development (OECD) (1996) *Integrating Environment and Economy: Progress in the 1990s*. Paris: OECD.

Organisation for Economic Cooperation and Development (OECD) (2001) *Public Sector Leadership for the 21st Century*. Paris: OECD.

Ormerod, P. (1994) *The Death of Economics*. London: Faber & Faber.

Ottewill, R. and Wall, A. (1990) *The Growth and Development of Community Health Services*. Sunderland: Business Education Publishers.

Owen, D. (1965) *English Philanthropy 1660–1960*. Cambridge, MA: Harvard University Press.

Page, D. (2000) *Communities in the Balance: The Reality of Social Exclusion on Housing Estates*. York: York Publishing Services.

Pan American Health Organization (2000) *Essential Public Health Functions* www.paho.org/english/gov/cd/cd42_15-e.pdf (accessed 2 December 2002).

Pareto, V. (1935) *Mind and Society*. New York: Harcourt Brace Javanovich.

Partners in Change (2001) *Communities and Health – Report from Outcomes Workshop*. Edinburgh: Partners in Change.

Patterson, I. and Judge, K. (2002) Equality of access to healthcare, in J. Mackenbach and M. Bakker (eds) *Reducing Inequalities in Health: A European Perspective*. London: Routledge.

Patterson, W.J. and Painter, M.J. (1999) Bovine spongiform encephalopathy and new variant Creutzfeldt-Jakob disease: an overview, *Communicable Disease and Public Health*, 2: 5–13.

Pawson, R. (2002a) Evidence-based policy: in search of a method, *Evaluation*, April, 8(2): 157–81.

Pawson, R. (2002b) *Evidence Based Policy: II. The Promise of 'Realist Synthesis'*. Working paper 4. London: ESRC Centre for Evidence Based Policy and Practice, University of London.

Pawson, R. (2002c) *Does Megan's Law work? A Theory-driven Systematic Review*. Working paper 8. London: ESRC Centre for Evidence Based Policy and Practice, University of London.

Pawson, R. and Tilley, N. (1997) *Realistic Evaluation*. London: Sage.

Payne, N. and Saul, C. (1997) Variations in use of cardiology services in a health authority: comparison of coronary artery revascularisation rates with prevalence of angina and coronary mortality, *British Medical Journal*, 314: 257–61.

Pearce, N. (1996) Traditional epidemiology, modern epidemiology and public health, *American Journal of Public Health*, 86(5): 678–83.

Pearce, I.H. and Crocker, L.H. (1943) *The Peckham Experiment: A Study of the Living Structure of Society*. London: Allen & Unwin.

Pearce, D., Barbier, E. and Markayanda, A. (1990) *Sustainable Development*. London: Earthscan.

Peckham, S. and Exworthy, M. (2003) *Primary Care in the UK: Policy, Organization and Management*. Basingstoke: Macmillan/Palgrave.

Pencheon, D., Gust, C., Melzer, D. and Muir Gray, J. (eds) (2001) *Oxford Handbook of Public Health Practice*. Oxford: Oxford University Press.

Pereira, J. (1993) What does equity in health mean? *Journal of Social Policy*, 22(1): 19–48.

Petersen, A. and Lupton, D. (1996) *The New Public Health*. London: Sage.

Pfeffer, J. (1992) *Managing with Power: Politics and Influence in Organizations*. Boston: Harvard Business School Press.

Phillips Report (2000) *BSE Enquiry Report*. London: HMSO.

Pickard, S. (1998) Citizenship and consumerism in healthcare: a critique of citizens' juries, *Social Policy and Administration*, 32: 226–44.

Pilisuk, M. and Parks, S.H. (1986) *The Healing Web: Social Networks and Human Survival*. Hanover, NE: University Press of New England.

Pill, R. and Stott, N.C.H. (1982) Concept of illness causation and responsibility, *Social Science and Medicine*, 16: 43–52.

Plsek, P.E. and Greenhalgh, T. (2001) The challenge of complexity in health care, *British Medical Journal*, 323: 625–8.

Policy Action Team 17 (2000) *Joining it up Locally, National Strategy for Neighbourhood Renewal*. London: Department of the Environment, Transport and the Regions.

Pollitt, C. (1993) *Managerialism and the Public Services*, 2nd edn. Oxford: Blackwell.

Pollock, A. and Price, D. (2000) Globalisation? Privatisation! *Health Matters*, 41: 12–13.

Pollock, A., Shaoul, J., Rowland, D. and Player, S. (2001) *Public Services and the Private Sector: A Response to the IPPR*. A catalyst working paper. London: Catalyst.

Popay, J. (ed.) (2001) *Regeneration and Health: A Selected Review of Research*. London: King's Fund.

Popay, J., Williams, G., Thomas, C. and Gatrell, T. (1998) Theorising inequalities in health: the place of lay knowledge, *Sociology of Health and Illness*, 20(5): 619–44.

Porter, M. and MacIntyre, S. (1984) What is, must be best: a research note on Conservative or deferential responses to antenatal care provision, *Social Science and Medicine*, 19: 1197–200.

Portes, A. (1998) Social capital – its origin and applications in modern society, *Annual Review of Sociology*, 24: 1–24.

Powell, M. (1998) *New Labour, New Welfare State? The 'Third Way' in British Social Policy.* Bristol: Policy Press.

Powell, M. (2000) New Labour and the third way in the British welfare state: a new and distinctive approach? *Critical Social Policy*, February, 20(1): 39–59.

Powell, M. and Exworthy, M. (2001) Joined-up solutions to address health inequalities analysing policy, process and resource streams, *Public Money and Management*, January–March, pp. 21–6.

Powell, M. and Exworthy, M. (2002) Partnerships, quasi-networks and social policy, in C. Glendinning, M. Powell and K. Rummery (eds) *Partnerships, New Labour and the Governance of Welfare*. Bristol: Policy Press.

Powell, M. and Glendinning, C. (2002) Introduction, in C. Glendinning, M. Powell and K. Rummery (eds) *Partnerships, New Labour and the Governance of Welfare*. Bristol: Policy Press.

Power, A. and Tunstall, R. (1995) *Swimming Against the Tide: Polarisation or Progress on 20 Unpopular Council Estates*. York: Joseph Rowntree Foundation.

Pratt, J. (1995) *Practitioner and Practices: A Conflict of Values*. Oxford: Radcliffe Medical Press.

Pratt, J., Plamping, D and Gordon, P. (1998) *Partnership Fit for Purpose?* London: King's Fund.

Price, C. and Tsouros, A. (eds) (1996) *Our Cities, Our Future*. Copenhagen: WHO.

Price, D., Pollock, A.M. and Shaoul, J. (1999) How the World Trade Organisation is shaping domestic policies in health care, *Lancet*, 354: 1889–91.

Pugh, G. (ed.) (1997) *Partnerships in Action*. London: NCB.

Purdue, D., Razzaque, K., Hambleton, R. and Stewart, M. (2000) *Community Leadership in Urban Regeneration*. Bristol: Policy Press.

Putnam, R. (1993) *Making Democracy Work: Civic Traditions in Modern Italy*. Princeton, NJ: Princeton University Press.

Putnam, R. (2000) *Bowling Alone – The Collapse and Revival of American Community*. London: Simon and Shuster.

Radford, G., Lapthorne, D., Boot, N. and Maconachie, M. (1997) Community development and social deprivation, in G. Scally (ed.) *Progress in Public Health*. London: FT Healthcare.

Ranade, W. (1998) *A Future for the NHS? Health Care for the Millennium*. Harlow: Longman.

Randall, E. (2001): *The European Union and Health Policy*. Basingstoke: Palgrave.

Raphael, D. and Bryant, T. (2002) The limitations of population health as a model for a new public health, *Health Promotion International*, 17(2): 189–99.

Rawles, J. (1972) *A Theory of Justice*. Oxford: Oxford University Press.

Rawles, J. (1989) Castigating QALYs, *The Journal of Medical Ethics*, 15: 143–7.

Rawnsley, A. (2001) *Servants of the People: The Inside Story of New Labour*. London: Penguin.

Rees, W. (1992) Ecological footprints and appropriated carrying capacity: what urban economics leaves out, *Environment and Urbanisation*, 4(2): 121–30.

Rees, W.E. (1998), Is 'sustainable city' an oxymoron? *Local Environment*, October, 2(3): 303–10.

Refugee Council (2002) *Government Announcement and Proposal Since its White Paper on Asylum: A Summary*. London: Refugee Council.

Regan, M. (1999) Health protection in the next millennium: from tactics to strategy, *Journal of Epidemiology and Community Health*, 53: 517–18.

Richards, S., Barnes, M., Coulson, A. *et al.* (1999) *Cross-cutting Issues in Public Policy and Public Services*. London: DETR.

Richardson, A. and Goodman, M. (1983) *Self Help and Mutual Care: Mutual Aid Organisations in Practice*. London: Policy Studies Institute.

Richardson, L. and Mumford, C. (2002) Community, neighbourhood and social infrastructure, in J. Hills and J. Le Grand (eds) *Understanding Social Exclusion*. Oxford: Oxford University Press.

Ritzer, G. (1993) *The McDonaldization of Society*. London: Sage.

Roberts, E. (1992) *Healthy Participation: An Evaluative Study of the Hartcliffe Health and Environment Action Group – A Community Development Project in South Bristol*. London: South Bank Polytechnic.

Roberts, H. (2000) *What Works in Reducing Inequalities in Child Health*. Barkingside: Barnardo's.

Roberts, V., Russell, H., Harding, A. and Parkinson, M. (1995) *Public/Private Voluntary Partnerships in Local Government*. Luton: Local Government Management Board.

Robinson, T.P. (2000) Spatial statistics and geographical information systems in epidemiology and public health, *Advances in Parasitology*, 47: 81–128.

Robson B., Brodford, M. and Deas, I. (1994) *Assessing the Impact of Urban Policy*. London: HMSO.

Rose, G. (1985) Sick individuals and sick populations, *International Journal of Epidemiology*, 14: 32–8.

Rostow, W.W. (1966) *The Stages of Economic Growth: A Non-communist Manifesto*. Cambridge: Cambridge University Press.

Rowntree, S. (1901) *Poverty: A Study of Town Life*. London: Macmillan.

Rowson, M. (2000) Blueprint for an unequal world, *Health Matters*, 41: 10–11.

Rowson, M. and Koivusalo, M. (2000) Who will inherit the earth? *Health Matters*, 41: 16–17.

Royal Society (1992) *Risk: Analysis, Perception and Management*. London: The Royal Society.

Rummery, K. and Glendinning, C. (1997) *Working Together: Primary Care Involvement in Commissioning Social Care Services. Debates in Primary Care No2*. Manchester: NPCRDC, University of Manchester.

Russell, H. (2001) *Local Strategic Partnerships: Lessons from New Commitment to Regeneration*. Bristol: Policy Press.

Russell, H. and Killoran, A. (1999) *Public Health and Regeneration: Making the Links*. London: Health Education Authority.

Rychetnik, L., Frommer, M., Hawe, P. and Shiell, A. (2002) Criteria for evaluating evidence on public health interventions, *Journal of Epidemiology and Community Health*, 56: 119–27.

Sachs, J. (2000) A new map of the world, *Economist*, 355(8176): 81–3.

Saffron, L. (1993) The consumers perception of risk, *Consumer Policy Review*, 3(4): 213–21.

Samuelson, P. (1976) *Economics: An Introductory Analysis*. Tokyo: McGraw-Hill.

Sandford, I. (2001) *Mainstreaming of HAZ Projects in LSL*. Lambeth. Southwark and Lewisham: HAZ.

Santillo, D., Johnstone, P. and Singhofen, A. (1999) *The Way Forward – Out of the Chemical Crisis*. Stockholm: Greenpeace International.

Sassi, F., Archard, L. and Le Grand, J. (2001) Equity and health care economic evaluation, *Health Technology Assessment*, 5(3).

Scally, G. (ed). (1997) *Progress in Public Health*. London: Financial Times Healthcare.

SCDC (Scottish Community Development Centre) (2001) *Achieving Better Community Development* http://www.scdc.org.uk/abcd_summary.htm (accessed 20 July 2002).

Schein, E. (1993) On dialogue, culture, and organisational learning, *Organisational Dynamics*, autumn, 22(3): 40–51.

Schuller, T., Baron, S. and Field, J. (2000) Social capital: a review and critique, *Social Capital: Critical Perspectives*. Oxford: Oxford University Press.

Schwartz, S. (1994) The fallacy of the ecological fallacy: the potential misuse of a concept and the consequences, *American Journal of Public Health*, 84(5): 819–24.

Scott, T. (2002) *Report of the First Meeting of the Joint NHS Leadership Centre and Faculty of Public Health Medicine, Public Health Leadership Thinking and Planning Group*, 16/17 May. Oxford: NHS Leadership Centre.

Scottish Executive (1998) *Working Together for a Healthier Scotland*, Cm 3854. Edinburgh: The Stationery Office.

Scottish Executive Health Department (2001) *Our National Health: A Plan for Action, a Plan for Change*. Edinburgh: Scottish Executive Health Department.

Scottish Office Department of Health (1999) *Towards a Healthier Scotland*. Edinburgh: The Stationery Office.

Scott-Samuel, A. (1998) Health impact assessment – theory into practice, *Journal of Epidemiology and Community Health*, 52: 704–5.

Scott-Samuel, A., Birley, M. and Arden, K. (eds) (2001) *The Merseyside Guidelines for Health Impact Assessment* (2nd edn). Liverpool: International Health Impact Consortium.

Scriven, A. and Orme, J. (2001) *Health Promotion: Professional Perspectives*, 2nd edn. Basingstoke: Palgrave/Open University.

Secretary of State for Health (1992) *The Health of the Nation. A Strategy for Health in England*, Cm 1986. London: HMSO.

Secretary of State for Health (1999) *Saving Lives: Our Healthier Nation*, Cm 4386. London: The Stationery Office.

Secretary of State for Health (2000) *The NHS Plan: A Plan for Investment, a Plan for Reform*, Cm 4818. London: The Stationery Office.

Secretary of State for Northern Ireland (1998) *Fit for the Future: A Consultation Document on the Government's Proposals for the Future of Health and Personal Social Services in Northern Ireland*. Belfast: The Stationery Office.

Secretary of State for Wales (1998) *NHS Wales: Putting Patients First*, CMB 3841. Cardiff: The Stationery Office.

Sefton, T., Byford, S., McDaid, D., Hills, J. and Knapp, M. (2002) *Making the Most of It: Economic Evaluation in the Social Welfare Field*. York: York Publishing Service.

Senge, P. (1999) *The Dance of Change: The Challenge of Sustaining Momentum in Learning Organisations*. London: Nicholas Brealey.

Service Users Advisory Group (2001) *Nothing About Us Without Us*. London: Department of Health.

Shaper, A.G., Pocock, S.J., Phillips, A.W. and Walker, M. (1987) A scoring system to identify men at high risk of heart attack, *Health Trends*, 19: 37–9.

Shapiro, S. (1994) Meta-analysis/schmeta-analysis, *American Journal of Epidemiology*, 140: 771–8.

Shaw, S. and Abbott, S. (2002) Too much to handle? *Health Service Journal*, 27 June, pp. 28–9.

Shaw, M., Dorling, D., Gordon, D. and Davey Smith, G. (1999) *The Widening Gap: Health Inequalities and Policy in Britain*. Bristol: Policy Press.

Sherman, L.W., Farrington, D.P., Welsh, B.C. and Mackenzie, D.L. (eds) (2002) *Evidence-based Crime Prevention*. London: Routledge.

Shiell, A. and Hawe, P. (1996) Health promotion, community development and the tyranny of individualism, *Health Economics*, 5: 241–7.

Shiva, V. (2000) *Respect for the Earth: Globalisation*, http://news.bbc.co.uk/hi/english/static/events/reith_2000/lecture5.stm

Silburn, R., Lucas, D., Page, R. and Hanna, L. (1999) *Neighbourhood Images in Nottingham*, JRF Area Regeneration Series. York: York Publishing Services.

Silverman, D. (1998) The quality of qualitative health research: the open-ended interview and its alternatives, *Social Sciences in Health*, 4(2).

Singleton, C. and Aird, B. (2002) As good as new: will the primary care infrastructure deliver the public health agenda? *Health Service Journal*, 27 June, pp. 28–9.

Skeffington, A. (1969) *People and Planning*. London: HMSO.

Skelcher, C., McCabe, A. and Lowndes, V. with Nanton, P. (1996) *Community Networks in Urban Regeneration*. Bristol: Policy Press.

Skills for Health (2002a) *National Occupational Standards/Competencies for Public Health Practice*. Bristol: Skills for Health.

Skills for Health (2002b) *Functional Map of Public Health Practice*. Bristol: Skills for Health.

Skinner, S. and Wilson, M. (2001) *Assessing Community Strengths*. London: Community Development Foundation.

Smaje, C. (1996) The ethnic patterning of health: new directions for theory and research, *Sociology of Illness and Health*, 18(2): 139–71.

Smithies, J. and Adams, L. (1990) *Community Participation in Health Promotion*. London: Health Education Authority.

Smithies, J. and Webster, G. (1998) *Community Involvement in Health: From Passive Recipients to Active Participants*. Aldershot: Ashgate.

Social Exclusion Unit (1998) *Bringing Britain Together: A National Strategy for Neighbourhood Renewal*. Cm 4045. London: HMSO.

Social Exclusion Unit (2000) *National Strategy for Neighbourhood Renewal*. London: HMSO.

Social Exclusion Unit (2001a) *A New Commitment to Neighbourhood Renewal: National Strategy Action Plan*. London: Cabinet Office.

Social Exclusion Unit (2001b) *National Strategy for Neighbourhood Renewal: A Framework for Consultation*. London: Cabinet Office.

Social Exclusion Unit (2002) *Transport and Social Exclusion*. London: Cabinet Office.

Solesbury, W. (2002) The ascendancy of evidence, *Planning Theory and Practice*, 3(1): 90–6.

Spear, S. (2003) Terrorism contingency planning saved lives during last legionnaires outbreak, *Environmental Health News*, 16 January.

Spencer, K. (1982) Comprehensive Community Programmes, in S. Leach and and J. Stewart (eds) *Approaches to Public Policy*. London: Allen & Unwin.

Spiegelhalter, D.J., Myles, J.P., Jones, D.R. and Abrams, K.R. (1999) An introduction to Bayesian methods in health technology assessment, *British Medical Journal*, 319: 508–12.

Stacey M, (1960) *Tradition and Change: A Study of Banbury*. Oxford: Oxford University Press.

Stacey, M. (1969) The myth of community studies, *British Journal of Sociology*, 20(2): 134–47.

Stacey, M. (1976) The health service consumer: a sociological misconception, in M. Stacey (ed) *Sociology of the NHS*, Sociological Monograph no 22. Keele: University of Keele.

Stafford, M., Bartley, M., Wilkinson, R. *et al.* (2002) *Healthy Neighbourhoods: Investigating the Role of Social Cohesion*. Paper presented to the Health Development Agency conference Social Action for Health and Wellbeing: Experiences from Policy, Research and Practice, 20–1 June, London.

Standing Conference for Community Development (SCCD) (2001) *Strategic Framework for Community Development*. Sheffield: SCCD.

Starfield, B. (1998) *Primary Care: Balancing Health Needs, Services and Technology*. New York: Oxford University Press.

Starkey, F., Taylor, P. and Means, R. (2001) Coming to terms with primary care trusts: the views of PCG board members, *Managing Community Care*, 9(2): 22–9.

Stein, Z., Susser, M., Saenger, G. and Marolla, F. (1975) *Famine and Human Development: the Dutch Hunger Winter of 1944–45*. New York: Oxford University Press.

Stephens, C. (2000) La globalisacion nos matan – globalisation is killing us, *Health Matters*, 41: 6–8.

Stewart, M. (2000) Local action to counter exclusion: a research review, *Joining It Up Locally – The Evidence Base*, report of Policy Action Team 17, volume 2. London: DETR.

Stewart, M. (2002) *Systems Governance: Towards Effective Partnership Working*. Paper to the HAD Seminar Series on Tackling Health Inequalities, September, London.

Stewart, M., Goss, S., Clarke, R. *et al.* (1999) *Cross-cutting Issues Affecting Local Government*. London: DETR.

Stewart-Brown, L. and Prothero, L. (1988) Evaluation in community development, *Health Education Journal*, 4447(4): 156–61.

Stewart-Brown, S., Shaw, R. and Morgan, L. (2002) *Social Capital in the Home and Health in Later Life*. Paper presented to the Health Development Agency conference Social Action for Health and Wellbeing: Experiences from Policy, Research and Practice, 20–1 June, London.

Strachey, L. ([1918] 1948) *Eminent Victorians*. London: Penguin.

Sullivan, H. (2001) Maximising the contributions of neighbourhoods – the role of community governance, *Public Policy and Administration*, 16(2): 29–48.

Sullivan, H., Root, A., Moran, D. and Smith, M. (2001) *Area Committees and Neighbourhood Management*. London: Local Government Information Unit.

Summerton, N. (1999) Accrediting research practices, *British Journal of General Practice*, 49(438): 63–4.

Susser, M. and Susser, E. (1996a) Choosing a future for epidemiology: I. Eras and paradigms, *American Journal of Public Health*, 86(5): 668–73.

Susser, M. and Susser, E. (1996b) Choosing a future for epidemiology: II. From black box to Chinese boxes and eco-epidemiology, *American Journal of Public Health*, 86(5): 674–7.

Swann, C. and Morgan, A. (2002) *Social Capital: Insights From Research*. London: Health Development Agency.

Swann, C., Falce, C., Morgan, A. and Kelly, M. (2002) *HDA Evidence Base. Work in Progress. Process and Quality Standards Manual for Evidence Briefings*. Health Development Agency (http://194.83.94.80/hda/docs/evidence/eb2000/corehtml/ebmanual.pdf).

SWPHO (South West Public Health Observatory) (2002) *Waste Management and Public Health: The State of the Evidence. A Review of the Epidemiological Research on the Impact of Waste Management Activities on Health*. London: SWPHO.

Tarrow, S. (1994) *Power in Movement: Social Movements, Collective Action and Politics*. Cambridge: Cambridge University Press.

Taylor, M. (1995) *Unleashing the Potential: Bringing Residents to the Centre of Regeneration*. York: Joseph Rowntree Foundation.

Taylor, M. (1997) *The Best of Both Worlds: The Voluntary Sector and Local Government*. York: Joseph Rowntree Foundation.

Taylor, M. (2000) Communities in the lead: organisational capacity and social capital, *Urban Studies*, 37(5–6): 1019–35.

Taylor, P. (2002) *Understanding the Policy Maze*. Glasgow: Community Health Exchange, Glasgow Healthy City Partnership and Health Education Board for Scotland.

Taylor, L. and Blair-Stevens, C. (eds) (2002) *Introducing Health Impact Assessment (HIA): Informing the Decision-making Process*. London: Health Development Agency.

Taylor, R. and Guest, C. (2001) Protecting health, sustaining the environment, in D. Pencheon, C. Guest, D. Melzer and J.A. Muir Gray (eds) *Oxford Handbook of Public Health Practice*. Oxford: Oxford University Press.

Taylor, M. and Hoggett, P. (1994) Trusting in networks? The third sector and welfare change, in P. Vidal and I. Vidal (eds) *Delivering Welfare: Repositioning Non-profit and Co-operative Action in Western European Welfare States*. Barcelona: Centro de Iniciativas de la Economia Social.

Taylor, P., Peckham, S. and Turton, P. (1998) *A Public Health Model of Primary Care – From Concept to Reality*. Birmingham: UK Public Health Association.

Terry, F. (1999) The impact of evidence on transport policy-making: the case of road construction, *Public Policy and Management*, January–March.

Thompson, H., Pettrigrew, M. and Morrison, D. (2002) *Housing Improvement and Health Gain: A Systematic Review*. Occasional paper no. 5. Glasgow: MRC Social and Public Health Sciences Unit, Glasgow.

Tilley, N. and Laycock, G. (2002) *Working Out What to Do; Evidence-based Crime Reduction*. Crime reduction research paper 11. London: Home Office Policing and Reducing Crime Unit.

Titmuss, R.M. (1943) *Birth, Poverty and Wealth*. Philadelphia, PA: University of Pennsylvania Press.

Tones, K. (2001) Health promotion: the empowerment imperative, in A. Scriven and J. Orme (eds) *Health Promotion: Professional Perspectives*. Basingstoke: Palgrave.

Towner, E., Dowswell, T. and Jarvis, S. (1993) *The Effectiveness of Health Promotion Interventions in the Prevention of Unintentional Childhood Injury: A Review of the Literature*. London: Health Education Authority.

Townsend, P. (ed) (1988) *Inequalities in Health*. London: Penguin.

Townsend, P., Davidson, N. and Whitehead, M. (eds) (1992) *Inequalities in Health*. London: Penguin.

Tudor-Hart, J. (1988) *A New Kind of Doctor*. London: Merlin Press.

Turner, B. (1985) *Health and Illness*. London: Allen & Unwin.

Turner, B.S. (2001) Risks, rights and regulation: an overview, *Health, Risk and Society*, 3(1): 9–17.

Ukoumunne, O.C., Gulliford, M.C., Chinn, S. *et al.* (1999) Evaluation of health interventions at area and organisation level, *British Medical Journal*, 319: 376–9.

UNCED (United Nations Conference on Environment and Development) (1992a) *Agenda 21*. Rio de Janeiro: UNCED.

UNCED (United Nations Conference on Environment and Development) (1992b) *The Rio Declaration on Environment and Development*. Rio de Janeiro: UNCED.

United Nations (UN) (1992) *Earth Summit. Agenda 21: The United Nations Programme of Action from Rio*. New York: UN Department of Information.

United Nations (UN) (1996) *World Urbanization Prospects Database – 1996 Revision*. New York: UN Department of Economic and Social Affairs, Population Division.

United Nations (UN) (1998) *World Population Estimates and Projections – 1998 Revision*. New York: UN Department of Economic and Social Affairs, Population Division.

United Nations Development Programme (1999) *Human Development Report 1999: Globalisation With a Human Face*. Oxford: Oxford University Press.

United Nations Development Programme (2001) *Human Development Report 2001* http://www.undp.org/hdr2001/

Vaill, P. (1999) *Spirited Leading and Learning: Process Wisdom for a New Age*. Englewood Cliffs: Prentice-Hall.

Von Korff, M., Koepsell, T., Curry, S. and Diehr, P. (1992) Multi-level analysis in epidemiologic research on health behaviors and outcomes, *American Journal of Epidemiology*, 135(10): 1077–82.

Von Pettenkofer, M. ([1873]1941) The value of health to a city: Two lectures delivered in 1873. Baltimore: The Johns Hopkins Press.

Walker, P., Lewis, J., Lingayah, S. and Sommer, F. (2000) *Prove it! Measuring the Effect of Neighbourhood Renewal on Local People*. London: New Economics Foundation.

Wallerstein, I. (1979) *The Capitalist World Economy*. Cambridge: Cambridge University Press.

Wallerstein, N. (1993) Empowerment and health: theory and practice of community change, *Community Development Journal*, 28: 218–27.

Walsh, J.A. and Warren, K.S. (1979) Selective primary care: an interim strategy for disease control in developing countries, *New England Journal of Medicine*, 301: 967–74.

Walt, G. (1998) Globalisation of international health, *Lancet*, 351: 429–33.

Wanless, D. (2001) *Securing our Future Health: Taking a Long-Term View.* Interim Report. London: HM Treasury.

Wanless, D. (2002) *Securing our Future Health: Taking a Long-Term View. Final Report.* London: HM Treasury.

Wanless Report (2002) *NHS Funding and Reform: The Wanless Report.* Research paper 02/30 http://www.parliament.uk/commons/lib/research/rp2002/rp02–030.pdf (accessed 17 July 2002).

Warren, R., Rose, S. and Bergunder, A. (1974) *The Structure of Urban Reform.* Lexington, MA: Lexington Books.

Waters, M. (1995) *Globalisation.* London: Routledge.

Webster, B. (1982) Area management and responsive policy-making, in S. Leach and J. Stewart (eds) *Approaches to Public Policy.* London: Allen & Unwin.

Weinstein, M. and Stason, W. (1977) Foundations of cost-effectiveness analysis for health and medical practices, *New England Journal of Medicine*, 31 March, 296(13): 716–21.

Weiss, C.H. (1995) Nothing as practical as good theory: exploring theory-based evaluation for comprehensive community initiatives for children and families, in J. Connell *et al.* (eds) *New Approaches to evaluating Community Based Initiatives: Concepts, Methods and Contexts.* Washington, DC: Aspen Institute.

Welford, R. (1995) *Environmental Strategy and Sustainable Development: The Corporate Challenge for the Twenty-First Century.* London: Routledge.

Wellman, B. (1979) The community question: the intimate networks of East Yorkers, *American Journal of Sociology*, 84: 1201–31.

Welsh Assembly Government (2002) *Well-being in Wales: Consultation Document.* Cardiff: Public Health Strategy Group, Office of Chief Medical Officer, Welsh Assembly Government.

White, A.K. and Johnson, M. (2000) Men making sense of chest pain – niggles, doubts and denials, *Journal of Clinical Nursing*, 9: 534–41.

Whitehead, M. (1995) Tackling inequalities: a review of policy initiatives, in M. Benzeval, K. Judge and M. Whitehead (eds) *Tackling Inequalities in Health: An Agenda for Action.* London: King's Fund.

Widgery, D. (1991) *Some Lives! A GP's East End.* London: Sinclair-Stevenson.

Wilkin, D., Gillam, S. and Coleman, A. (eds) (2001) *The National Tracker Survey of Primary Care Groups and Trusts 2000/2001: Modernising the NHS?* Manchester: National Primary Care Research and Development Centre, University of Manchester.

Wilkin, D., Coleman, A., Dowling, B. and Smith, K. (2002) *The National Tracker Survey of Primary Care Groups and Trusts 2001/2002: Taking Responsibility?* Manchester: National Primary Care Research and Development Centre, University of Manchester.

Wilkinson, R. (1996) *Unhealthy Societies: The Affliction of Inequality.* London: Routledge.

Wilkinson, R.G. (1997) Health inequalities: relative or absolute material standards? *British Medical Journal*, 314: 591–5.

Wilkinson, R. (2000) *Mind the Gap: Hierarchies, Health and Human Evolution.* London: Weidenfield.

Wilkinson, R. and Marmot, M. (eds) (1998) *The Solid Facts: Social Determinants of Health.* Copenhagen: Regional Office for Europe, WHO.

Williams, A. (1985) The economics of coronary artery bypass grafting, *British Medical Journal*, 291: 326–9.

Williams, A. (1999) Calculating the global burden of disease: time for a strategic reappraisal? *Health Economics*, 8: 1–8.

Williams, G. and Popay, J. (2002) Lay knowledge and the privilege of experience, in J. Gabe, D. Kelleher and G. Williams (eds) *Challenging Medicine*. London: Routledge.

Williams, C. and Windebank, J. (2000) Helping each other out? Community exchange in deprived neighbourhoods, *Community Development Journal*, 35(2): 146–56.

Williamson, O. (1975) *Markets and Hierarchies: Analysis and Antitrust Implications*. London: The Free Press.

Williamson, C. (1992) *Whose Standards? Consumer and Professional Standards in Health Care*. Oxford: Oxford University Press.

Willmott, P. and Young, M. (1960) *Family and Class in a London Suburb*. London: Routledge and Kegan Paul.

Wilson, G. (1998) Staff and users in the postmodern organisation: Modernity, postmodernity and user marginalisation, in M. Barry and C. Hallett (eds). *Social Exclusion and Social Work: Issues of Theory, Policy and Practice*. Lyme Regis: Russell House.

Winkler, F. (1987) Consumerism in health care: beyond the supermarket model, *Policy and Politics*, 15: 1–8.

Wistow, G. and Barnes, M. (1993) User involvement in community care: origins, purposes and applications, *Public Administration*, 71: 279–99.

Wong, K. and Butler, G. (2000) *Taking Asylum: A Guide to Community Safety Partnerships on Responding to the Immigration and Asylum Act 1999*. London: National Association for the Care and Rehabilitation of Offenders.

Wood, M. and Vamplew, C. (1999) *Neighbourhood Images of Teesside JRF Area*, Regeneration Series. York: York Publishing Services.

Woodhead, D., Jochelson, K. and Tennant, R. (2002) *Public Health in the Balance: Getting it Right for London*. London: King's Fund.

World Commission on Environment and Development (1987) *Our Common Future (The Brundtland Report)*. Oxford: Oxford University Press.

WHO (World Health Organisation) (1946) *Constitution*. Geneva: WHO.

WHO (World Health Organisation) (1978) *Report on the International Conference on Primary Care, Alma Ata, 6–12 September*. Geneva: WHO.

WHO (World Health Organisation) (1981) *Global Strategy for Health for All by the Year 2000*. Geneva: WHO.

WHO (World Health Organisation) (1985) *Health For All in Europe by the Year 2000, Regional Targets*, Copenhagen: WHO.

WHO (World Health Organisation) (1986) *Ottawa Charter for Health Promotion: An International Conference on Health Promotion, November 17–21*. Copenhagen: WHO.

WHO (World Health Organisation) (1991) *Health For All Targets: The Health Policy for Europe*. Copenhagen: Regional Office for Europe, WHO.

WHO (World Health Organisation) (1997) *Health and Environment in Sustainable Development: Five Years after the Earth Summit*. Geneva: WHO.

WHO (World Health Organisation) (2000) *Evaluation and Use of Epidemiological Evidence for Environmental Health Risk Assessment: Guideline Document*. Copenhagen: Regional Office for Europe, WHO.

WHO (World Health Organisation) (2003) *SARS Affected Areas* http://www.who.int/csr/sarsareas/en/ (accessed 20 May 2003).

WHO (World Health Organisation)/UNICEF (1978) *Primary Health Care: The Alma Ata Conference*. Geneva: WHO.

Yach, D. and Bettcher, D. (1998) The globalization of public health, I: threats and opportunities, *American Journal of Public Health*, 88(5): 735–8.

Yen, I. and Syme, S. (1999) The social environment and health: a discussion of the epidemiological literature, *Annual Review of Public Health*, 20: 287–308.

Yorkshire Forward (2001) *Active Partners*. York: Yorkshire Forward.

Young, K., Ashby, D., Boaz, A. and Grayson, L. (2002) Social science and the evidence based policy movement, *Social Policy and Society*, 1(3): 215–24.

Zakus, J.D.L. and Lysack, C.L. (1998) Revisiting community participation, *Health Policy and Planning*, 13(1): 1–12.

Zwi, A.B. and Yach, D. (2002) International health in the 21st century: trends and challenges, *Social Science and Medicine*, 54: 1615–20.

Index

ABCD (Achieving Better Community
    Development), 282–3, 284, 291–2
accountability partnerships, 64
Acheson, Sir Donald
    report on health inequalities (1998), 9,
        16–17, 18, 67, 101–2, 166, 168, 169–70
    report on public health in England (1988),
        8–9
action planning, and community health and
    well being, 293–5
age, and attitudes to health, 135–6
ageing population, 192, 195
Agenda, 21–8, 202, 207, 208
air pollution, 120, 254
animal disease outbreaks, 109
antenatal screening, 122
Arblaster, L., 175
Arts for Health Movement, 77
asylum seekers, 79, 87–92
    public health needs of, 87–9
    strategies to meet needs of, 89–92
Audit Commission, 60, 91, 189

Bayesian approaches to epidemiology, 255,
        256–8, 260
Bentham, Jeremy, 274
biomedical model, *see* medical model
bioterrorism risks, 109, 113
Black Report on health inequalities, 165–6,
        166–7, 168
Blair, Tony, 33, 34
Blair-Stevens, C., 302
Blears, Hazel, 18, 27

Bradford HAZ, 190
Bringing Britain Together (Social Exclusion
        Unit), 181
British Medical Association, 300, 307
British Medical Journal, 212
Brown, Gordon, 21
Brundtland Report (1987), 193
Bryson, J.M., 51
BSE (bovine spongiform encephalitis), 55,
        109, 110, 126
built environment, and community
        networking, 159
Butler, Josephine, 133

Cabinet Office
    and emergency planning, 124
    and health protection, 111, 115
    and national partnerships, 73
    Performance and Innovation Unit, 25
Campbell collaboration, 232, 261
cancer, and European Union health strategy,
        56
capacity and capability in public health, 57–8,
        79–92
    asylum seekers case study, 79, 87–92
    and the public health professional project,
        83–6
    and the public health workforce, 80–1
    skills and competencies, 81–3, 86
    and training needs, 82–3
capitalism, and globalization, 213
carers
    attitudes to health, 136

and government modernization agenda,
42–3
carrying capacity, and sustainable futures in
cities, 201
central-local partnerships, 64
Chadwick, Edwin, 7, 133
change management, and future public health
policy, 29–30
Chapman, J., 29–30
Chemical Releases Inventory, 122
Chief Medical Officer
Getting Ahead of the Curve, 113, 121
report on the public health function
(2001), 18, 20
children
asylum seeking, 88, 89
and community health and well being,
279–80, 283–4
cholera, 6, 221
cities, *see* sustainable futures in cities
City Challenge, 179
civil contingency planning, 54
CJD (new variant Creutzfeldt-Jacob
Disease), 109, 221
climate change, 109, 222
clinical audit, 49
Cochrane collaboration, 231–2, 261
cognitive continuum framework, in health
impact estimation, 303–6
collaborative partnerships, 59, 60, 61–3
and asylum seekers, 91
Cochrane and Campbell collaborations,
231–2, 237, 261
and health protection, 127
and primary care, 99, 100
Commission on Environmental Health,
Agendas for Change, 119
Commission for Health Improvement,
Nothing About Us Without Us, 42
Commission for Patient and Public
Involvement in Health, 40, 42–3
common good doctrine, 274
Communicable Disease Surveillance Centre,
122
communicable diseases, 47, 52–3, 54, 108,
109
and European Union health strategy, 56,
110
and globalization, 221
communication, and asylum seekers, 91

communities
and partnerships in public health, 69–70,
71
and primary care, 98, 99
communities of interest, health inequalities in,
186
Community Chests, 39
Neighbourhood Renewal, 182
community connectedness, 293
community development
and community health and well being, 279,
285–7
and networking, 145–60
and the 'community' dimension to
health, 148–52
community and voluntary sectors, 154–5
factors influencing community
networking, 159
health effects of community networks,
155–6
in practice, 156–9
skills of networking, 157–8
and social capital, 146, 148, 149
strategies, 158–9
tackling health inequalities through, 173
'weak ties' and 'strong ties', 147, 150
community development projects, 178–9
Community Empowerment Fund, 39, 182
community focus, and government
modernization agenda, 43–4
community health councils, 131
community health movements, 96–7, 134–5
community health and well being, 226,
278–95
ABCD model of, 282–3, 284, 291–2
action, 279
and action planning, 293–5
fields of, 280–1
Labonte's model of, 287–9, 292
LEAP (Learning Evaluation and Planning)
model of, 284, 289–95
measurable outcomes from, 283–4
and public health programme evaluation,
284–9
and strong communities, 291–2
value systems, 279–80
community nurses, 96, 97, 100, 131
community partnerships, 76–8
conservative governments, and health
inequalities, 167

consumerist approach to public involvement, 140
Consumers in NHS Research, 132
context dependence/independence, and evidence-based public health, 240, 241
cost–benefit analysis, 268, 276
cost–consequences analysis, 268, 269, 275
cost–effectiveness analysis, 268, 269, 275
cost–utility analysis, 268, 269, 275, 276
counterfactuals, and evidence-based public health, 230
Creating a Health Protection Agency (Department of Health), 113, 114
Critical Appraisal Skills Programme, 242
Crosby, B.C., 51

Davey Smith, G., 171
deterministic modelling, and health impact analysis, 306
devolution
    and national partnerships, 73
    and public health policy, 22–3
directors of public health, 51
    in health authorities, 131
    and partnerships, 68
    and primary care trusts, 102–3, 118
disabled people
    and community health and well being, 279–80
    and community-based activities, 154–5

Earth Summit debate (Johannesburg, 2002), 223
Eastern Europe, globalization and health inequalities in, 219
eco-epidemiology and population level approaches, 252–3
ecological fallacy arguments, and epidemiology, 253
ecological modernization, 202
economic evaluation, 226, 264, 265–6, 268–77
    and equity, 275
    framework for public health, 269–73
        piloting, 271–2
        strengths of, 273–4
    and health impact analysis, 307
    systematic review of, 268

types of, 268–9
    see also health economics
Economic and Social Research Council, evidence network, 232–3
educational priority areas, 178–9
efficiency and equity, in health economics, 266, 275
emergency planning and response, 54, 108, 117, 123–6
empiricism, and theory in evidence-based public health, 244
employment, neighbourhood policies on, 183–4
Environment Agency, 111, 114, 115, 118, 122
environmental hazards, and health protection, 53–4, 108, 109
environmental health officers, 130–1
epidemiology, 225, 246–62
    Bayesian approaches to, 255, 256–8, 260
    classical and public health, 248–51
    and community health and well being, 286
    eco-epidemiology and population level approaches, 252–3
    and evidence-based medicine, 261–2
    future developments in, 255–61
    genetic, 253–4
    history of, 251–2
    life course approaches to, 258–60
    medical versus lay, 137–8
    and meta-analysis, 253, 255–6, 258, 260
    multilevel approaches to, 260–1
    scope of, 247–8
equity
    efficiency and, 266, 275
    and primary care, 98, 99
ethics, and health economics, 274
European cities, 198–201, 206
European Sustainable Cities, 198, 199–200
European Union (EU)
    'Europe of the Regions', 47, 55
    future public health policy, 28–9, 47, 55–6
    and health protection, 110
    and international partnerships, 72
    Sixth Environmental Action Programme, 113
    and urban growth, 198
evidence and evaluation, 5, 225–309
evidence-based public health, 6, 83
    and community health and well being, 286
    and epidemiology, 261–2

and government modernization agenda, 33
and health impact analysis, 308
multidisciplinary, 10–11, 225, 227–45
    defining, 229–31
    development of, 231–7
    and different research traditions, 240–3
    problems of, 237–43
    role of theory in, 243–4
and the professional project, 84–5
and public health policy, 17–18
evidence-informed policy and practice, 231

families, and partnerships in public health, 71
Farr, William, 164
fertility rates, global, 195
Fifth Framework for Research in the
        European Union, 200
food implicated health threats, 108, 109, 114
Food Standards Agency (FSA), 110, 111,
        115, 118, 122
food-borne disease, 221–2
foot and mouth disease, 109, 115, 118, 124
Frenk, Julio, 24
future of public health policy, 14, 26–30,
        47–56
    health protection, 52–4
    management and leadership, 50–1
    and public health history, 48–50
    and public health services, 51–2
    regionalism, 54–6

garden cities, 178
General Agreement on Trade in Services,
        216, 218
genetic epidemiology, 253–4
Geographic Information Systems (GIS), 123
Getting Ahead of the Curve, 113, 121
globalization
    and emerging public health risks, 220–2
    global trade policy, and the UK health care
        context, 217–18
    and the 'global village', 210
    the globalization debate, 211–12
    and health, 1, 5, 110, 162, 210–24
    and health care organizations, 222
    and health inequalities, 214, 218–20
    positive and negative impacts on public
        health, 213–14, 223–4
    promoters of economic globalization,
        214–17

and sustainable futures in cities, 198, 201,
        202
Göteborg, sustainable development in, 203–4
governing partnerships, 64
Government Interventions in Deprived Areas
        (HM Treasury), 181
GPs (general practitioners)
    and asylum seekers, 88–9
    and epidemiology, 249–50
    and health inequalities, 174
    and lay involvement in public health, 138–9
    and primary care, 95, 97, 100, 105
Green Paper on the Urban Environment
        (Commission of the European
        Communities), 199

Hannerz, U., 211
HAZs, see Health Action Zones (HAZs)
health action zones (HAZs), 9, 17, 20, 178,
        182, 186–7
    and evidence-based public health, 244
    and mainstream services, 189–90
    and partnerships, 64, 65, 66, 67, 70, 73, 74,
        152
    and primary care, 103
Health for All movement, 93, 96, 97, 103, 135
health authorities, 131
Health Development Agency (HDA), 17, 18,
        85, 91, 119
    evidence-based public health database,
        233–5
health economics, 263–77, 297
    defining economics, 264–5
    discipline of, 265–6
    efficiency and equity in, 266, 275
    opportunity cost in, 267
    and public health action, 264, 274–6
    quality adjusted life years (QALYs), 266–7,
        275, 276
    role of, 264
    see also economic evaluation
Health Education Authority, 182
health impact, 226, 296–309
    assessment, 296, 297–302, 308–9
        paradigms and disciplines, 300–1
        robust quantitative, 306–8
    estimation and analysis, 297, 303–8, 309
        and the cognitive continuum framework,
            303–6
Health Improvement Fund, 76

health inequalities, 1, 5, 9, 11
  Acheson Report on, 9, 16–17, 18, 67,
    101–2, 166, 168, 169–70
  addressing, 67–8
  and asylum seekers, 87–9, 91
  causes of, 164–6
  and the 'community' dimension to health,
    148–9
  and community health and well being, 280
  and economics, 264, 275
  and evidence-based public health, 239–40
  and future public health policy, 26
  and globalization, 214, 218–20
  and government modernization agenda, 32
  and health action zones, 74
  improving access to health care, 174–5
  and inequity, 164
  and lay involvement in public health, 129
  and local government, 28
  and neighbourhood policies, 183–7
  new directions in tackling, 161, 163–76
  New Labour policy on, 167–9
  and new technology, 210, 219–20
  and the *NHS Plan*, 19, 20
  and partnerships, 67–8, 73, 78, 172–3
  potential policies for reducing, 170–5
  and primary care, 95, 99, 101–2, 103–4
  in Scotland, 75–6
  socio-economic, 165–7
  Tackling Health Inequalities reports, 18, 20,
    22
  targets, 19, 20, 52, 67
  UK policy effectiveness, 169–70
  Vision to Reality report on (2001), 18, 21
  and the WHO (World Health
    Organisation), 8, 216–17
The Health of the Nation (Department of
    Health), 16, 17, 66, 97, 172
health professionals, 80
  challenging the dominance of, 84
  and community focus, 43–4
  ethical stance of, 274
  and lay involvement in public health,
    138–40, 141, 144
  and leadership, 44–5
  and networks, 147, 153
  partnerships, 70–2
  tackling health inequalities, 170–5, 176
health promotion
  campaigns, 229

  and community health and well being,
    288–9
  'in the community', 149–50
  and primary care, 97
  promoting healthy behaviours, 173–4
  and public health policy, 24
health protection, 24, 52–4, 58, 107–27
  and contemporary health threats, 108–10
  Department of Health policies for, 127
  emergency planning and response, 54, 108,
    117, 123–6
  emerging policy and organization, 110–13
  hazards and risk assessment, 119–21, 126
  historical development in the UK, 113–14
  and local authorities, 118–19
  organizations and structures for, 113–19
  scope of, 108
  surveillance and prevention, 121–3, 126
Health Protection Agency (HPA), 54, 103,
    111, 114–15, 116, 118
Health and Safety Executive (HSE), 111,
    114, 115, 118, 126
health visitors, 96, 130–1
Healthy Cities movement, 93, 96, 135
healthy living centres (HLCs), 9, 17
  and partnerships, 63, 64, 65, 66, 67, 70, 73,
    78
  and primary care, 103
hierarchy of evidence, and multidisciplinary
    public health, 237–40
history of public health, 5–9, 48–50
  early twentieth century, 7, 133–4
  and epidemiology, 251–2
  and health protection, 113–14
  lay perspectives in, 132–5
  and New Labour, 9
  and 'new' public health, 8–9
  and the NHS, 7–8
  nineteenth century, 6–7, 48, 49, 133
  urban policy and neighbourhood renewal,
    178–9
HIV/AIDS, 53, 72, 109, 195
HLCs, *see* Healthy Living Centres (HLCs)
hospitals, transport to, 184
House of Commons Health Committee,
    critical report on public health (2001),
    18, 20
housing
  and asylum seekers, 88
  neighbourhood policies on, 184

HPA, *see* Health Protection Agency (HPA)
HSE, *see* Health and Safety Executive (HSE)
Human Genome Project, 253–4
Huxham, C., 68

Ibsen, Henrik, *An Enemy of the People*, 1, 2, 7
IMF (International Monetary Fund), 215, 216
immunisation, 133
  and asylum seekers, 89, 91
  and European Union health strategy, 56
  MMR (Measles, Mumps and Rubella), 121
individualism, pitfalls of, 68
individuals, and partnerships in public health, 71
inequalities, *see* health inequalities
infectious diseases, 52–3, 107, 109
  and globalization, 221, 222
  monitoring, 117
  responses to incidents, 126
  secondary prevention of, 122
influenza virus, 53
  'Avian Flu', 109
Institute of Psychiatry, Health Economics Unit, 269
Integrated Prevention and Pollution Control regime, 122–3
interest group approach to public involvement, 141
international partnerships, 72
International Statistical Classification of Diseases and Related Health Problems, 254–5
Internet
  and epidemiology, 254
  and globalization, 214
  sources on tackling health inequalities, 175
Introducing Health Impact Assessment (Health Development Agency), 302
Involving Patients and the Public in Healthcare (Department of Health), 42

'joined up policy', 16, 18, 25, 26
  and change management, 29–30
  and government modernization agenda, 32
  and neighbourhood renewal, 180
  and partnerships, 69, 72–3, 78
  and public health training needs, 82–3

Kavanagh, D., 72

Labonte, R., model of community health and well being, 287–9, 292
Labour movement, 133
Larson, M., 83
lay contribution to public health, 58, 128–44
  case study of, 142–3
  and community networks, 153–4
  history of, 132–5
  importance of, 129–30
  and lay knowledge vs. medical knowledge, 136–7
  medical perspectives on, 137–40
  in the NHS, 130–2
  promoting, 140–3
  understanding the lay perspective, 135–7
leadership
  and future public health policy, 50–1
  and government modernization agenda, 44–5, 46
  strategic leadership and asylum seekers, 91
LEAP (Learning Evaluation and Planning), model of community health and well being, 284, 289–95
learning organizations, and community health and well being, 282
Legionnaires Disease, 117, 126
life course approaches to epidemiology, 258–60
Ling, T., 65
lobbying, as a policy for reducing health inequalities, 171–2
local authorities/government
  and future public health policy, 28
  and government modernization agenda, 38, 41, 180
  and health protection, 118–19
  loss of power, 50
  and the NHS, 103, 130–1
  and partnerships, 64
  and sustainable futures in cities, 207
Local Exchange Schemes, 77
local health protection structure, 116
local partnerships, 73–6
  community partnerships, 76–8
local politics, and public health action, 1–2, 7
Local Strategic Partnerships (LSPs), 21, 38–9, 40, 65, 67, 69, 74–5, 78
  and neighbourhood renewal and regeneration, 181–2, 190

Local Voices (National Health Services Management Executive), 131
localization, and sustainable futures in cities, 201
Lock, K., 297, 299
London, Greater London Authority, 28
London School of Economics, Centre for Social Exclusion, 269

Macdonald, D., 68
'McDonaldization', 212
Macintyre, Professor Sally, 233
malaria, 221, 222
Malmö, sustainable development in, 204–5
management
    and future public health policy, 50–1
    see also leadership
Manchester, joint health unit, 28
media, and public health lobbying, 171–2
medical model, 66
    and lay involvement in public health, 138–40, 143–4
    and primary care, 99
medical officers of health, 130–1
men, and health inequalities, 164, 166, 174
meta-analysis
    and epidemiology, 253, 255–6, 258, 260
    and evidence-based public health, 238
miasma theory of disease, 6, 244, 251
Milburn, Alan, 22, 32, 43, 76, 101, 129
Mindell, J., 306–7
minority ethnic groups
    and community health and well being, 279–80
    and health inequalities, 164, 188
mixed economy of welfare, 40–1
MMR (Measles, Mumps and Rubella) vaccinations, 121
Modernization Agency, 45
Mooney, G., 274
mortality rates
    and AIDS, 195
    and epidemiology, 252
    fall in, 165
    inequalities in, 164, 169
multidisciplinary public health, 9–11
    evidence-based, 10–11, 225, 227–45
    and health impact assessment, 298–9, 300–1

and partnerships, 57, 59, 67
    networking, 152–3
    and the professional project, 83–4
    and public health policy, 16
    and the public health workforce, 81
    and sustainable futures in cities, 201
multilevel approaches to epidemiology, 260–1

National Commission for Patient and Public Involvement, 132
National Radiological Protection Board (NRPB), 112, 114, 115, 122
National Standards for Specialist Practice in Public Health, 3, 81–2
National Strategy Action Plan, 181
Navarro, V., 218
neighbourhood effect, 188
Neighbourhood Renewal Community Chests, 182
Neighbourhood Renewal Fund, 182, 183
Neighbourhood Renewal programme, 9, 64, 75, 77, 103, 132
neighbourhood renewal and regeneration, 161, 177–91, 229
    and evidence-based public health, 239, 242, 243, 244
    and health, 182–3
    historical context, 178–9
    main programmes, 189–90
    neighbourhood policies and health inequalities, 183–7
    public health and the neighbourhood, 187–91
    re-emergence of the neighbourhood, 180–2
    in Sweden, 203
Neighbourhood Renewal Unit, 179
neighbourhood wardens, 182, 183
networks
    Economic and Social Research Council evidence network, 232–3
    and the neighbourhood effect, 188
    network approach to public involvement, 141–2
    networking for health gain, 58
    and partnerships in public health, 71
    and sustainable futures in cities, 207
    see also community development, and networking
New Commitment to Regeneration, 182–3

New Deal for Communities, 9, 17, 77, 103, 177, 182, 183, 186, 187, 188, 189
  modernization agenda, and community health and well being, 278
New Labour government
  and lay involvement in public health, 132
  modernization agenda, 13–14, 19, 31–46
    and collaboration, 46
    common threads of, 40–5
    as a container, 35–6
    democratic institutions, 36–40
    and economics, 275
    key principles of reform, 33
    and the legacy of Thatcherism, 34–5
    and 'old Labour', 34
  public health policy, 13, 15–30
    constraints on implementation, 23–6
    and 'decisionless decision-making', 20, 26
    and devolution, 22–3
    future of, 26–30
    and 'joined up policy', 16, 18, 25, 26
    and partnerships, 57–8, 65–6, 72–3
    and primary care, 94
    state of, 16–23
    see also health inequalities
The New NHS, 101
'new' public health (1980s), 8–9
new social movements, 134
new technology
  and health inequalities, 210, 219–20
  uncertain hazards of, 109
new towns movement, 178
NHS (National Health Service)
  and asylum seekers, 88–9
  changing nature of public involvement, 130–2
  and community partnerships, 77
  emergency planning and response, 117
  and epidemiology, 249
  and globalization, 214, 217–18
  and government modernization agenda, 36
  and health inequalities, 168, 170
  and the Health Protection Agency, 115
  internal market, 35
  and the LEAP model, 290–1
  and local partnerships, 75, 103
  management, 51
  partnerships with local authorities, 64
  patient forums in NHS trusts, 43

Patient's Charter, 131
patients as consumers, 131
  and primary care, 94, 96, 100, 101
  and public health history, 7–8, 48, 49, 50
  and public health policy, 16, 18–19, 21
    constraints on implementation, 23, 24
   and local government, 28
  public health in primary care, 9
  and public health services, 51–2
  public health spending, 26
  and regionalism, 54
  and the welfare state, 133–4
  workforce skills and competencies, 81
NHS Plan, 18, 19, 20, 21
  and devolution, 22, 23
  and health inequalities, 168
  and healthy living centres, 63
  and the Modernization Agency, 45
  and partnerships, 69
  and primary care, 101, 104
  and quality of services, 45
  and regionalism, 27
nicotine replacement therapy, 256–7
Nightingale, Florence, 244
Northern Ireland
  Community Development and Health Network, 280
  Joint Irish Institute for Public Health, 73
  primary care, 95, 105, 106
  public health policy in, 23
  Regional Strategy for Health and Social Well-being, 280–1
nuclear threats, 54, 109, 114
Null hypothesis, 256, 257
nurses
  community nurses, 96, 97, 100, 131
  overseas trained in the UK, 222

OECD (Organisation for Economic Cooperation and Development), 201, 214
offenders, epidemiology and the treatment of, 250–1
O'Keefe, E., 215
opportunity costs, 267, 302
option appraisal, *see* economic evaluation

Pareto, Vilfredo, 274

participation, 5
  and community health and well being, 283,
    284, 289, 292
  lay contribution to public health, 58,
    128–44, 153–4
  and primary care, 99
  public participation and neighbourhood
    renewal, 178
partnerships, 5, 59–78
  and community health and well being, 279
    LEAP model of, 289–90
  community partnerships, 76–8
  defining, 60–1
  and evidence-based public health, 239
  and government modernization agenda,
    33, 36, 41–2
  and government policy, 57–8, 69
  and health inequalities, 67–8, 73, 78, 172–3
  and health protection, 119
  international, 72
  levels of, 63–4
  local, 73–6
  and multidisciplinary public health, 57, 60,
    67
  national, 72–3
  and neighbourhood renewal and
    regeneration, 183, 190–1
  and networking for health, 152–4
  organizational issues, 68–9
  partnership working, 42
  and primary care, 96, 103–4, 104–5
  reasons for, 65–70
  types of, 64–5
  working with the public and communities,
    69–70
  see also collaborative partnerships; Local
    Strategic Partnerships (LSPs)
Patient's Charter, 131
PCGs (primary care groups), 95, 100, 101,
  102
PCTs (primary care trusts), 9, 26, 58, 95,
  100, 101, 106
  and directors of public health, 102–3,
    118
  and local partnerships, 75, 78
  moving public health to, 104–5
  patient forums, 43
  and social services, 101
  and training in public health, 86
Pettenkofer, Max Von, 48

police officers, and the public health
  workforce, 80
Policy Appraisal and Health (Department of
  Health), 301–2
pollution
  air pollution, 120, 254
  and health protection, 112–13, 120, 121
population change, and urbanization, 192,
  194–7
poverty
  and asylum seekers, 91
  in European cities, 198
  and health inequalities, 148–9
    and neighbourhoods, 183–4, 185
    upstream policies for tackling, 170–1
  policies to tackle, 168
  Rowntree surveys on, 133
power relationships, and networks, 151, 153
Pratt, J., 68–9
pregnancy
  antenatal screening, 122
  and life course epidemiology, 259, 260
  Teenage Pregnancy Unit, 72, 168
primary care, 93–106
  and community health movements, 96–7
  defining, 95
  and health inequalities, 95, 99, 101–2,
    103–4
  new connections with public health, 97–9
  and partnerships, 96, 103–4, 104–5
  re-evaluating, 94–5
  see also PCTs (primary care trusts)
primary care organizations, 95
professional closure, 81
professional project, 83–6
public health action, 1–2, 4, 130
  and economics, 264, 274–6
  and local politics, 1–2, 7
  scope of, 3
Public Health Alliance (now the UK Public
  Health Association), 98
Public Health Laboratory Service (PHLS),
  112, 114, 117, 122
Public Health Observatories, 261–2
public health professionals, see health
  professionals
public health resources, 1, 4
  and economics, 264
public services, globalization and the reform
  of, 215, 218

purchaser-provider partnerships, 64

quality adjusted life years (QALYs), 266–7, 275, 276, 300
quality of life, and community health and well being, 290–1, 292–3
quality of services, and government modernization agenda, 45
quantitative/qualitative research, and evidence-based public health, 240, 241

randomized controlled trials
    and epidemiology, 253
    and evidence-based public health, 238
Rathbone, Eleanor, 133
Rawls, J., 275
Reducing Health Inequalities: An Action Report, 168
Regional Coordination Unit, 181
regional health protection structure, 116
    emergency planning and response, 117
regionalism, 54–6
    elected regional assemblies in England, 37–8, 40, 54–5
    and future public health policy, 27–8
    and neighbourhood renewal and regeneration, 180–1
representative approach to public involvement, 140–1
Research and Development Strategy for Public Health, 83
reverse colonization, 212
Revitalising Health and Safety, 114
Richards, D., 72
Rio Declaration on Environment and Development, 112
risk assessment, and health protection, 119–21
risk factor analysis, and epidemiology, 247–8, 250, 253
robust quantitative health impact assessment, 306–8
Rogers Report on urban life (2000), 180
rough sleepers initiative, 72
Rushey Green Time Banks, 77

Samuelson, Paul, 264–5, 267
SARS (Severe Acute Respiratory Syndrome), 109, 110

Saving Lives: Our Healthier Nation, 17, 19, 21, 22, 63, 69, 76, 168
    and evidence-based public health, 233, 235, 239
    and primary care, 101
scoping public health practice, 3
Scotland
    NHS Plan, 23
    partnerships and public health, 67, 73, 75–6
    primary care, 95, 105, 106
    Working Together for a Healthier Scotland, 76
Scottish Community Development Centre, 279, 281, 289
Scottish Environmental Protection Agency, 114
self-help organizations, 134, 141, 155
service users, and government modernization agenda, 42–3, 45
Shifting the Balance of Power: Next Steps (Department of Health), 9, 18, 19, 27, 39, 41, 42, 190
    and community focus, 44
    and primary care, 75, 101, 102
Single Regeneration Budget, 179, 181
smoking, and nicotine replacement therapy, 256–7
Snow, John, 6
social capital, 146, 148, 149, 219
    and neighbourhoods, 188–9
social class, and health inequalities, 166, 184
social exclusion, 11
    in European cities, 198
    and networks, 157
    and the *NHS Plan*, 69
    policies to tackle, 168
Social Exclusion Unit, 73, 167, 181, 183, 184, 185
social model of health, 279
social services, and primary care trusts, 101
social workers, 80, 130–1
Soviet Union (former), globalization and health inequalities in, 219
Standard Regeneration Budget, 77
stochastic modelling, and health impact analysis, 306
Stockholm, sustainable development in, 202–3
Strachey, Lytton, *Eminent Victorians*, 244
strategic leadership, and asylum seekers, 91

structural adjustment policies, 215
Sure Start projects, 9, 17, 19, 64, 72, 73, 75,
        103, 132, 188
    and inequality, 170
    Rose Hill, 76
sustainability and health, 113
sustainable futures in cities, 1, 5, 161–2,
        192–209
    and the concept of sustainable
        development, 193–4
    European cities, 198–201
    multidisciplinary policy issues in, 201
    strategic issues, 205–6
    Swedish cities case study, 202–5
    world population and urban growth, 192,
        193–201
*Sustainable Urban Development in the
        European Union* (Commission of the
        European Communities), 200
Swedish cities, sustainable futures in, 202–5
systematic reviews, and evidence-based
        public health, 238

Tackling Health Inequalities reports, 18, 20, 22
targets
    and government modernization agenda, 33
    health inequalities, 19, 20, 52, 67
        and primary care trusts, 102
    and leadership, 44
    and national partnerships, 73
Taylor, L., 302
teachers, and the public health workforce, 80,
        81
teamwork, and the professional project, 84
Teenage Pregnancy Unit, 72, 168
terrorism threats, 109, 113, 115, 125
Thatcherism, and New Labour government
        modernization agenda, 34–5
TIABIM decision making, and health impact
        estimation, 304
Time Banks, 77
tobacco related diseases, and globalization,
        220–1
tourism, and infectious diseases, 221
*Towards an Urban Agenda in the European
        Union* (Commission of the European
        Communities), 200
trade liberalization
    and globalization, 215–16
        and health inequalities, 218, 220

trade union movement, 133
training in public health
    integrating and financing, 85–6
    needs, 82–3
transport
    neighbourhood policies on, 184
    in Stockholm, 203
tuberculosis (TB), 126, 219, 221

unemployment, in European cities, 198
United Nations
    Conference on Environment and
        Development (Rio, 1992), 193, 202
    Development Programme report (2001),
        219, 221
United States
    National Public Health Performance
        Standards Program, 50
    Public Health Organization, 52
upstream policies, for tackling health
        inequalities, 170–1
Urban Summit (2002), 180
urbanization and urban development, 192,
        193–201
    emerging policy on urban management,
        206–7
    European cities, 198–201, 206
    and world population change, 192, 194–7
utilitarianism, and health economics, 274,
        275

Vision to Reality (2001), 18, 21
voluntary sector, 133, 134
    and community-based activities, 154–5

Wales
    local health groups, 95, 105
    NHS Plan, 23
    partnerships and public health, 73, 75
Wanless Report (2002), 18, 21–2, 26
wardens, neighbourhood, 182, 183
Warren, R., 60
waste management activities, 120
welfare state, and the NHS, 133–4
Wellington, Duke of, 56
Welsh Public Health Service, 52
WHO (World Health Organisation), 8, 64,
        216–17
    and collaboration, 66
    and European cities, 198

and global policy on tobacco control,
220–1
and health protection, 110
and international partnerships,
72
and primary care, 93, 96, 98
women's movement, 134, 135
workforce, *see* capacity and capability
in public health
workplace hazards, 114
World Bank, 214, 215, 216, 218
World Commission on Environment
and Development, 193

world population growth, 194–5
urban, 195–7
WTO (World Trade Organisation), 214,
215–16, 218, 223
and health protection, 110, 112
Trade Related Intellectual Property Rights
Agreement, 222

Yach, D., 223
young people, peer pressure and social
networks, 156

Zwi, A.B., 223